NURSING IN THE 1980s

CRISES, OPPORTUNITIES, CHALLENGES

EDITED BY **Linda H. Aiken,** RN, PhD, FAAN

Vice president for research
The Robert Wood Johnson Foundation
Princeton, NJ

Susan R. Gortner, RN, PhD, FAAN

Associate Editor
Professor and associate dean for research
School of nursing
University of California
San Francisco, CA

33 Contributors

AMERICAN ACADEMY OF NURSING

J. B. LIPPINCOTT COMPANY
Philadelphia • Toronto

NURSING IN THE 1980s

CRISES, OPPORTUNITIES, CHALLENGES

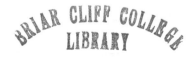

The American Academy of Nursing proudly dedicates this volume to the million practicing nurses in recognition of their essential contributions to the health of the American people.

1 2 3 4 5 6

Library of Congress Cataloging in Publication Data
Main entry under title:

Nursing in the 1980s.

Includes index.
1. Nursing — United States.   2. Medical care — United States.   I. Aiken, Linda H.
II. Gortner, Susan R.   III. American Academy of Nursing.
RT4.N83   362.1'7   81-20829
ISBN 0-397-54406-5   AACR2
ISBN 0-397-54413-8 (pbk.)

CONTENTS

v

PART **3**

THE CHALLENGES OF LONG–TERM CARE

PART **4**

THE CONTRIBUTION OF NURSE PRACTITIONERS
TO AMERICAN HEALTH CARE

CONTRIBUTORS

LINDA H. AIKEN, RN, PHD, FAAN is a nurse sociologist and vice president for research for The Robert Wood Johnson Foundation in Princeton, New Jersey. Dr. Aiken has practiced as a clinical nurse specialist in cardiovascular nursing in teaching-hospital settings. She is the author of numerous papers on health policy issues and is editor of *Health Policy and Nursing Practice*. Dr. Aiken is a member of the Institute of Medicine of the National Academy of Sciences and past president of the American Academy of Nursing.

GENROSE J. ALFANO, RN, MA, FAAN joined Lydia E. Hall in starting the program at Loeb Center for Nursing and Rehabilitation in 1962. For the past 12 years she has served as its director. Ms. Alfano brought to Loeb a background in public health nursing; general medical-surgical nursing; and nursing education in medical-surgical out-patient nursing. She has served on numerous committees and lectured extensively on the importance of clinically well-prepared generalists in nursing to carry out all phases of the process of nursing.

J. GRAHAM ATKINSON, DPHIL is a mathematician and chief rate analyst at the Maryland Health Services Cost Review Commission. His interest is the development and implementation of incentive payment systems for hospitals.

VIRGINIA Z. BARHAM, RN, EDD, FAAN is a nursing consultant for the California Board of Registered Nursing and the Kaiser-Permanente medical care program. She has served on numerous state and national committees and has been a frequent speaker in this country and abroad.

VIRGINIA CLELAND, RN, PHD, FAAN is a professor of nursing at Wayne State University College of Nursing. Dr. Cleland has conducted several large studies that relate to nurse employment, most particularly the problems of dual-career women. She has served on the American Nurses' Association (ANA) and Michigan Nurses' Association commissions on economic and general welfare and their task forces on reimbursement. She also served on the ANA Task Force on Human Resources and the ANA Commission on Nursing Services Task Force on characteristics of a professional practice climate.

JOYCE C. CLIFFORD, RN, MS, FAAN is vice president for nursing at the Beth Israel Hospital, Boston and clinical associate professor at Boston University. Ms. Clifford is a nationally recognized leader in nursing service administration. She is president of the American Society for Nursing Service Administrators.

DONNA DIERS, RN, MSN, FAAN is dean and professor at Yale University School of Nursing. She is currently involved in health policy, research on systems of care, nurse-midwifery, and the expanding nursing role.

JO ELEANOR ELLIOT, RN, MA, FAAN is director of the Division of Nursing, Bureau of Health Professions, Health Resources Administration. She is former director of nursing programs at the Western Interstate Commission for Higher Education and chief executive officer of the commission's Western Council on Higher Education for Nursing. She has been president of the American Nurses' Association, chairman of the American Journal of Nursing Company, and a member of the Board of International Council of Nurses.

CARROLL L. ESTES, PHD is a sociologist and professor in the Department of Social and Behavioral Sciences and director and chairperson of the Aging Health Policy Center at the school of nursing at the University of California in San Francisco. She is author of *The Aging Enterprise* and is currently directing a major national study of long term care.

CLAIRE M. FAGIN, RN, PHD, FAAN is dean of the University of Pennsylvania School of Nursing. She is a member of the Institute of Medicine and the National Board of Health Examiners. She is editor of several books in the fields of psychiatric and pediatric nursing and author of numerous articles on health policy. She currently serves on the Private Sector Task Force on Competition and Health Delivery.

LORETTA C. FORD, RN, EDD, FAAN is dean, school of nursing and director of nursing, University of Rochester Medical Center, Rochester, New York. Dr. Ford, an internationally known nursing leader, has devoted her career to practice, education, consultation and influencing health services inquiry. Her practice of nursing has spanned inpatient and outpatient services, community health, and military nursing. Dr. Ford's studies on the nurse's expanded role in health care delivery in community health nursing, her specialty area, led to the creation of the first nurse practitioner model at the University of Colorado; more recently she provided administrative leadership for the unification of practice, education, and research in nursing at the University of Rochester.

SUSAN R. GORTNER, RN, PHD, FAAN is professor of nursing and associate dean for research in the school of nursing, University of California, San Francisco. She also is an affiliated faculty member of the Institute of Health Policy Studies in the school of medicine and the Aging Health Policy Center in the school of nursing. Prior to coming to the university, she had twelve years of federal service with the Division of Nursing, Public Health Service, where she served as chief of the nursing research branch. Dr. Gortner designed the first inter-agency agreement between the Bureau of Health Manpower and the Veterans Administration, which resulted in a study extending the work of Lewis and Resnick on the scope of practice and nurse practitioners in ambulatory care settings. Her primary research interests are in science and health policy, family health, and cardiovascular surgery.

ADA JACOX, RN, PHD is a nurse who has worked in clinical and academic settings throughout her career. She presently holds joint appointments as a professor of nursing at the University of Maryland (where she teaches in the doctoral program in nursing) and at Saint Joseph Hospital in Towson, Maryland (where she serves as director of research and evaluation). Her current interest is to develop roles through which nurses in academic settings can be more closely involved in the day-to-day operation of clinical agencies, including acute care hospitals. She presently is a member of the American Nurses' Association board of directors and the American Nurses' Foundation board of trustees. Her major research interests have been with the pain experience and organizational structures designed to promote greater autonomy for nurses in practice.

ELLA KICK, RN, MSN is a gerontological nurse specialist and assistant professor of nursing at the Medical College of Akron. She was the recipient of a Robert Wood Johnson Faculty Fellowship in Primary Care, which included a year of study at the University of Colorado. She is chairperson of the ANA Council for Nursing Home Nurses and serves on the ANA task force on the White House Conference on Aging. Her other gerontological experiences include director of nursing service in a nursing home; Medicare/Medicaid surveyor/consultant; and primary care in a community center. In addition to teaching Ms. Kick provides consultation to nursing homes and speaks at workshops and seminars on various aspects of gerontological nursing.

TERRY S. LATANICH, JD was the lead attorney on the Federal Trade Commission's Eyeglasses Rule, which was the first FTC rule in the health manpower area. That rule permitted eye care professionals to advertise their services notwithstanding state laws that banned that practice. Since 1979, Mr. Latanich has been the program advisor for the Commission's Occupational Deregulation Program. In that capacity he oversees the Commission's investigations of commercial dental practice, disputes between dentists and denturists over the fitting of dentures, disputes between and among ophthalmologists, optometrists, and opticians over who should be permitted to fit contact lenses, and the Bureau of Consumer Protection's investigation into restrictive practice requirements, reimbursement limitations, and access to hospital privileges questions.

LAUREN LeROY, CPHIL is assistant director of the Institute for Health Policy Studies (IHPS) at the University of California, San Francisco. Ms. LeRoy worked on health legislation in the office of the secretary, Department of Health, Education and

Welfare and spent several years directing the Washington office of the Health Policy Program (now the IHPS). Among her publications are *Primary Care in a Specialized World, Deliberations and Compromise: the Health Professions Educational Assistance Act of 1976* (co-authored with Philip R. Lee), and *The Costs and Effectiveness of Nurse Practitioners.*

EUGENE LEVINE, PHD recently retired from the United States Public Health Service after serving for 30 years in the fields of health manpower research, analysis and planning. He is now a consultant to various governmental agencies and to private and professional organizations concerned with the solution of health manpower problems. Dr. Levine was deputy director of the Division of Health Professions Analysis of the United States Public Health Service where he directed a number of national studies on nursing turnover and job satisfaction, nurse staffing and productivity, and patient and personnel satisfaction with care. Also, he has directed studies on the methodology for health manpower planning, developed management information systems for health agencies, and is currently analyzing the manpower implications of programs of disease prevention and health promotion.

CHARLES E. LEWIS, MD, SCD is professor of medicine, professor of nursing, and professor of public health at the University of California, Los Angeles. He is chief of the Division of General Internal Medicine and Health Services Research. Dr. Lewis has been involved in research and practice with nurses for many years. In the mid-1960s he conducted the first randomized clinical trial of nurses in extended roles. He subsequently has been involved in assessing the impact of school nurse practitioners and the development and evaluation of programs preparing family nurse practitioners. In 1980 he received the Rosenthal Award from the American College of Physicians in recognition for his studies of nurses in extended roles. His recent research interests have included studies of the development of children's health-related beliefs and behaviors and the impact of teaching self-care to children.

HAROLD S. LUFT, PHD is a health economist and associate professor of health economics at the Institute for Health Policy Studies, University of California, San Francisco. His research covers a wide range of areas including applications of benefit cost analysis, studies of medical care utilization, relationship between volume of surgery in hospitals and postoperative mortality, regionalization of hospital services, duplication of health insurance coverage, competition in the medical care market, and health maintenance organizations. In addition to numerous articles in scientific journals, he recently authored *Health Maintenance Organizations: Dimensions of Performance*, a comprehensive review of studies of HMOs.

MARGARET L. McCLURE, RN, ED, FAAN is executive director of nursing at New York University Medical Center in New York City. She has spent her entire professional career in hospital nursing and has held a variety of staff and administrative positions during that time. In addition, she has authored numerous articles regarding critical issues facing the profession in general and hospital nursing in particular.

DAVID MECHANIC, PHD is university professor and dean of the faculty of arts and sciences at Rutgers University in New Jersey. He is one of the most prominent medical sociologists in the world. Dr. Mechanic is author of *Medical Sociology, Mental Health and Social Policy*, and numerous other books dealing with health and health issues. He is a recognized scholar in the field of mental health and he chaired the president's commission on Mental Health Panel on Problems, Scope and Boundaries in 1977 to 1978.

EVELYN B. MOSES, acting chief, data collection and analysis branch, Division of Health Professions Analysis, has specialized in the study of the nurse supply characteristics and the requirements for nurses during her professional career. She worked for the American Nurses' Association in the research and statistics department with a major focus on the background data and research for the economic and general welfare programs as well as issues and data on nurse supply and requirements. She joined the staff of the division of nursing, Bureau of Health Manpower Education, Public Health Service in 1972 where she developed the projects that led to the design and the undertaking of the Sample Surveys of Registered Nurses and the revisions in the methodologies used to project the supply of nursing personnel. She also participated in the projects developed to determine national requirements for nursing personnel.

M. JANICE NELSON, RN, EDD is associate administrator for nursing at State University Hospital, Upstate Medical Center, Syracuse, New York. She is the author of a number of papers, publications, and presentations including workshops in staffing and budgeting in nursing.

DOROTHY S. ODA, RN, DNSC, FAAN is associate professor, school of nursing, University of California, San Francisco; nursing director, The Robert Wood Johnson Foundation National School Health Program; and vice president, Nursing Dynamics Cooperates, Mill Valley, California. Her preparation and professional experience are in community health nursing with a special interest in school health.

GRETCHEN A. OSGOOD, RN, MS is associate director of the Division of Nursing in the Health Resources Administration's Bureau of Health Professions. She was one of the staff involved in implementing the Nurse Training Act of 1964 and each successive modification of that legislation.

PATRICIA A. PRESCOTT, RN, PHD is an associate professor at the University of Maryland School of Nursing where she is currently the principal investigator of two three-year national studies of nurse staffing issues—"Temporary Service Agencies, Nurses and Hospitals" and a "Study of Nursing in Hospitals." In addition to her research grants, Dr. Prescott teaches research methods in the doctoral program at the University of Maryland.

LAURA REIF, RN, PHD is a nurse sociologist. She is assistant professor of Family Health Care Nursing and faculty associate, Aging Health Policy Center, at the School of Nursing of the University of California at San Francisco. For the past twelve years Dr. Reif has studied populations in need of long term care. Her research has focused on the impact of chronic illness on patients and their families, factors which affect the organization and delivery of services to individuals with chronic functional impairments, and in-home and other community-based services for the elderly and disabled. Dr. Reif is the co-editor of *Home Health Care Services Quarterly*.

CARL J. SCHRAMM, PHD, JD is a lawyer and labor economist. He is director of the Center of Hospital Finance and Management at the Johns Hopkins University

School of Hygiene and Public Health. He is also vice chairman of the Maryland Health Services Cost Review Commission. He is a former Robert Wood Johnson Foundation Health Policy Fellow and is currently Director of the Foundation's Municipal Health Services Program.

PATRICIA SCHULTHEISS, JD is a staff attorney working on the Federal Trade Commission's nurse practitioner/nurse-midwife investigation. She is a former participant of the Women's Rights Litigation Clinic at Rutgers University where she worked on a case involving the New Jersey Council of Nurse-Midwives.

ELDONNA M. SHIELDS, RN, MSN is a gerontological nurse specialist and assistant professor of nursing at the Medical College of Ohio. She is also chairperson of the Division of Gerontological Nursing Practice of the American Nurses' Association. Ms. Shields currently operates an independent practice in gerontological nursing.

NANCY J. STEIGER, RN, MS is a lecturer at the University of California, San Francisco, where she teaches courses in family health, self care, and health assessment. Her clinical work includes care of clients with end-stage renal disease and, more recently, supervision of nursing students in the ambulatory care clinics of Kaiser–San Francisco. In addition, she teaches a stress management series to the San Francisco community through the health promotion series of Kaiser.

BRUCE C. VLADECK, PHD is a political scientist and assistant commissioner for Health Planning and Resources Development, New Jersey State Department of Health. He has been responsible for implementation of the system of hospital reimbursement on the basis of case-mix (DRGs) as well as other hospital and nursing home reimbursement activities and day-to-day management of the State Health Planning and Development Agency. *Unloving Care: The Nursing Home Tragedy* is one of his many publications.

DUANE D. WALKER, RN, MS, FAAN is associate administrator of the hospital and clinics, and director of nursing service at Stanford University Hospital. Mr. Walker also has a variety of teaching responsibilities as a lecturer at the Stanford University School of Medicine and as associate clinical professor of the University of California, San Francisco, School of Nursing. He holds several executive positions in professional organizations including the American Academy of Nursing Task Force on Public Relations, the California Nurses' Association Nursing Administration Commission (vice chairperson), the Western League for Nursing Forum Planning Committee, and the California League for Nursing Association (vice president). Mr. Walker also serves on the U.S. Pharmacopeia Committee of Revision for the Advisory Panel of Nursing Practice.

PREFACE

Over the past forty years, rapidly increasing knowledge and new technologies have reshaped nursing practice. Nurses, traditionally concerned with the provision of comfort, psychological support, and assistance with activities of daily living, are increasingly involved in the direct application of complex modern medical technologies to patient care.

The institutions where most nurses practice have also been transformed, and nurses' roles and responsibilities have changed accordingly. Hospitals, the major employer of nurses, have evolved from small community institutions managed by nurses or voluntary groups to multimillion dollar enterprises employing a broad array of personnel and providing a wide range of medical and social services. The nursing home, a relatively new health care institution that emerged over the past 25 years, also will present an increasing challenge to the nursing profession.

Disease patterns have shifted from a predominance of acute infectious diseases to chronic illnesses. New organizational arrangements are required to provide appropriate long term care for these illnesses. As a result of this need, more autonomous roles have emerged for nurses, particularly in ambulatory settings, in the provision of care to the chronically ill and the increasing numbers of frail elderly.

These shifts in the patterns of medical care have occurred in the context of dramatic social change. Changing attitudes regarding women's participation in careers outside the home have resulted in significant modification of nurses' career expectations. Many nurses now view their employment as lifelong career commitments rather than as temporary work to generate a second income, and consequently many are seeking identification as professionals with career advancement opportunities.

Given these many changes in health care and society, it is not surprising that nursing is in a state of ferment. New responsibilities for nurses, new career expectations, and the changing needs of sick people all require modifications not only in the traditional relationships between nurses and physicians, but also within the institutions in which nurses work. These changes will not come easily. Relationships between health professionals and organizational arrangements for the provision of health care are deeply embedded in traditions not easily modified.

The challenge for nursing in the 1980s will be whether nurses can reaffirm their commitment to clinical excellence and demonstrate its importance with sufficient persuasiveness to cause health care institutions and ambulatory settings to restructure nursing responsibilities in ways that keep pace with nurses' career expectations. In the long run, new opportunities for nursing to play a broader, more satisfying role in the totality of health care seem good. Health care is a growing industry. The demand for nursing care can only increase in contrast to a decline in the demands for other kinds of trained people. Changing disease patterns, technological advancements in health care, and the need for continuing health surveillance for those with long term chronic illnesses should mean that nurses and nursing will be of even greater importance in the future.

The American Academy of Nursing commissioned the papers included in this volume to provide nurses and others with the basis for informed decisions on health care issues of importance in the 1980s. The academy is committed to identifying issues in nursing and in society that require the development of new approaches or alternative strategies for the improvement of patient care. Further, it is the mission of the academy to influence the future direction of the practice of nursing and the nursing profession so that the full potential of nursing's contribution to society will be realized. This volume is the eighth in a series of academy publications that have focused on changes in society at large and in patterns of health care offering readers the opportunity to reflect on nursing roles and the interrelationships between nurses and other health care providers.

This volume examines the issues, dilemmas, and challenges facing nurses in the 1980s. It is an interdisciplinary analysis with contributed papers by leading experts in nursing and health care. The major purpose of the book is to lay the groundwork for the formulation of goals and priorities for nursing in the 1980s. The papers explore in depth not only the dilemmas faced by nurses today, but also the likely consequences of their actions, or inactivity, for the future of the profession.

This project was supported by a grant from The Robert Wood Johnson

Foundation to the American Nurses' Foundation. We are grateful to both foundations for their assistance.

We would also like to acknowledge the important contributions made by Fellows of the American Academy of Nursing and the Governing Council of the Academy. Margaret Carroll and Bette Mitchell provided professional staff assistance and Katherine Parker managed the manuscript preparation. Our special thanks to David Miller of J. B. Lippincott Company for his personal interest in the book.

Linda H. Aiken, RN, PHD, FAAN
Susan R. Gortner, RN, PHD, FAAN

Acknowledgments

The officers and members of the Governing Council of the American Academy of Nursing for the years 1978 through 1981 made major contributions to this volume.

Linda H. Aiken

Genrose J. Alfano

Kathryn E. Barnard

Ann W. Burgess

Mary Elizabeth Carnegie

Shirley S. Chater

Mary E. Conway

Donna Diers

Vernice Ferguson

Susan R. Gortner

Helen K. Grace

Crystal M. Lange

Janetta MacPhail

Ingeborg G. Mauksch

Barbara B. Minckley

June S. Rothberg

Sally Galbraith Thomas

Harriet H. Werley

Marie J. Zimmer

P A R T 1

NURSES: A NATIONAL RESOURCE

Nurses are the largest single group of health professionals in the United States. In 1980, there were close to 1.6 million nurses, and well over a million were actively practicing.

Nurses are very versatile professionals. Preparation in physiology and pathology and their application to clinical practice, as well as background in the social and behavioral sciences, sets nurses apart from other health disciplines. This unique combination of knowledge and expertise enables nurses to assume broad responsibilities in all aspects of health care. They care for critically ill patients with life support systems as well as counseling the well on health promotion and disease prevention. In the care of the chronically ill, they combine clinical management of the disease process with counseling, social support, and patient teaching in a way that is both unique and successful as measured by health outcomes.

Nurses' versatility has made them essential in the day-to-day operation of our major health care institutions. Nurses are the only professional presence around-the-clock in hospitals and nursing homes. Therefore their astuteness in clinical assessment and their anticipation of impending crises are essential to the well-being of patients. Furthermore, nurses have major roles in managing the operation of these institutions. In hospitals, for example, nurses coordinate and manage all hospital services at the ward level. They are held accountable for ensuring that patients are fed, units are clean, equipment is available, patients are transported to the proper location at the appointed time, and a host of other managerial responsibilities in addition to their direct responsibility for nursing care.

Nurses have traditionally been designated as a national resource in wartime. However, only in the past 25 years have nurses also achieved national prominence at home in peacetime. Since the mid-1950s, government at all levels has been concerned about maintaining an adequate supply of nurses. The current acute shortage of nurses in hospitals and nursing homes has been an issue of congressional debate and study and a frequent topic covered by the news media. There is widespread and growing public awareness that nurses are indeed an essential component of American health care.

The papers in Part I examine nursing as a national resource. The first chapter, written by Aiken, examines both what nurses have hoped to achieve from federal health policy and the realities of what has been accomplished. Fagin, a nurse, and Schramm, a labor economist, present their perspectives on the causes and consequences of the current shortage of nurses. Although their frame of reference is necessarily different, they agree on many of the underlying issues. The papers in Part I provide a basic understanding of the nursing labor market, how it works or fails to work, and identifies strategies for consideration in the 1980s. These papers provide a framework that should be useful in helping the reader evaluate the issues raised in subsequent chapters.

The chapter by Moses and Levine, which appears at the end of this volume, presents data from the most recent (1980) national survey of registered nurses. Readers may wish to refer to that chapter first since it provides updated information on nurses and their practices, which will be a useful background for other chapters.

LINDA H. AIKEN

1

THE IMPACT OF FEDERAL HEALTH POLICY ON NURSES

Over the past 20 yr, nurses have become increasingly interested in public policy, especially federal health policy. Their interests stem from perceptions that the day-to-day professional activities of nurses are significantly influenced by federal policies and programs.

The purpose of this paper is to examine what nurses have hoped to gain through federal health policy and the realities of what has been accomplished. The intent is to seek a better understanding of the potentials and limitations of federal policy in order to more effectively target nurses' collective energies in the 1980s on those strategies that are most likely to be effective in achieving nurses' professional goals.

PUBLIC POLICY

Public policy in health is the continuous process whereby health professionals, institutions, and industry interact with legislators, the executive branch of government, and the judiciary to determine the role government will play in the health sector. The process and products of federal health policy are aimed at improving the health care of the public and shaping the environment of those who work in health care.

Public policy formulation includes the following: the way issues are raised on the public agenda; the process by which laws are passed commit-

The opinions, conclusions, and proposals in the text are those of the author and do not necessarily represent the views of The Robert Wood Johnson Foundation.

ting resources to programs that affect people; the development of rules and regulations that interpret statutes; the actual process of program implementation; and the evaluation of the usefulness of the program that provides the basis for continuing program revisions.[1-3] Policymakers are not faced with a *given* problem; rather, they have to identify and formulate each problem to be addressed.[4] The interaction that results in the formulation of the problem is a critical stage in the public policy process. Once the problem is formulated and moved to the public agenda, the resulting programs are incremental in nature rather than total reformulations of previous programs or policies.

> Decisions effecting small or incremental change and not guided by a high level of understanding . . . are the decisions typical of ordinary political life. . . . It is decision-making through small or incremental moves on particular problems rather than through a comprehensive reform program. It is also endless; it takes the form of an indefinite sequence of policy moves.[5]

The formulation of federal health policy as we know it today grew out of the collapse of the American economy in the Great Depression of 1929 and the resulting social chaos that affected millions.[6] The social and economic consequences of the Depression were of such magnitude that individuals and communities were powerless to affect the economy or to prevent the human tragedies associated with widespread unemployment. At first the burden of economic relief to the unemployed was carried by local tax revenues. However, as unemployment increased and local relief budgets escalated, municipalities exhausted their capacity to respond.

The public began to look to Washington for a national solution to the problems crippling every state and locality in the nation.

> With signs of disaster on all sides and with millions in desperate straits, attitudes toward destitution were momentarily reversed. Many began to define their hardships, not as an individual fate, but as a collective disaster, not as a mark of individual failure, but as a fault of "the system."[7]

Having defined the collapse of the national economy as a "system" failure, the federal government was charged with the responsibility and authority to relieve both the economic and social deprivation that plagued the country and to prevent the recurrence of such problems in the future; and the events and circumstances of the Depression had a definite, centralizing effect upon governmental activity. The federal government, in response to the collapse of local governments, assumed not only a larger role in public spending, which undercut the preeminence of local governments, but also moved toward centrally defined goals and standardized programs across the states.[8]

Franklin Roosevelt's New Deal brought the federal government for the first time into economic security programs on a broad front. There was recognition that health care was essential to rebuilding the social and economic fabric of American life and that the provision of health care was an issue that would have to be addressed on a national scale.

The historic report of the Committee on Economic Security, which led to the Social Security Act of 1935, endorsed the principle of national health insurance.[9] Although national health insurance was not included in the Social Security Act, the stage had been set, and the federal government's role in health care continued to expand in an incremental fashion. The old age insurance provisions of the Social Security Act involved the federal government in the care of the indigent and infirm elderly, which necessarily included health services. In 1950 amendments to the Social Security Act permitted, for the first time, benefits for the disabled and support for direct payments by state and local welfare agencies to providers of health services for impoverished Social Security beneficiaries. Thus, between 1935 and 1965 the federal government gradually assumed greater and greater responsibility for financing health services.[10] In 1965 and 1966, with the enactment of Medicare and Medicaid, federal health policy became explicit and Washington assumed major responsibility for the provision of health care to all of the elderly and many of the poor.

Once the federal government began to pay for health care for so many Americans, it necessarily became a federal commitment to ensure that adequate health resources were available, including physicians, nurses, and hospitals. Since 1965 the process of how Washington has attempted to implement this commitment is generally described as federal health policy.

The federal government's broad and growing commitment to health care is apparent from the rapid escalation of federal health expenditures since 1965. As indicated in Figure 1-1, federal health expenditures grew from $3 billion a year, or 11% of total national health expenditures, in 1960, to $61 billion, or 29% of total expenditures, by 1979.[11] Given the magnitude of federal health expenditures, it is not at all surprising that those working in the health sector have increasingly looked to Washington to provide solutions to problems affecting both health services and improvements in the day-to-day working conditions of health care providers.

Yet, nurses may overestimate the capacity of the federal government to affect nursing practice. In a federal form of government such as ours, the constituent units are separate, and—to a large extent—independent political powers. Under the Federal Constitution, the states retain for themselves all powers not specifically conferred upon the federal government. In the case of nursing, states define nursing practice, license nurses, and establish requirements for nursing schools.

Aside from the broad powers that states have traditionally held, there is increasing public support in the 1980s for a diminishing federal role in American life. The "new federalism" advocated by the Reagan administration is a plan to significantly expand the role of the states in domestic spending pro-

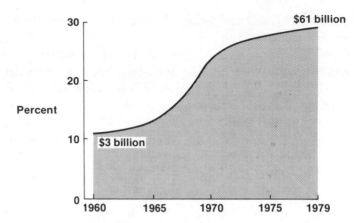

FIGURE 1-1 Percent of national health expenditures financed by federal funds, 1960–1979 (Freeland MS, Schendler CE: National health expenditures: Short-term outlook and long-term projections. Health Care Financing Review, Winter 1981, 2[3]: 97–138).

grams. The proposal includes the payment of federal grants directly to state governments, who would in turn make allocation decisions. The role of the states will also be strengthened by the federal government relinquishing control over certain programs such as Medicaid through substantive changes in law.

In addition to the strong, traditional role of states and any new influence accrued by their increased responsibility for domestic programs, the importance of private industry in health care should not be minimized. The federal government has set general ground rules for industry's behavior by establishing federal legislation in the areas of antitrust, consumer protection, and labor–management relations. However, beyond the broad framework established by these laws, the federal government does not become involved in the outcomes of negotiations within private industry. Many of the policy decisions made by industry have a greater impact on the day-to-day practice of nursing than do government public policy decisions.

The decade of the 1980s holds many challenges for nurses. How these challenges are met may determine the quality of health care received by the public and nursing's future role in health care. The following analysis will attempt to shed new light on the issues of concern to nurses and the extent to which those issues have or will be addressed by federal health policy.

PROMINENT CONCERNS OF NURSES

Federal health policies affect health care providers in four ways. The first and most important is that the federal government pays for health care for the poor and the elderly. Second, federal health manpower programs support the training of health care providers in order to influence the supply, composition, or distribution of the work force.[12] Third, many of the new ideas and innovations in clinical care come from federally supported research, and fourth, federal programs provide capital support for new and renovated health care facilities, including nursing and medical schools, hospitals, community health centers, and rural clinics.

The nursing profession has attempted to leverage these four types of federal strategies to bring about improvements in areas of prominent concern to nurses. Six issues that have been the focus of concern are as follows:

1 *Removing financial barriers to health care.* A major public policy goal of nurses has been to achieve universal health insurance coverage so that no American is denied access to health services because of the inability to pay for needed care.

2 *Improving the quality of nursing care available.* The primary strategy advocated by nurses to improve quality has been to broaden the education of nurses, and change the mix to include a higher proportion of nurses with baccalaureate and higher degrees.

3 *Ending the shortage of hospital nurses.* Since World War II there has been a persistent shortage of hospital nurses that has in recent years become more acute despite a doubling of the number of nurses in practice. Given the failure of local institutions or state groups to resolve the shortage, nurses (and other providers) have looked to the federal government for assistance in finding a national solution.

4 *Improving nurses' economic rewards.* Nurses' incomes have not kept pace with incomes of comparable professional groups. Low relative incomes are associated with high levels of dissatisfaction, problems with nurse retention, and declining enrollments in nursing schools.

5 *Expanding nurses' independent roles within hospitals.* The rapid growth of knowledge and technology and changing medical practice patterns have made the traditional social contact between nurses, physicians, and hospitals incompatible with nurses' changing responsibilities in hospitals.

6 *Developing new professional roles outside the hospital.* National concerns about the delivery of effective and affordable health care have resulted in the evolution of new roles for nurses in ambulatory care and research.

IMPACT OF FEDERAL POLICY ON NURSES

To what extent over the past 20 years has the federal government been able to address nursing's major concerns?

REMOVING FINANCIAL BARRIERS TO HEALTH CARE

Nurses for many years have had a major commitment to remove the financial barriers that impede the public's access to health care. The American Nurses' Association (ANA) was the first major provider group to publicly support Medicare. "The American Nurses' Assocation had endorsed the proposal quite early, when such an independent position took considerable courage."[13] Nurses have also supported universal coverage for all Americans through comprehensive national health insurance.

Although national health insurance legislation has not been passed, insurance coverage has been extended to the elderly and some of the poor. About 90% of Americans are now covered by some form of public or private health insurance. However, in addition to the 20 million persons not protected by health insurance, only 68% of expenditures for the insured are actually covered. A large proportion of ambulatory services are not covered by insurance, and it is estimated that as many as half of all American families are not protected against the costs of catastrophic illness.[14]

Increased insurance coverage of the poor and elderly since 1965 has substantially improved these groups' access to health care.[15] The poor now see physicians more often than the affluent, which is entirely appropriate considering their higher burden of illness. The traditional differences in use of health services between racial and ethnic groups have narrowed as have the differences between urban and rural residents.[16]

Despite these gains, national health insurance remains an important item on nursing's agenda for the future. Inadequate insurance coverage of ambulatory care and catastrophic illness creates major constraints to the delivery of essential nursing care.

IMPROVING THE QUALITY OF NURSING CARE

There has been a virtual revolution in the education of nurses over the past 20 yr.[17] Before 1960 most nurses were trained in hospitals, where the focus was primarily on training bedside nurses for acute care settings.[18] The expansion of ambulatory services, the growth of nursing homes, the evolution of hospitals into complex institutions requiring special clinical and nursing management expertise, and the increasing numbers of the elderly and people with chronic illness all demanded nurses with broader education who were qualified to assume greater autonomy in the delivery of health services.

Nurses, therefore, began to move nursing education into colleges and universities where a broader general education could be combined with clinical expertise.[19, 20] As indicated in Figure 1-2, there has been a major shift from hospital-based programs to those in colleges and universities. In 1960

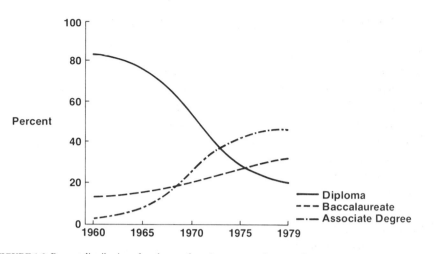

FIGURE 1-2 Percent distribution of graduates of nursing programs by type of program, 1960–1979 (National League for Nursing, NLN Nursing Data Book, 1980. New York: National League for Nursing, 1981).

83% of new graduates were trained in hospitals.* In 1980 83% of new graduates had been educated in colleges and universities — a dramatic reversal in the short period of 2 decades.

In addition to generic nursing education, registered nurses have pursued college degrees in large numbers. In 1977 one out of every ten nurses was pursuing a post-RN college degree.[21] By 1980 almost one-third of all practicing nurses had at least a baccalaureate degree — the goal set in 1963 by the Surgeon General's Consultant Group on Nursing.[22]

Graduate nursing education has also expanded very rapidly. Between 1964 and 1979 there was a 335% increase in the number of graduations from master's programs. In addition, between 1960 and 1980 the number of nurses enrolled in doctoral programs increased by over 500%.[23]

Federal policy played a major role in improving the educational qualifications of nurses. During the period 1965 through 1981, the federal government, through the Nurse Training Act and research programs, appropriated a total of $1.5 billion.[24] Over $834 million was invested in institutional support of schools of nursing. Most of these funds were deployed to improve the quality of nursing education. Federal funds were particularly important to the growth of collegiate programs and graduate programs where there were no patient revenues to offset the expansion of programs. Special projects and construction funds (totaling $382 million) contributed to curricula development and improvements in the physical plant of schools in colleges and universities. Formula and capitation grants (totaling $329.9 million) enabled schools to employ additional faculty, provide audiovisual equipment, enlarge

*Unless otherwise specified, all educational data were obtained from *NLN Nursing Data Book 1980*. New York: National League for Nursing, 1981.

library collections, and support a host of other activities that contributed to improved nursing education.

ENDING THE SHORTAGE OF HOSPITAL NURSES

For more than 30 yr there has been a chronic shortage of nurses. The nation's output of nurses has more than doubled since 1950, and the increase in employed nurses has outstripped population growth by 139%. Paradoxically, the nursing shortage now seems worse than ever.

The only time during the past 30 yr when the national shortage of hospital nurses eased and vacancy rates in hospitals declined was during the period 1968 to 1971. As indicated in Figure 1-3, hospital nursing vacancy rates dropped rather dramatically from over 23% in 1961 to 9% in 1971, a decline that corresponded to the rapid increases in nurses' salaries (as compared to teachers' salaries, Fig. 1-3), which accompanied improved reimbursement to hospitals by Medicare. During this period, a significant number of inactive nurses came back to active practice either in response to relative wage increases or as part of the general movement of American women into the labor force. Over one-third of the net increase in the number of employed nurses from 1966 to 1972 – an increase that profoundly reduced hospital vacancy rates – came from the existing pool of inactive nurses.[25, 26]

In an occupation made up predominantly of women, labor force participation is one of the most important factors affecting the national supply.[27] For example, between 1960 and 1980 the labor force participation rate for nurses jumped from 55% to over 75%. If the current activity rate was still at 1960 levels, there would be 300,000 nurses less in active practice today!

The primary federal strategy to ease the hospital nursing shortage has

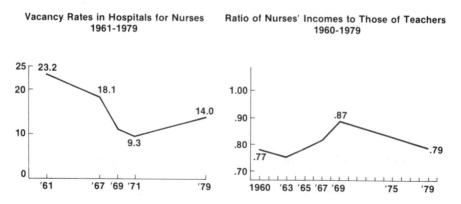

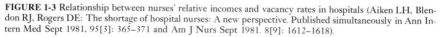

FIGURE 1-3 Relationship between nurses' relative incomes and vacancy rates in hospitals (Aiken LH, Blendon RJ, Rogers DE: The shortage of hospital nurses: A new perspective. Published simultaneously in Ann Intern Med Sept 1981, 95[3]: 365–371 and Am J Nurs Sept 1981. 8[9]: 1612–1618).

been to increase enrollments in nursing schools. Yet, increased enrollments had little to do with the alleviation of the shortage during the few years following the introduction of Medicare.[28] Furthermore, when nursing school graduations were at an all time high in 1978 (78,000 nurses a year), the hospital shortage had reappeared and was more severe than ever.

The federal government through various manpower training programs can increase the number of people trained in any given occupation if sufficient resources are invested. However, in the case of nursing, there is no direct association between numbers of graduates from nursing schools and hospital vacancy rates. The complexity of the factors that determine how many nurses work in hospitals and how many nurses hospitals would like to employ (represented by vacancy rates) limit the extent to which federal policy can resolve this problem.

Health economists have observed that the labor market for nurses does not respond to changes in supply and demand.[29-32] In most occupations, shortages are self-correcting. Increased competition among employers for the available workers leads to increased wages. As wages rise relative to other occupations, more students elect to come into the field and inactive persons return to active employment. Eventually the shortage is resolved, and relative wages may stabilize or even decline, which usually acts to avert a subsequent surplus.

The market for nurses is not self-correcting. Despite a persistent shortage, salaries have not risen. Nursing is affected by an economic market phenomenon known as monopsony (or, technically, oligopsony), which refers to the presence of only a few employers. Sixty-six percent of nurses work in hospitals. Some communities have only one or two hospitals, and most have fewer than ten. If nurses want to work in health care, they must, for the most part, work in those hospitals. Further, the nature of nurses' education is such that it does not seem to allow them to move easily out of nursing or health care into other positions of comparable status. In short, nurses are in a captured labor market. As a result, nurses' salaries and working conditions have not kept pace with other groups.

There is strong evidence that limiting the growth of nurses' salaries relative to others is the single most important factor contributing to the current perceived national shortage of nurses.[33] Because the salaries of nurses are low relative to other hospital workers, hospitals can afford to substitute nurses for non-nurses. Where we would expect to see hospitals reacting to a critical shortage of nurses by substituting other personnel for nurses, just the opposite seems to be occurring. Given the low relative salaries of nurses, there is evidence that many hospitals are stockpiling nurses, which results in real shortages in other hospitals, particularly those in less desirable locations. The evidence suggests that adjustments in nurses' incomes to make them more compatible with those of other professionals with comparable responsibilities may be the best way of swiftly overcoming the perceived shortage.

Increasing the incomes of nurses is not a national priority or a federal responsibility. Also, some federal policies could conceivably make the shortage worse. Efforts to increase the number of graduates from nursing schools or importing foreign trained nurses will further depress incomes and exacerbate the perceived shortage.

There are two possible strategies for resolving the shortage. The first would be an effort by leaders in nursing and the hospital industry to come to some consensus about the cause of the shortage and identify strategies for its resolution. If the answer is allowing nurses' salaries to rise, offsetting savings will have to be achieved by reallocation of resources. Hospital expenditures exceed $100 billion a year. Most hospital budgets are large enough to permit reallocation without impairing essential hospital services. Community hospitals, for example, spend close to $6 billion annually on equipment and renovation or construction of the physical plant. In fact, since 1968 the growth of nonsalary hospital expenses has outstripped salary expenses rather significantly.[34]

The second alternative is collective bargaining. The evidence to date indicates that collective bargaining has a favorable effect on nurses' salaries even in states with strong hospital cost containment programs, further evidence that hospitals do have flexibility in the allocation of resources.[35, 36] In the absence of other solutions, collective bargaining is likely to increase in the 1980s.

IMPROVING NURSES' ECONOMIC REWARDS

The depression of nurses' relative incomes has not only been a major contributing factor to the perceived shortage of hospital nurses, it has also been a primary source of dissatisfaction among nurses, and has contributed to high staff turnover rates in hospitals and nursing homes. Nurses' current incomes do not compare well with those in other occupations predominantly filled by women (Fig. 1-4). Nurses' salaries are on par with the national average salaries for secretaries, even though the educational preparation is considerably greater for nurses. Teachers and female professional, technical, and kindred workers earn more than nurses in the current market. Health professionals whose work and general responsibilities are roughly similar to those of nurses — social workers, physical therapists, and pharmacists — all appear to be faring better than nurses.[37] As illustrated in Figure 1-5, nurses' incomes in 1974 dollars have actually declined over the past 5 yr.

Nursing home salaries are even less competitive than those of hospitals. Despite the desperate need for nurses in nursing homes, the average salaries

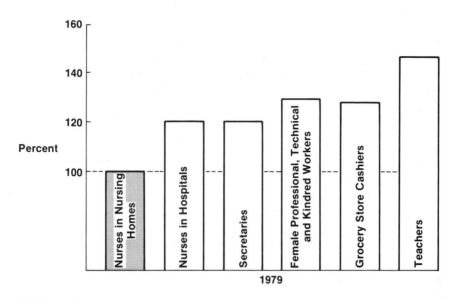

160

140

120

Percent

100 -- --

Nurses in Nursing Homes

Nurses in Hospitals

Secretaries

Female Professional, Technical and Kindred Workers

Grocery Store Cashiers

Teachers

1979

FIGURE 1-4 Comparison of nurses' salaries to other salaries (Aiken LH, Blendon RJ. Rogers DE: The shortage of hospital nurses: A new perspective. Published simultaneously in Ann Intern Med Sept 1981, 95[3]: 365–371 and Am J Nurs Sept 1981, 81[9]: 1612–1618).

for nurses in nursing homes are 10% to 20% below hospital nurses' salaries. The noncompetitive salary structure in nursing homes creates a major problem in attracting and retaining nurses to care for the 1.3 million nursing homes residents.

The salary structures for nurses in hospitals and nursing homes are based on the assumption that most nurses are temporary workers. Thus, the salary structures are relatively flat with modest increases for administrative responsibilities but almost no differential for experience. A recent national survey of nurses found that there was only a $2,000 a year difference in average salaries of beginning nurses and those of nurses with 20 yr of experience.[38] All recent national surveys of nurse employment patterns, however, indicate that nurses are staying in the labor force longer than ever before. The lack of recognition of experience in salary increments is a major source of dissatisfaction among nurses with hospital employment.

In addition, the development of benefits based on seniority is almost totally absent in hospitals. The types of retirement packages common in the teaching profession that act to increase retention of teachers within school districts or states are not found in health care institutions. Nurses have nothing to lose from changing jobs frequently because seniority has no advantages. It is surprising, given the high reported costs of nurse recruitment and inservice education for new graduates, that hospitals have not tried strategies used successfully by other industries to retain their most experienced and productive employees.

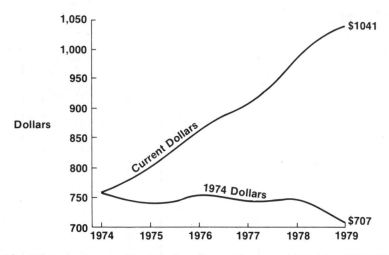

FIGURE 1-5 National average monthly salaries for staff nurses in current and 1974 dollars, 1974–1979 (University of Texas Medical Branch at Galveston. National surveys of Hospital and Medical School Salaries).

An examination of hospital nurse vacancy statistics reveals that most vacancies are in intensive care units (ICUs) and the undesirable hours on nights and weekends. Yet the economic incentives are almost negligible for nurses to work in the physically and emotionally demanding ICUs or during unpopular hours.

Can the federal government play a role in the improvement of the employment conditions in health care institutions? Hospitals and nursing homes in the United States are primarily private employers subject only to those labor relations laws that now affect most other private industries. The federal role in private employment has been limited to establishing general ground rules for the operation of the private marketplace, that is, minimum wage, worker safety, civil rights, and general parameters to guide employee–employer collective bargaining.

Beyond setting the ground rules for collective bargaining, the federal role has never been to determine the outcome of negotiations. The opportunity to negotiate working conditions is available to employees in private industries under the protection of federal law but the outcomes are not protected or determined by federal policy. Thus, only private agreements between nurses and hospitals or nursing homes collectively negotiated could alter current working conditions.

EXPANDING NURSES' INDEPENDENT ROLES WITHIN THE HOSPITAL

There are fundamental incompatibilities in the present social contract between nurses and physicians.[39] In reality, this contract is reflected in licensure laws. The difficulties of broadening the interpretation of nurses' roles as specified in existing licensure laws, and clarifying the clinical decision-making authority of the nurse and how it should relate to that of the physician in the hospital context, has lead to conflict between individual nurses and physicians and antagonism between the two professions.

There are four major reasons why nurses believe that the social and legal contract between nurses and physicians regarding clinical decision-making should be modified.

1   Nurses are now in command of much of the available clinical expertise to care for the seriously ill and are expected to make judgments about its appropriate use. No change has taken place, however, in the nurses' sphere of authority in the care of patients.

2   Despite the fact that hospitalized patients are sicker than ever before and require constant professional surveillance and timely intervention to prevent crises, there has been little formal recognition of the importance of the nurse's role in the new level of clinical decision making required by very sick patients.

3   Physicians, like other professionals, now work fewer hours, and there are extended periods when physicians are not present in the hospital or easily accessible for direct consultation. Despite this reality, the authority of the nurse to act in the absence of the physician has not been redefined.

4   The shift in medicine from general to subspecialty practice has resulted in the involvement of multiple physicians in the care of a single patient. Fragmentation of care can result in costly and dangerous duplication or omission. The role of the nurse has not changed to recognize this need for continuing synthesis of the prescriptions of many physicians and professional surveillance of multiple diagnostic and treatment regimens.

Nurses have hoped that federal policy would more explicitly address the need for a greater independent role for nurses in hospitals, particularly because the federal government has supported the training of nurses with broader education and expertise. However, the licensure of health professionals has been a traditional state responsibility, one that federal policy would not preempt. Thus any change in licensure laws or interpretation of existing laws must be pursued in a state-by-state fashion in the state government policy arena.

DEVELOPING NEW PROFESSIONAL ROLES OUTSIDE THE HOSPITAL

Federal health policy has effectively assisted nurses in the development of new and challenging roles outside the hospital that more fully use nurses' advanced education and clinical expertise. Federal support has been a major catalyst in the development of new career opportunities in ambulatory care and in nursing research.

The federal government has been the major source of support for nursing research. Federal monies were essential to enable students to enroll in doctoral programs, for the start-up funds for new doctoral programs in nursing, and for research grants to qualified nurse researchers.

The evolution of new roles for nurses in ambulatory care — nurse practitioners and nurse midwives — provided many nurses the opportunity to embark upon different career paths. Although nurse practitioner programs supported initially by private foundations, the federal government made a major contribution in the 1970s, investing $64 million in nurse practitioner and nurse midwife education.

Despite subsidies of nurse practitioner education, however, federal policy on nurse practitioners can be characterized as ambivalent. Federal expenditures for nurse practitioners were justified on the basis of a shortage and maldistribution of physicians. In addition to increasing the supply of nurse practitioners, however, federal policy is responsible for a massive increase in the supply of physicians (Fig. 1-6). Federal programs encouraged medical schools and medical educators to increase the number of first year students, of medical schools, and of physicians in general care specialties. These efforts were so successful that the number of practicing physicians will increase by one-third in the 1980s alone, leading to predictions of a physician "excess" by 1990.[40] The success of federal manpower policy in the production of nurse practitioners on the one hand has been thwarted on the other by the concurrent increase in the physician supply.

Federal government reimbursement policy also reflects the ambivalence of health manpower policy regarding nurse practitioners. One of the greatest

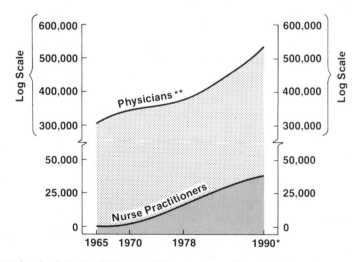

FIGURE 1-6 Supply of physicians** (includes DOs) and nurse practitioners, 1965–1990* (projected). (Graduate Medical Education National Advisory Committee. Report to the Secretary. Washington, D.C.: U.S. Dept. of Health and Human Services, September 30, 1981).

barriers to the effective use of nurse practitioners has been the lack of third party reimbursement even by federal programs.

The evolution of the nurse practitioner concept has had many direct and indirect effects on the nursing profession. It has opened new, intellectually challenging career options for nurses outside of the restraining bureaucracy of the hospital, encouraged closer collaborative relationships with physicians, and developed new types of ongoing relationships between nurses and the public. But the nurse practitioner movement has also generated confrontation with physicians in office-based practice who are concerned about declining office visits. There appears to be a growing backlash against nurse practitioners that is primarily economic in nature. Although the federal government has established antitrust laws to protect the rights of individuals or groups to pursue their chosen work, these laws will not preempt state nurse practice acts. The future of nurse practitioners will be largely determined by state level policy decisions on the definition and scope of nursing practice.

CONCLUSIONS

Federal health policy over the past 20 yr has been sensitive to some of nurses' major concerns. Indeed, the federal government has provided important leadership in removing financial barriers to health care, one of nursing's highest priorities for years. Even though national health insurance remains on the agenda for the future, major improvements have been made in broadening health insurance coverage for the elderly and the poor.

Federal policies have also improved the quality of nursing care available to the public by broadening the educational preparation of nurses and increasing the proportion of nurses with baccalaureate and higher degrees. In addition, federal policy was central in the development of new professional roles for nurses outside the hospital, particularly nurse practitioners and nurse midwives in ambulatory care and nurse researchers in clinical and academic settings.

Nursing's other concerns have simply not been on the public agenda at the federal level either because they were not seen as national priorities or, more importantly, they were not defined as federal responsibilities.

Health policy in the United States operates in the context of federalism. The primary responsibilities for policies that most directly affect nurses are not held by the federal government but by the individual states. In addition, many of the concerns of nurses involve private sector institutions such as hospitals and nursing homes. The federal government has established a broad framework to govern private industry and has a very limited direct role in setting private sector policies. Also, some of nurses' concerns cannot be addressed by legislation. Some complex interactions between professions do not lend themselves to legislative solution.

Over the past decade nurses have tended to overestimate the federal government's capacity to influence issues directly related to the practice of nursing and to underestimate the extent to which responsibility and power in American life is diffused among multiple groups. Many of the issues of greatest concern to nurses cannot be resolved by federal intervention. Instead, public policy at the state level, collective bargaining with industry, and joint negotiations between nurses, physicians, and health care institutions represent strategies that may bring about solutions over the next decade.

The one definitive contribution the federal government could make to broadening the responsibilities of nurses in hospitals and nursing homes, and facilitating the development of improved working environments, is to support special projects to demonstrate the effectiveness and feasibility of new and innovative approaches. Many institutions are not opposed to change. Rather, the day-to-day complexities and demands of hospitals and nursing homes militate against the investment of front-end time and resources necessary to find creative, new solutions. To date, no federal agency has been given the mandate to fund demonstrations of this kind. Targeting some of the existing federal nursing resources on timely and innovative demonstrations in the settings were nurses practice could have a far more beneficial effects on the future quality of health care than efforts to increase enrollments in basic nursing programs.

REFERENCES

1   Anderson, J.E. *Public policy-making*. New York: Praeger, 1975.

2   Jenkins, W.I. *Policy analysis*. New York: St. Martin's Press, 1978.

3   Starling, G. *The politics and economies of public policy*. Homewood, IL: Dorsey Press, 1979.

4   Lindblom, C.E. *The policy-making process*. Englewood Cliffs, NJ: Prentice-Hall, 1968.

5   Braybrook, D. and Lindblom, C.E. *A strategy of decision*. New York: Free Press, 1963.

6   Ripley, R.B. *American national government and public policy*. New York: Free Press, 1974.

7   Piven, F.F. and Cloward, R.A. *Regulating the poor: The functions of public welfare*. New York: Random House, 1972, p. 61.

8   Hofferbert, R.I. *The study of public policy*. Indianapolis: Bobbs-Merrill, 1974.

9   Somers, A.R. and Somers, H.M. *Health and health care: policies in perspective*. Germantown, Md.: Aspen Systems Corporation, 1977.

10   Vladeck, B. *Unloving care: The nursing home tragedy*. New York: Basic Books, 1980.

11   Freeland, M.S. and Schendler, C.E. National health expenditures: Short-term outlook and long-term projections. *Health Care Financing Review*, Winter 1981, 2(3):97–138.

12   Fein, R. and Bishop, C. *Employment impacts of health policy developments*. Washington, D.C.: National Commission for Manpower Policy, Special Report No. 11, October 1976.

13   Somers, A.R., and Somers, H.M., *op. cit*, p. 165.

14   Aiken, L.H. Alternative care models: The impact of financing constraints. *Nursing's influence on health policy for the eighties*. Kansas City, MO: American Academy of Nursing, 1979.

15   Davis, K. and Schoen, C. *Health and the war on poverty: A ten-year appraisal*. Washington, D.C.: Brookings Institution, 1978.

16   Rogers, D.E., Aiken, L.H., Blendon, R.J. *Personal medical care: Its adaptation to the 1980's*. Washington, D.C.: Institute of Medicine, National Academy of Sciences Occasional Paper, 1980.

17   Kalisch, P.A. and Kalisch, B.J. *The advance of American nursing*. Boston: Little, Brown and Co., 1978.

18   Ashley, J. *Hospitals, paternalism, and the role of the nurse*. New York: Teachers College Press, 1976.

19   American Nurses' Association. *Educational preparation for nurse practitioners and assistants to nurses: A position paper*. New York, 1965.

20   American Nurses' Association. *A case for baccalaureate preparation for nursing*. Kansas City, Mo., 1979.

21   Moses, E. and Roth, A. What do statistics reveal about the nation's nurses? *American Journal of Nursing*, 1979, *79*, 1745–1756.

22   Department of Health, Education and Welfare. *Toward quality in nursing*. Report of the Surgeon General's Consultant Group on Nursing. Washington, D.C.: U.S. Government Printing Office. PHS Publication No. 992, 1963.

23   American Nurses' Association. *Directory of nurses with doctoral degrees*. Kansas City, Mo.: American Nurses' Association, 1980.

24   Institute of Medicine. *Six-month interim report by the Committee of the Institute of Medicine for a Study of Nursing and Nursing Education*. Washington, D.C.: National Academy Press, 1981, Appendix 1.

25   Yett, D.E. *An economic analysis of the nurse shortage*. Lexington, Mass.: D.C. Heath & Company, 1975.

26   Feldstein, P. *Health care economics*. New York: John Wiley and Sons, 1979.

27   Freeman, R.B. The evolution of the American labor market, 1948–80. In M. Feldstein (ed.) *The American economy in transition*. Chicago: University of Chicago Press, 1980.

28   Yett, D.E., *op. cit*.

29   Altman, S. *Present and future supply of registered nurses*. (DHEW Pub. No. (NIH) 72–134), 1971.

30   Yett, D.E., *op. cit*.

31   Sloan, F.A. *Equalizing access to nursing services*. (DHEW Pub. No. HRA 78–51). Washington, D.C.: Government Printing Office, 1978.

32   Feldstein, P., *op. cit*.

33   Aiken, L.H., Blendon, R.J., Rogers, D.E. The shortage of hospital nurses: A new

perspective. Published simultaneously in *Annals of Internal Medicine*, September 1981, *95*(3):365–371, and *American Journal of Nursing*, September 1981, *81*(9): 1612–1618.

34   Michela, W.A. Changes in the distribution of selected hospital expenses. *Hospitals, Journal of the American Hospitals Association*, February 1, 1979, 28–29.

35   Feldman, R., Lee, L. and Hoffbeck, R. Hospital Employees' Wages and Labor Union Organization. Final Report, Grant Number 1-R03-HSO3649-01, National Center for Health Services Research, OASH, November, 1980.

36   Miller, R.U. Hospitals. In G.G. Somers (ed.) *Collective bargaining: Contemporary American experience*. Madison, WI: Industrial Relations Research Association, 1980.

37   Aiken, L.H., Blendon, R.J., Rogers, D.E., *op. cit.*

38   Donovan, L. Survey of nursing incomes, part 2. What increases income most? *RN*, February 1980, *43*:27–30.

39   Aiken, L.N. Nursing priorities for the 1980's: Hospitals and nursing homes. *American Journal of Nursing*, February 1981, *81*(2):324–330.

40   Graduate Medical Education National Advisory Committee. *Report to the Secretary*. Washington, D.C.: U.S. Dept. of Health and Human Services, September 30, 1980.

CLAIRE M. FAGIN

2

THE NATIONAL SHORTAGE OF NURSES: A NURSING PERSPECTIVE

A critical shortage of nurses that is both qualitative and quantitative exists in the United States.[1] While the issue of a shortage of nurses has been discussed for 3 decades, the problem seems less amenable to solution now than it did in previous years. The maturity of the nursing profession will be tested by the manner in which it grapples with and proposes solutions to this problem. Nursing's professional maturity expressed in assertive stances toward a variety of other nursing and health care issues, while appropriate, must not divert attention from developing proposals to ameliorate the nursing shortage. This problem affects several other groups whose solutions to the nursing shortage may be antithetical to both the continued progress of the profession and long-term solutions to health care deficits.

In 1980 the number of registered nurses was almost twice that of 1960.[2] The 1.4 million nurses holding the registered nurse license were surveyed in September 1977 by the American Nurses' Association (ANA).[3] Of this group it was found that 73% were in the nursing labor force. Despite this high percentage of working nurses, there are between 90,000 and 100,000 vacant, budgeted registered nurse positions in hospitals alone; serious nursing shortages in nursing homes, and unfilled nursing positions in community health agencies.[4] A review of current enrollment data indicates a decreasing number of high school graduates and a declining proportion of graduates entering nursing programs.[5]

Permission has been granted by the *Journal of Public Health Policy* for this edited, updated version of article published in Vol. 1, No. 4, 1980.

This paper reviews the background of this potential crisis in health care, presents some interpretations of how it happened, and makes recommendations for the future with regard to restructuring employment for nurses. These recommendations have implications for attracting men and women to the profession. Since more than 60% of employed RNs work in hospitals the paper emphasizes these settings.

BACKGROUND OF THE PROBLEM

The question of the nation's supply of nurses has been discussed widely since World War II. Initial governmental intervention to encourage expansion of the nursing supply occurred in the mental health field in 1946 and in general nurse training in the mid-1950s.

The Health Professions Education Assistance Act of 1963 was a major step by the federal government to commit funds to health professions training. This act was the result of numerous studies conducted in the late 1940s and 1950s that stressed the inadequate supply of health manpower. Following the Report of the Surgeon General's Consultant Group on Nursing, which recommended increased support to nursing education, the Nurse Training Act of 1964 was passed. During the subsequent decade, a significant increase in both the nation's supply of nurses and in nurses' educational preparation occurred.

From 1971 to the present, the question of federal support to nursing has been debated in the executive and legislative branches of government. The Nixon administration's attempt to impound nursing appropriations was followed by President Ford's pocket veto of the Nurse Training Act, followed again by President Carter's pocket veto in 1978 and his proposal to rescind monies already approved. President Reagan in 1981 also requested rescissions in nursing appropriations and markedly reduced new funding.

In early 1980 President Carter and his staff at the Department of Health and Human Services — formerly Health, Education and Welfare (HEW) — justified their request for a $78 million reduction in the support of nursing education programs by claiming the adequacy of the aggregate supply of nurses and anticipating by 1985 a balance of supply and need.

This projection was based on two studies supported by HEW that modeled data around a prospective national health insurance and Health Maintenance Organization utilization.[6,7] Other studies focusing on demographic and morbidity changes and the prospective needs for acute, chronic, and long-term care postulated a much larger number of nurses, but these were seen to be inflated projections.[8] However, the current experience supports the validity of the latter approach.

It is possible also that the Carter Administration's viewpoint was formed by a belief on the part of some observers that a surplus of nurses was on the horizon. From a 30-yr perspective on the "shortage" issue, it is interesting to note that the present hysteria follows, by only a few years, a report stating that signs of a surplus of nurses were appearing and that "heightened awareness" needed to occur in relation to this possibility.[9] Regional variations in nursing employment were occurring in 1977, particularly in relation to employment of graduates of associate degree programs. However, these variations were characterized as "frictional" with no significant surpluses but with "regional differences in the severity of shortage."[10]

These views are supported by the 1977 ANA survey that found that 70%, or 978,324 registered nurses, were in active practice. About 43,000 or 3% were seeking employment in nursing, a figure well within the "frictional unemployment" range; 23% were not employed nor looking for employment. About 4% or 46,780 nurses were employed in other fields. More than 60% of employed nurses were working in hospitals.[11]

The participation rate of nurses is significantly higher than for professions such as social work and teaching, which report lower active employment levels.[12] Blaming the inactive "pool" for the nursing shortage* does not take into account several other findings of the 1977 survey: 34.5% of the inactive nurses have children under the age of 17; a significant decrease in activity rates occurred in nurses with children under the age of 6; more than one-third of the inactive group were nurses over the age of 50, more than 80% of this group have no credential higher than the diploma. The physical demands of the staff-nurse role and the increased complexities of technologic nursing care make it virtually impossible to expect a significant number of these nurses to return to the nursing work force.

The anticipated balance of supply and need for registered nurses over this decade was based both on projections of health services and nursing school enrollment data. We now know that enrollment projections made in the early 1970s were overly optimistic. National League for Nursing (NLN) data show that the "supply of new nurses has not increased significantly since 1974 and in 1978 a decline in admissions was recorded; the first since the 1960s."

> The decline in aggregate RN graduations is predicted to be about 2 to 3 percent-per-year. . . . The smallest decline will be registered among baccalaureate programs, with a modest increase actually occurring in 1980 and 1981, followed by slight yearly declines to 1985. Associate degree programs are predicted to display a slightly accelerating decline. . . and diploma programs will continue in a long range pattern of decline.[13]

*The Reagan administration currently uses this excuse for recommending cutbacks in funds for nursing.

The present shortage of nurses, coupled with the declines in enrollment in nursing programs, provides the backdrop for predicting a major crisis in health and illness care in the coming decades. In addition, the percentage of registered nurses in the nursing force suggests that an increased demand for nurses has occurred. The following section explores this phenomenon.

THE DEMAND FOR NURSES

Several factors have caused an increased demand for registered nurses. These are (1) increased acuteness of the condition of hospitalized patients of all ages; (2) increased degree of illness of long-term-care patients of all ages; (3) increased sophistication of treatment in and out of hospitals; (4) increased pressure on nurses from changes in physician specialization in hospitals; (5) demographic changes in population, with growth in absolute number and percentage of persons over 65; (6) focus on community-based care and home health care; (7) emphasis on health and health maintenance.

Changes in the degree of patient illness in hospitals and the technological revolution are probably the most dramatic and have occurred more quickly than the others. They were also unexpected since, as is common with the nursing experience, the resultant need for nurses was completely omitted from considerations of cost containment and of shortening patients' stays in hospitals. Note that the expansion of hospital beds that occurred after the Hill–Burton Act also ignored the question of nursing resources. Thus, while factors 5, 6, and 7 have contributed to an increased need for nurses in that they imply predominantly "caring" *versus* "curing" functions, the extreme changes in acute and long-term care have caused the near hysteria characterizing our current mood.

A simple comparision of the increased number of critical care beds in the past decade (16,000 to about 40,000) explains why hospitals nationwide have changed their staffing patterns to rely more heavily on registered nurses. The following statistics were reported in 1976–77 for a 14-bed pediatric intensive-care unit; one head nurse, one clinical nursing specialist, 18 registered nurses, 10 nursing technicians. In 1980 the projection for this unit is one head nurse, one clinical nursing specialist, and 36 registered nurses. Shortening the hospital stay heightens the nursing problems caused by the increased acuteness of illness in that there is little or no convalescent time in the hospital. This change increases the requirements for nurses and concomitantly for more sophisticated registered nurses. Numerous examples could be given of "step-down" units whose population resembles the intensive-care units of a decade ago, and nursing homes whose populations were in hospitals 10 yr ago.

These changes have not only created a marked increase in the demand for registered nurses but have also changed the nature of the routine day — increasing the emotional and physical demands on nurses and heightening the need for nurses to be technologically and interpersonally competent. It should be recognized that changes in the nature of graduate medical education, the elimination of the internship, and the decrease in the number of residents in several subspecialties have had enormous impact on the role of the nurse. The expanded role perceived as pertaining to ambulatory care is the *sine qua non* for the nurse in a tertiary care setting. The nurse working in a hospital where there are insufficient numbers of nursing colleagues can be expected to "burn-out" very rapidly and, at the least, seek nursing employment elsewhere.

It should be clear that the factors identified are important indicators of nursing requirements at present and in the future but that some are the dominant causes of our present and future problems.

CHARACTERISTICS OF NURSING WORK AND EDUCATION THAT INHIBIT IMPROVEMENT OF THE NURSING SHORTAGE

The factors identified as causing the present shortage of nurses also create conditions that inhibit long-term employment. In addition, other factors such as economic conditions, status problems, career mobility, rotation of hours, and power to effect change contribute to the frustration and unhappiness in many nurses. Since another position is always available and, since for some nurses the life-long *career* is less important than the *job*, leaving one job for another is common. Further, problems such as those listed inhibit interest in nursing as a career among women and men. A few words about each is in order before we consider some recommendations for improvement in the present and future supply of nurses. The factors I am discussing are overlapping and not mutually exclusive.

ECONOMIC CONDITIONS

Much data support the view that a nursing shortage does exist. Yet economic theory holds that in a competitive market, price is determined by supply and demand. Short supply and high demand ought to affect price but the principles of supply and demand and market pricing have not yet affected the shortage of nurses. While labor markets may not be perfectly competitive since employers have some control over wages, wage policy generally is conditioned by the available supply of labor.[14]

Those workers most highly paid in our country have benefited from a protectionist organization (*e.g.*, union), which keeps supply down and wages up.[15] Unions that have been most successful cover workers who are in skilled occupations. Workers who have only one possible employer do not benefit from this kind of protection.

Using principles of supply and demand alone and examining average nursing salaries at the staff nurse level – the level considered at national crisis proportions – we must conclude that *the nursing shortage is a shortage at a price*. The previous "so-called shortages" occurred during the 1950s. The question of real *versus* artificial shortage – if market principles apply – was no more apparent then than now. We are beginning to see upward movement in the beginning salary levels in some hospitals and health facilities, in some areas. We are also noting salaries of faculty and deans with doctorates responding to the market as well as salaries of nursing administrators with doctoral degrees. An examination of salaries of the past few years, however, indicates negligible increases in view of inflation. In 1977 the ANA reported the mean national salary for all workers as $13,000 per year. The national mean salary for staff nurses (entry level) was $11,172 at that time.[16] A 1979 national survey[17] indicated that the mean annual entry level salary was $12,816, approximately a 7% increase per year, which is regressive in real dollars. Regional and local differences from the mean were and are apparent.

For example, in Philadelphia and New York recent advertisements indicate that many hospitals start the new bachelor degree graduate at approximately $18,000 per year. According to the *New York Times*, however, the 1980 agreement with uniformed services in New York provided $21,000 as the beginning salary for sanitation workers and $23,000 for policemen and firemen.

These anecdotal indications of variation in mean salaries should not, therefore, mask the main point, which is that nurses' salaries and fringe benefits do not offer fair value for skills, education, and conditions of employment. A 1975 complaint in Denver by a group called Nurses, Inc., to the Equal Employment Opportunity Commission, and subsequently to federal court as a class action suit, asked that salaries of nurses in the city be comparable with male city employees including sign painters, tree trimmers, and tire servicemen. The mean starting salary for male classifications at that time was $1,592.81, compared with $1,090.77 for female classifications, including nurses. In April 1980 a federal appeals court ruled against Nurse, Inc., on the basis that the law recognizes discrimination against people only not jobs.

It is important to identify possible reasons for the fact that nurses' salaries have not risen sufficiently to create a balance of supply and demand. Among the possibilities are the following:

- The nature of nurses' services are not viewed as critical and the quality of nursing care does not directly affect bed occupancy and income.
- "Need" for nurses is a value judgment related to quality and does not convert to "demand," which relates to economic factors.
- Employers are, *de facto*, united as *one*, although numerous; the market for nurses has been called a monopsony since it is dominated by one employer, the hospital.
- "Unions" (*e.g.*, state nurses associations) are too weak and too egalitarian to affect the employers sufficiently.
- Nurses, for the most part, do not have a direct relationship with the payer-patient, and their services are not recognized as carrying large decision-making responsibilities.
- Women, even for the same work, are paid less than men. Thus, in a predominantly female field low salaries have both a historical and sociologic basis.
- Finally, and perhaps most important, nurses themselves have been late in demanding financial rewards for their work, thus perpetuating all the aforementioned problems.

These factors among others have created a situation that, over time, has stymied market forces, kept salaries down, and inevitably contributed to creating the shortage now loudly decried. The nursing shortage does exist, and its measure must eventually be taken in the quality of nursing services performed by hurried, overworked, underpaid, and largely unappreciated nurses.

It should be clear that whether or not salaries are the prime motivators for entry into the profession, recruitment, and retention, they play a major role in understanding the problem and require major consideration.

STATUS PROBLEMS

Nursing suffers a lower social status and deference than other professions because of a variety of social, educational, and historical factors. The connotation of "service" or "calling," the predominance of women in a world controlled by men, and the daily conscious and unconscious put-downs nurses receive by being excluded from the decision-making process imply a lower status than that accorded to other professionals. Nurses are expected to comply with physicians' and administrators' priorities and desires whether or not these differ from the nurses' or patients needs and priorities. When nurses do not fulfill the others' expectations they set themselves up for an often hostile relationship. When they do, they frequently experience a sense of guilt and frustration since they have not fulfilled their own nursing (and human) goals; the latter is shown to be the major determinant of whether a nurse remains in a position.

The various educational programs preparing nurses also contribute to the status problem. Since the majority (20%) of nurses are prepared at the baccalaureate level and above, nurses are treated according to what their hospital colleagues consider the lowest possible denominator. The interpersonal behaviors observed in most hospital settings indicate a deprecation of women and nurses. An *RN* magazine survey noted "three out of four doctors regard nurses as their assistants — and nothing more."[18] Yet approximately 60% of physicians under 36 believe nurses require a bachelor of science degree at entry, an indication of the low esteem accorded to the baccalaureate degree in our society. It seems that it is treated as a PhD only as it concerns nurses.

CAREER MOBILITY

Tied to if not integral in the status problem is the question of career mobility. This question is perhaps as relevant to the public image of nursing as to nurses themselves and, therefore, is particularly important as we consider dropping nursing enrollments. The public image of the nursing career is that of the staff nurse in a medical or surgical setting who is prepared in the hospital school. Frequently nurses in other fields or positions are asked such questions as "When did you leave nursing?" and "Were you ever a real nurse?" Few people recognize that nursing is a life-long career with an infinite variety of stopping points — including the role of staff nurse.

While the baccalaureate entry level provides for vertical and horizontal mobility, all nurses have some degree of horizontal mobility. The largest percentage of nurses *not* employed in nursing are those whose highest educational credential was received in a hospital school.[19] This finding is in sharp disagreement with a commonly held belief that hospital school graduates serve as the most stable work force in nursing. It is, however, important as we examine the problem of career mobility over a working lifetime and the relative lack of mobility in the hospital school graduate.

Adding to the mobility problem for the hospital-school and associate degree nurses are the current expectations of employers concerning nurses' roles and functions. In settings as varied as community health agencies, nursing homes, and teaching hospitals, many nurses are performing in expanded roles required by the changes in the roles of others and the needs of patients.

The *1977 National Sample Survey of Registered Nurses* commented on these changes in nursing roles and functions as follows:

> Several tasks were performed more often by nurses with higher levels of formal education than by nurses with less education. A significantly higher

percentage of registered nurses with baccalaureates than with diplomas or associate degrees obtained health histories, performed some portions of physical examination, selected a plan of treatment as a result of interpreting laboratory test results, developed therapeutic plans, instructed patients in management of a defined illness, instructed and counseled patients and families in health promotion and maintenance, implemented therapy, and had primary responsibility for providing follow-through on patient care routinely or often. In addition, a significantly higher proportion of nurses with master's degrees or doctorates than with baccalaureates or less routinely or often performed each of three tasks related to development of health care plans, instructed and counseled patients and families in health promotion and maintenance, and had primary responsibility for providing follow-through on patient care.[20]

In contrast, there was a tendency for two tasks to be performed more often by registered nurses with less than a baccalaureate educational preparation. These tasks were assisting the physician during physical examinations and administering medications.

These findings make it clear that reality is quite different from the mythology concerning nursing education and practice—mythology that is extremely resistant to change. Perhaps the technique of denial is used to lessen the discomfort of cognitive dissonance created by the conflict between the real world and the myths of the "good old days." It should be clear at this time that the myths of the nursing field are *not* conducive to attracting capable students in the numbers needed.* In both associate degree and baccalaureate programs a decline in the enrollment of men occurred in 1978 as compared with 1975. Since a marked increase had occurred between 1972 and 1975, this decline must be carefully examined. On the other hand an increase in percentage and absolute numbers of male and other minorities enrolled in hospital schools occurred during this period. Hospital schools had a poor record in attracting such students before the 1975 report. Coupled with the decline in the number of hospital schools and in their total enrollments, this finding may have negative implications concerning the qualifications of students. From the standpoint of career mobility, it should be clear that the hospital school offers the least advantages.

HOURS ROTATION

How many professionals other than nurses work on rotating shifts? It is clear to all young nurses that nursing is 24 hr a day, 7 days a week. This is at once a positive and negative characteristic of the work. It is positive because it provides the continuity necessary to plan and implement nursing care. The

---

*The good myths tend to prevail in war time when nursing programs have always attracted persons who at other times might not select the field.

24-hr nursing for the institutional patient includes monitoring, assessing, treating, and coordinating care, which all nurses see as basic to their interests in the field — that is, of course, providing that they can do it successfully. Nonetheless the disadvantages from the social, psychological, and physiological standpoints of rotating from days to evenings to nights should be clear.

Data are accumulating that show the hazards of shift work and most specifically of three shifts on an irregular basis.[21] Studies of physiological, psychological, chronobiologic, and social reactions revealed increases in stress, social problems, sleep problems, and digestive disturbances.[22]

Even without these disturbances it must be acknowledged that under-staffing on evenings and nights contributes to even greater tension and exhaustion than on other shifts. Lack of support services and personnel and the relative absence of physicians place excessive burdens on nurses already taxed by their own work. It should be very clear that the consideration of most appropriate styles of rotation for all services should be uppermost in the minds of all administrators. While there is need for further research in this area, there are data indicating that interference with physiological and psychological functions is greater on some shift rotations than on others. Despite the obvious importance of this factor, relatively little attention is given to the information presently available and its use in developing some improvement. This is particularly surprising in view of the creativity of management in other fields.

ETHICAL CONFLICTS

That ethical dilemmas are a major factor in the frustration of nurses has become very clear in the past few years. The numbers of nurses who have focussed on ethics in doctoral and postdoctoral work has increased greatly over the past 5 yr. There are now several journals devoting full attention to this topic. Ethical conflicts usually have to do with questions about nurses' rights to inform patients of alternative treatments; the abuse of patients in hospitals and other health care facilities; policies of institutions with regard to the supervision of nurses' work by physicians when such does not occur; nurses' interpretation of clinical findings and their alteration of actions in accordance with these; communication with families about the condition of patients; disagreements with the physician's mode of treatment and provision of information. There is considerable ambiguity in the guidelines affecting nurses in most health care agencies. For the most part these guidelines describe the physician's function quite carefully and in the process exclude the nurse's. The fear of transcending the line separating nurses' rights and responsibilities from physicians' rights and responsibilities in ethical areas prevents many nurses from taking actions for the benefit of patients. It also may lead to severe distress on the part of nurses when their views differ sharply from those prevailing in the power structure.

POWER TO EFFECT CHANGE

Before delineating the reasons why nurses often feel powerless to effect change I must comment that these pertain to the aggregate. On a personal level many nurses have found that change in small and large systems is possible. However, the factors identified as inhibitors to improvement in the nursing shortage contribute to building a system that limits the development of power.

Power to effect change in one's work includes the ability to influence the conditions of work; the ability to interact with others in decision making when it involves areas of knowledge and responsibility; the authority consonant with responsibilities; the continuity to see problems through; sufficient security and group support to make problems manifest; considerable autonomy in one's work; and accountability. It should be clear that few of these characteristics prevail at this time. In survey after survey nurses tell of their concerns and stress their lack of participation in determinations concerning their work lives. In a study done in Texas and being replicated in several other states, the data show that

> nurses are dissatisfied with employment when job conditions do not allow them to administer professional nursing care to patients. These conditions are due to hospital policies and administrative attitudes that fail to accommodate the following professional prerogatives:
>
> - Autonomy of practice and respect for the judgment of the professional.
> - Determination of standards of quality of care and determination of staffing needs and work schedules to achieve the standards.
> - Educational programs and support (financial and time) for updating knowledge and skills.
> - Participation with full vote in establishing policy related to patient care, personnel benefits, and working conditions.
> - Work responsibilities that are nursing related, with elimination of requirements for nurses to perform tasks that are the responsibility of other services.
> - Recognition and personnel benefits comparable to those accorded other health care professionals."[23]

The expansion, contraction, and change in hospitals that have had such a marked effect on nursing all occurred without any consideration of, or influence from, nurses. Status differences between nurses and members of other professions, as well as the real difference in educational preparation between nurses and their colleagues, also is antithetical to the development of power.

The small number of nurses on hospital boards is a vivid reminder of this point.

Most important in the absence of power, is the divisiveness within the nursing group itself with regard to its common cause. While there is considerable potential for power in such a large group, it is rarely exercised. A disproportionate percentage of the total working group views the term "professional" as their due but have "jobs" rather than "careers". This has a dramatic effect on nurses' assertiveness regarding salaries, since in many cases the nurse's salary is secondary to her husband's except at times of economic crisis. Thus, the kind of long-term commitment to goals, necessary in the exercise of power, is often missing. Although it is true that many nurses differ from this description, instituting real change would require improvement on a radical scale.

Finally, it should be noted that the *nursing shortage itself is a deterrent* to continuity in nurses' working patterns. Overwork, double shifts, stress in not being able to meet patients' needs, lack of supports from colleagues, time for the change in pace necessary to most people in a working day all contribute to turnover and lag time in replacement. Thus, the shortage problem becomes an everexpanding spiral in many inpatient health care facilities.

I hope in the next section to outline the steps needed to ensure an adequate and appropriate supply of nurses in the next 2 decades.

RECOMMENDATIONS FOR THE FUTURE

Recommendations for the future supply of nurses in the United States must address the present nursing population as well as appropriate changes to improve the profession's ability to recruit applicants. The foregoing has identified changes in the demands upon nurses having to do with the increasing complexity of patient care; the increase in morbidity with lowering of mortality; the increasing percentage of aged persons in the population; and changing roles in relation to physicians. Also identified were factors inhibiting the solution to the problem at present and in the future. Some of these factors can be grouped as "image" and are relevant both to optimization of the present nursing supply and to improvement of enrollment in programs in nursing education.

RECOMMENDATION 1

At present the responsibility for *improving conditions affecting nursing employment* rests principally with employers. As a matter of principle affecting every recommendation, it must be stated that nurses must have control over the changes that affect their destiny. Translated to the operational level, questions of salary, benefits, working conditions (including rotation, double shifts, floating from unit to unit or service to service), and adequate supports must be addressed by administrators but solved by nurses representing all the levels involved in the problems. Given the characteristics of the nonworking registered nurse population, it is highly unlikely that a large percentage of these nurses can be expected to return to nursing and ameliorate the shortage. Thus, it is exceedingly important to nurture the working group and help maintain continuity of employment. While salaries are only one part of this picture and will not alone suffice, they can be expected to affect the presently employed nurse to some degree, entice some nonworking nurses to return, and markedly influence enrollment as young women and men hear that nursing "pays well."

Earlier I indicated that nursing does not fit the market principle of short supply and high demand driving prices up. Paul Samuelson illustrates the function of supply and demand by contrasting the "case of a compulsory draft for the military services with the case where service pay is raised high enough to coax out a voluntary army. Although money costs appear greater, the real cost . . . may be less if re-enlistments cut out training needs and better use is made of . . . personnel."[24] The direct cost of replacing each nurse has been estimated to be from $2,500 and $12,000. A substitution of nurses in the Samuelson statement lets the reader draw his own conclusions.

I questioned earlier whether one reason nursing does not fit the supply–demand rules was that multiple employers tend to cooperate in setting levels of nurses' salaries. It is clear that market forces must be allowed to emerge for nursing to be considered a competitive profession.

Nurses' own recognition that salaries indicate values placed on their work is long overdue. Their conflict about supporting the internal organization or the economic and general welfare functions of the national organization has impeded the strength of this area. Responses to surveys are now showing that nurses are placing higher priority on salaries than in previous years, but agencies employing nurses do not seem to make a connection between salary levels and nursing shortages; thus they make little effort to compete with other nurse employers.

Studies have shown that job performance and the quality of patient care are at least as high a priority for nurses as is salary.[25] Thus, changes in the power structure that place value on nursing are important to retain and attract more practitioners to the field. Horizontal and vertical mobility for nurses in patient care roles must be recognized and rewarded. Sensitivity to nursing as a career must be shared by top administrators so that nurses in patient care roles as well as administrative roles are brought into the decision-making process. The increasing number of nurses choosing to work for "Rent-a-Nurse" agencies rather than directly for a hospital is a symptom of this problem. The factor identified as most important by agency-employed nurses was control over working conditions.

The Texas study described some hospitals that did not have nursing shortages. It is instructive to review the findings.

> Each unit has a staff of registered nurses with two or three assisting staff, all under the charge of a head nurse. The head nurse has at least a baccalaureate and frequently holds a master's; she bears full responsibility for the unit, including hiring of personnel. All nursing care is provided by registered nurses; the assisting staff fulfill secretarial, messenger, supply, patient transportation, and communication activities. The assigned staff plan for total coverage of the unit, shifts, days off, holidays, etc.
>
> On these units, primary nursing is practiced. Each nurse has three or four patients for whom she is responsible; she and a second primary care nurse share the responsibility for care of their patients on days off. Nurses on evenings and nights also have primary care assignments, so they have input equal to that of the nurses on the day shift into the total nursing care program of the unit.
>
> Planning for inservice education is done to provide opportunities for meeting everyone's learning needs. And a shift differential ensures that enough nurses choose to work the evening and night shifts so rotation is not a problem. There is collaboration among units in the hospital and among nearby hospitals for educational programs, so that nurses have a choice of opportunities to update their knowledge and skills. Staff nurses may participate in selected programs while on duty and may take advantage of additional programs on their own time at no cost. Tuition and fees are paid for continuing education, workshops, and courses taken for credit in degree programs.
>
> A quality assurance program provides evaluations of the quality of care provided patients and of performance of individual nurses. Salary increases are tied to performance. Nurses may have input into all policies affecting nursing practice, patient care, or personnel benefits. Nurses share planning for patient care with physicians, pharmacists, nutritionists, and other health care disciplines, and take part in decisions about patient discharge or movement to another care unit.[26]

It is clear that principles of automony, respect, recognition, and concern go a long way.

As far as rotation of hours is concerned, it must be recognized that around-the-clock requirements are difficult at best. Nurses must participate in the solutions chosen for this and other problems. Exploration of current research findings, gathering information about new ideas being tested, and the development of trials should be encouraged. Further, it must be noted that nurses spend considerable time in nonnursing functions on all shifts, but on evenings, nights, and weekends, this factor causes significant loss of hours for nursing care. Nurses on evenings, nights, and weekends often perform medical, housekeeping, clerical, messenger, social service, specialty therapist, admission, pharmacy, and other roles that should be assumed by those departments around the clock, 7 days a week. Not only would the proper assumption of responsibility enable the nurse to nurse but by providing appropriate supports the onus of shift and weekend work might be lessened.

Last, changes in the workplace in response to the fact that most nurses are married women with children are long overdue. Such changes should allow for part-time work, flexible schedules, and provision for, or at least sensitivity to, child care needs. Disincentives in the tax structure affecting married working women must also be examined.

Episodic answers (*i.e.*, filling jobs) to the question of supply of nurses will not be an effective solution in an environment that was never responsive to nurses and is now out of control.

RECOMMENDATION II

The question of career mobility must be dealt with in a variety of ways. First, *opportunities should be provided for educational advancement*. Given the salaries identified earlier, it is folly for state and federal governments to ignore or abandon support to nursing education. This paper has concentrated on the supply question without differentiation of types of preparation. It has been noted that 20% of the 1.4 million nurses hold the baccalaureate degree, some 5% hold the master's degree, and .02% the doctoral degree.

The preparation of nursing students is dependent on adequate numbers of teachers, administrators, and other supportive personnel. Schools need to devote resources to recruitment of all students, including minorities, and to remedial programs. Scholarship programs are essential if nursing is to have any edge on recruitment at undergraduate levels. It is important to recognize that hospital schools receive a significant portion of their budget from third party payers. This support is not available to other programs.

The need for support at graduate levels should be clear given the numbers cited earlier, the paucity of nursing research, and the inadequate preparation of most nursing administrators (directors of nursing), supervisors, and head nurses, a large percentage of whom hold no collegiate degree.

Support for graduate education must be followed by sufficient rewards in the clinical setting to enable improvement in patient care to follow advancement in nursing education. The availability of clinicians with masters degrees is crucial to the patient care support system. Their knowledge and skills supplement the primary nurse and provide a backup of strength, which will lessen frustration. Clearly economic rewards must ensure continuity of this level of preparation.

Support for continuing education is also important. If we are to respond to nurses' priorities in patient care, it is crucial to help them maintain and improve their knowledge and skills.

RECOMMENDATION III

Finally, *the question of entry level education for nurses must be addressed in a planned and logical manner.*

The recommendation that the baccalaureate degree should be the entry level requirement for registered nurse licensure, with "grandparenting" of present license holders, is an idea long overdue. A planned phase-out of hospital schools must occur in the next few years. Most of the problems we presently face have been exacerbated by the unwillingness of nurses, physicians, administrators, and the public to address this subject in a rational manner. As my viewpoint as a nurse educator may be seen as suspect, however, facts supporting this position may be enumerated briefly. To maintain continuity of employment, nurses require a career orientation rather than job training. Their education must provide possibilities for upward mobility. The patient public requires nurses able to synthesize knowledge from the physical and social sciences and act assertively on its behalf. Status problems affecting the present and future supply of nurses cannot be solved by the prebaccalaureate structure. Expanded role requirements in and out of hospitals can be prepared for at no less than the baccalaureate level. Hospital school graduates' participation in the nursing labor force is less than at any other educational level, and the present covert cost to the consumer of hospital school programs through third party support adds to hospitalization costs.

When we look at future enrollments it goes without saying that the educational polytype is a major deterrent to maintenance of enrollment and subsequently to nurse supply. Necessary changes in nursing's image must be fostered so that recruitment of men into the profession may compensate for the loss of women. At present we are faced with three interlocking variables affecting applications to nursing programs: population changes with reduced numbers of 18 yr olds; the availability for women of a multitude of career options that seem to have higher status; and the stereotype of nursing as a subservient, underpaid, and female field. The first two variables cannot be overlooked but are unalterable. It is therefore the third with which we must deal.

I have already discussed the question of competitive salaries. The other two characteristics of the nursing stereotype are tied to the way in which most nurses are educated and the subsequent mobility that results from this education. Can anyone argue that nursing can make itself appear more attractive a profession for men and women by maintaining a prebaccalaureate educational structure?

RECOMMENDATION IV

There have been recommendations for the baccalaureate as entry level to registered professional nursing since 1911. The recommendations and rhetoric have not been followed by *rational planning of nursing education on a state, regional, or national basis.* This must occur without delay and should include the following:

1 Examining implications for local, state, regional, and national nurse needs, if phase-out of hospital schools occurs.
2 Planning for the expansion of existing baccalaureate programs (and associate degree if indicated) and possible consortia of programs to handle areas unserved by colleges and universities.
3 Establishing new priorities for funding that will recognize the need for educational mobility for present license holders.
4 Establishing priorities for funding that will incorporate the recruitment and maintenance of minority students in baccalaureate programs.
5 Getting people to the right program initially.

The resolution of the educational dilemma in nursing is important to both nurses and the public. It is important to the public so that it may expect some consistency in a vital service. It is important to nurses if they wish to see the nursing profession attract able men and women and maintain self-direction or autonomy. Obtaining professional power and influence requires the unified support of the nursing body to the worth of a life-long commitment to nursing and health care. If nurses as a group, rather than individual innovators, are to perform major roles in primary care, gerontologic nursing care, and hospice care, as well as sophisticated technologic roles in tertiary care settings, educational programs must be at the minimum of baccalaureate for entry, with educational mobility possible and practical.

RECOMMENDATION V

I might recommend that the image of nursing discussed earlier be addressed in a *massive public relations campaign.* However, this cannot be done in a credible manner unless issues of salary and working conditions are improved and some agreement on entry is achieved. Ambiguity and exaggeration cannot be converted into a successfully persuasive campaign.

Nurses and the public cannot have it both ways. If it is acknowledged

- that professional nursing is a unique and essential component of health care;
- that nurses are the equals of other health care providers;
- that nurses have a place in the power structure;
- that they are accountable for their nursing acts; and
- that nursing practice is knowledge operationalized;

then nurses must be educationally qualified in a manner commensurate with these beliefs. If not, no amount of money spent on image changing will help, so this recommendation must be seen as subsidiary and dependent on the others.

Finally, *all governmental plans for change in health service should be required to address the implications for nursing resources in such plans.*

REFERENCES

1   Fagin, Claire M. The Shortage of Nurses in the United States. *Journal of Public Health Policy* 1:4 (December 1980), 293–311.

2   U.S. National Center for Health Statistics. *Health Resources Statistics.*(DHEW Publ. No. (PHS) 79–1509) Washington, D.C., U.S. Government Printing Office, 1979.

3   Roth, Aleda et al. *1977 National Sample Survey of Registered Nurses: A Report on the Nurse Population and Factors Affecting their Supply.* Springfield, Va., National Technical Information Service, 1979, 207.

4   American Hospital Association. Recruitment, retention become key goals in hospital's quest for more nurses. *Federation of American Hospitals Review.* Little Rock, Arkansas (April–May 1980), 12.

5   Johnson, Walter L. Supply and Demand for Registered Nurses: Some Observations on the Current Picture and Prospects to 1985. Part 2. *Nursing & Health Care* 1:11 (September 1980), 76, 79.

6   Doyle, Timothy C. et al. *The Impact of Health Systems Changes on the Nation's Requirements for Registered Nurses* in 1985. Division of Nursing. (DHEW Publ. No. (HRA) 78–9) Washington, D.C., U.S. Government Printing Office, 1978.

7   Gue, R.L. et al. A Micro Model for Assessing Nursing Manpower Demand and Supply, Final Report, Community Systems Foundation, Ltd., Washington, D.C. 1977.

8   Western Interstate Commission for Higher Education. *Analysis and Planning for Improved Distribution of Nursing Personnel and Service. A National Model of Supply, Demand, and Distribution, Final Report.* Boulder, 1977.

9   Ginzberg, Eli. Policy Directions in Millman, M.L. Ed., *Nursing Personnel and the Changing Health Care System.* Cambridge, Mass: Ballinger Publishing Co., 1978, 265.

10   Johnson, Walter. Supply and Current Demand for Nurses in Light of a Survey of Newly Licensed Nurses in Millman, M., *Op. Cit.*, 129.

11   Roth, Aleda et. al. *Op. Cit.*

12   *NLN Testimony. Op. Cit.*

13   Johnson W (1980) 73, 74.

14   Samuelson, Paul. *Economics.* New York: McGraw-Hill, 8th Ed, 1970. 569.

15   Friedman, Milton. *Free to Choose.* New York: Harcourt Brace Jovanovich, 1980.

16   Roth, Aleda et. al. *Op. Cit.*

17   University of Texas Medical Branch at Galveston, 1980. *1979 National Survey of Hospital and Medical School Salaries.*

18   Lee, Anthony A. How nurses rate with M.D.'s. Still the Handmaiden. *RN* (July 1979), 21–30.

19   Roth, Al et. al. *Op. Cit.*

20   *IBID*

21   Akerstedt, T., and Froberg, J.E. Shift work and health — interdisciplinary aspects in P.G. Rentos & R.D. Shaphard (Eds.); *Shift Work and Health, A Symposium.* (DHEW Publ. No. (NIOSH) 76–203). U.S. Department of Health, Education, and Welfare. National Institute for Occupational Safety and Health, 1976.

22   *IBID*

23   Wandelt, Mabel A., et. al. Why Nurses have Nursing and What Can be Done About It. *American Journal of Nursing* 81:1 (January 1981), 76.

24   Samuelson, Paul. *Op. Cit.*, 70

25   White, Charles H. Where Have all the Nurses Gone — and Why. *Hospitals:* May 1, 1980, 70.

26   Wandelt, Mabel A. *Op. Cit.*

CARL J. SCHRAMM

3

ECONOMIC PERSPECTIVES ON THE NURSING SHORTAGE

As the 1980s unfold, the issue of a shortage of nurses has emerged as the pre-eminent issue in health care manpower. Local newspapers cover the problem as it manifests itself in community hospitals that reportedly are forced to shut down services due to their inability to recruit adequate numbers of nurses.[1] Classified pages carry columns of want ads offering nurses employment not only in the local community but all over the country. Indeed, some hospitals in the United States routinely run ads in newspapers in England, Ireland, Scotland, and Australia.[2] Why has the shortage of nurses to staff our hospitals and nursing homes become an issue demanding so much attention?

This article presents an economic consideration of the problem. The first section outlines an analytic framework that will prove useful in examining several of the reasons offered for the acute shortage of nurses as well as the potential solutions. In the second section, we briefly consider what is meant by the term "nursing shortage." The third section presents an analysis of the various reasons for the shortage, with a view toward the solutions that might emerge for policymakers. Finally, we examine the dangers of manpower forecasting and caution against large-scale corrective measures involving major changes in training.

ECONOMIC CONSIDERATIONS

The shortage of nurses in this country is not a problem that has only recently been given attention. Since the end of World War II there has been a chronic perceived shortage of nurses, and the problem has been analyzed from an economic perspective, with efforts to eliminate the shortage couched, accordingly, in terms of economics. For example, the thrust of many of these efforts has been aimed at increasing the supply of nurses and, for the most part, it has not succeeded. Indeed, some say it may be aggravating the problem. Perhaps the fact that the market for nurses does not seem to be obeying the forces of supply and demand indicates that the market is somehow peculiar or perverse, and does not respond in the way classical economics would predict. Whatever the ultimate answer may be, the nurse should recognize that it will have its basis in economics, and for that reason appreciate the importance of a basic understanding of the workings of the nursing labor market. With that in mind, it is useful to begin by reviewing some fundamental economic concepts.

SUPPLY OF NURSES

The concept of a market for nursing labor and how this market functions in a purely competitive economy are best understood by examining the decisions that a nurse and an employer respectively make.

From the nurse's standpoint, the decision to work depends largely on the price, or wage, being offered for her services by employers. As the wage level of nurses goes up, the nurse interested in maximizing her income will offer more hours per week or more days per year. Some nurses who were previously not working will now likely decide to enter the market. This relationship between wages offered and number of hours supplied is intuitive, and it is referred to as the *supply* curve for the nursing labor market.

Lest it appear too simple, however, several considerations that complicate the matter should be introduced. The first point is that the individual nurse's decision to work may be influenced by other factors besides the wage paid. For example, leisure time can be viewed as a "commodity," and an individual nurse's decision to work can be viewed in much the same way as a choice between leisure and other commodities. As the hourly wage rises, the price of an hour of leisure becomes more expensive relative to that of other commodities, and the particular nurse may decide to substitute other commodities for leisure — in other words, the nurse may decide to work more hours. But at a certain point, at a high enough wage, the nurse may, because of the additional income, decide she wants more of all commodities *including the commodity, leisure.*

At this level of wage (point A on Fig. 3-1), the income effects dominate the substitution effects, and the individual nurse may actually cut back the number of hours worked. The existence of this phenomenon, known as the backward-bending supply curve, has been observed in other labor markets, and there is recent evidence that suggests it may be present in the nursing labor market as well.[3]

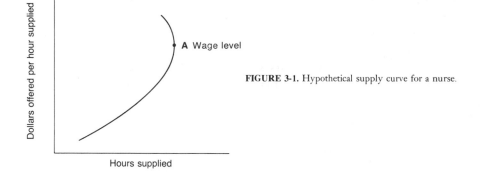

FIGURE 3-1. Hypothetical supply curve for a nurse.

A second factor that may affect the nurse's decision is the institutional constraints on the hours of work. In real life, the number of hours per week and the amount of vacation time per year may be fixed by the employer, and the individual nurse will face an "all or nothing" proposition. This is important because there is growing evidence that the employers of nurses are becoming more flexible in accepting part-time work and nontraditional work schedules. Finally, the nurse's decision to work may be influenced by certain nonpecuniary factors, such as the "psychic rewards" recieved from treating people who are ill.

The existence of the above-mentioned factors necessitates that two additional considerations be made before we can get an accurate picture of the supply curve for the nursing labor market. The first is that, while we have spoken of supply being measured in terms of the number of hours offered by an individual nurse, it is the *overall* picture of supply that we are interested in. Supply can be measured in a number of ways: We could, for example, examine the number of nurses who are working, or use that number as a percentage of the total number of people ever educated and licensed as nurses. But for the purpose of an aggregate market analysis, it is most useful to lump together all the individual nurses' supply curves, each reflecting unique personal influences, and consider the *total* quantity of labor supplied to the market, be it measured in terms of hours per year or days per year.

The final consideration to be made is the effect of time on the supply curve. At this point it is useful to introduce the concept of elasticity. Wage elasticity is a measure of the responsiveness of supply to changes in price; if a rise in the wage level causes only a slight increase in the quantity of labor supplied, then economists say that at that wage level, supply is inelastic. Conversely, if a rise in wage level brings about a proportionately greater increase in the quantity of labor supplied, then supply is elastic at that wage level.

In the very short run, say a few weeks, the quantity of nursing labor available in the economy as a whole may be virtually fixed. There is too little time for other workers to learn the skills of a nurse, and equally little time for nurses to retrain for other occupations. While an increasing wage may induce previously idle nurses to enter the market, and induce nurses who are presently working to offer more hours per week or more days per year, the short-run supply of labor is relatively inelastic. Over a period of several years, however, nurses may be able to shift into other occupations, and other workers will be able to learn the skills of a nurse. Thus, the long-run supply of labor is relatively elastic.

DEMAND FOR NURSES

The aggregate decisions of employers of nurses constitute the demand side of the nursing labor market. From the individual employer's standpoint, the decision to hire a nurse is based largely on two determinations.

The first, and most important, is a determination of whether the value of the nurse's services exceeds the cost (*i.e.*, the wage) of the nurse. In the parlance of economics, the profit-maximizing employer, in a competitive market, will hire any "factor of production" (*e.g.*, a nurse) up to the point where the value of its marginal product (*i.e.*, the value to the employer of the services of that additional nurse) is equal to the cost of the factor. Since this is an important concept and its common sense may not immediately be apparent, an example may help. Suppose that the value, to a hospital, of the marginal product of nurses was $15,000, and their wage was $12,000. Why wouldn't the hospital be satisfied with the number of nurses it employed? The answer is a simple matter of revenues and cost; hiring an additional nurse would bring $15,000 in additional revenue for the hospital, and it would cost the hospital only $12,000. The profit-maximizing employer in this position would therefore start hiring additional nurses.

Eventually, of course, as more and more nurses were hired, the value of their marginal products would diminish, and at some point would be less than the wage paid. At this point, the employer would cease hiring additional nurses.

From this marginal revenue product (MRP) schedule, as it is called, the employer can determine the number of nurses that can be profitably hired at various wage levels, and this, in essence, is the employer's demand curve for nurses. As one would expect, as the wage an employer must pay a nurse goes up, the quantity of labor that can profitably be hired decreases, and consequently the demand curve slopes downward from left to right.

The remaining determination an employer makes in the decision to hire is an analysis of the possibilities of substituting both machines and more-skilled or less-skilled personnel for nurses. As mentioned earlier, as with any other factor of production, this decision is a function of the cost of the substitute labor (*i.e.*, the price of the machine or the wage of the more-skilled or less-skilled worker), and the value of the marginal product of the substitute labor.

As these costs and values change over time, the demand for nurses varies, and this effect is particularly noticeable in the case of hospital employ- ers. Once, before the period of relatively higher wage levels (which have de- veloped during the last 15 yr) registered nurses were the principal providers of care and service within the hospital. As comparative wage costs for profes- sional nurses increased, substitute labor was employed, essentially diluting the numerical importance of the nurse in the overall functioning of the hos- pital. Recent evidence suggests that hospitals are reassessing previous deci- sions and are beginning to replace less-skilled labor with nurses (*see* Chap. 7). If this is so, then it reflects a deliberate analysis of the comparative wage levels of substitute labor and the observed or perceived differences in produc- tivity of professional nurses relative to other labor inputs.

In addition to the decision to substitute labor of one type for that of an- other, however, the hospital often may substitute labor with machines. Tech- nologic advances are generally adopted for their reputed ability to displace more costly labor. But, in the case of health care delivery, the expected machine–labor trade-off is not a certainty. Indeed, efforts at maintenance-free hospital design, a trend of the 1950s and 1960s, have been abandoned al- together. And, contrary to previous experience with technologic innovation in other sectors, the application of technology in hospitals has sometimes resulted in the employment of more nurses in absolute terms, and nurses of higher technologic competence in relative terms. The skill level and number of nurses working in an intensive care unit are evidence of this phenomenon.

Armed with an understanding of the supply and demand curves for nurse labor, we can now turn our attention to the workings of a competitive labor market. Suppose that, initially, the supply and demand curves (labeled S_0 and D_0 respectively) were as they appear in Figure 3-2a. At wage W_0, the quantity of labor supplied by nurses, Q_0, would be equal to that demanded by employers, also Q_0, and economists say that at this point the market "clears."

Now suppose that nursing services become more valuable to employers and the demand curve shifts outward from D_0 to D_1 (*i.e.*, at any given wage, employers will want to hire more nurses than previously), as shown in Figure 3-2b. At the old wage level, W_0, the quantity demanded by employers will be Q_1, but the quantity supplied will still be Q_0; thus, there will be a shortage of $Q_1 - Q_0$. But in a properly functioning competitive market this shortage will be temporary; employers will raise the wage level offered in an effort to at- tract more nurses, and at higher wages, presumably, more nurses will decide to work. Of course, at this higher wage, employers will demand a somewhat smaller quantity of nurses than they did at the old wage. After a period of time, then, these forces will produce a new wage, W_2, and quantity, Q_2, where the market clears, as shown in Figure 3-2c.

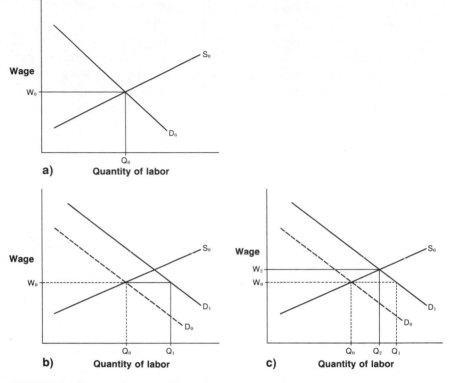

FIGURE 3-2. Adjustments in a competitive market.

INSTITUTIONAL FORCES

The market forces of supply and demand do not, however, always operate freely to set price in a market. In the nursing labor market, as in most other markets for labor, there are certain constraints on the free flow of labor and hence the ultimate free movement of price. Taken together, these constraints are referred to as institutional forces or "fixes," suggesting their role in impeding the pure forces of supply and demand.

One example of an institutional force is collective bargaining; concerted activity on the part of suppliers to improve the welfare of individual workers by, for example, bargaining for a wage increase will clearly affect the free movement of price. While many other examples of institutional forces exist, one in particular illustrates the point as it applies to the market for nurses. Historically, a majority of registered nurses received their training in 3-yr diploma schools. These schools were most often run by community hospitals, and were frequently administered by personnel reflecting the religious affiliation of the hospital to which they were attached. These schools were almost always founded and supported as an integral part of the hospital. From the perspective of labor market analysis, they produced nurses who had a special loyalty to the hospital sponsoring the school, in many cases made stronger by a sense of religious vocation. Such a sense was compounded by several factors inherent in a system of training that limited the nurse's mobility both occupationally and geographically. The training did not qualify one for a bachelor's degree. The nurses were constrained from moving to other occupations where the college-level liberal arts component of their education would be valued, and were barred even from civil service nursing where the bachelor's degree was often required for public health positions and school nursing. Geographic mobility was limited by the nature of the nonuniversity training experience. The reputations of all but a few 3-yr schools were, at best, regional; coupled with the great variety in state licensing standards, the portability of the training beyond the community in which the hospital was situated was limited.

HUMAN CAPITAL APPROACH

A somewhat different perspective on the traditional market analysis of supply, demand, and institutional forces emerges from the human capital approach to understanding labor market behavior.[4] The human capital approach offers several further dimensions useful in understanding worker and employer behavior. Regarding the supply side, human capital theory attempts to examine the threshold question of why people choose nursing as an occupation in the first place. Human capital theory suggests that people, when considering alternative career paths, seek to minimize their monetary and nonmonetary investments in the training necessary to enter a given occupation and to maximize the return on their training over their expected work lives. Of course, such considerations are affected by the person's aspirations, talent, background, and tastes – a person with acrophobia, for example, is not likely to consider a career as a window washer on a skyscraper.

Applying the human capital approach, one imagines the teenager, upon high school graduation, making a comparison among potential career paths. Some, quite obviously, yield much higher income streams through life. Some require more or less formal education. Some link rewards more to entrepreneurial ability than to formal training. Such considerations are gauged by the person in a manner similar to a business investment decision. Capital is expended only because the anticipated return is thought to exceed the present alternative uses of the capital. The person considering a bachelor's degree in nursing program, then, anticipates an investment–income profile similar to that set out in Figure 3-3. The person invests in education in two major ways: The first is the direct investment of tuition; the second is the opportunity costs of not working in another occupation during the training period. In Figure 3-3, these annual costs appear respectively as $4,000 and $10,000. The prospective nurse weighs these costs against the anticipated income stream,

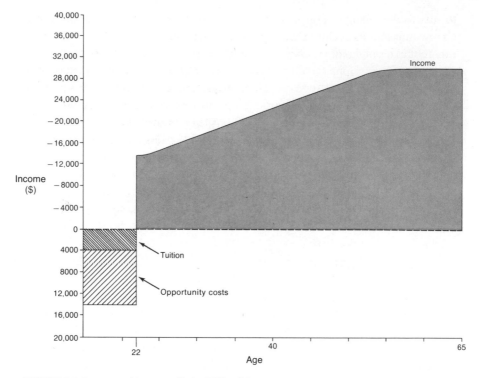

FIGURE 3-3. Investment/income profile for BSN training.

assuming no work-life hiatus, limited in Figure 3-3 to a starting salary of $14,000 and a maximum salary of $30,000 (in current dollars). The decision to take training in nursing as opposed to becoming a physician may depend on the amount of resources the person has to invest and the need to have income sooner as opposed to later in life. The choice of nursing over other occupations requiring bachelor's level training and enjoying a similar or higher lifetime income profile may reflect tastes, life-style preference, or some psychic income dimension, such as the sense of vocation mentioned previously.

Before examining the employer's human capital perspective, it is useful to understand one other aspect of nursing education. Because of the specific nature of the skills imparted during schooling, the transferability of the nurse's training investment to other occupations may be significantly lower than that of a person who acquires a more general, less specialized bachelor's degree. This is an important point to keep in mind for policy regarding the recapture of nurses who may have shifted to other occupations or who merely withdrew from the labor force altogether.

Human capital theory is equally useful in explaining employer behavior. Employers may be regarded as investing in every new employee. Substantial recruitment costs, lost productivity during the familiarization period, and formal on-the-job training programs amount to significant expenditures in almost all cases. During the initial months and, in some cases, years, the monetary value of the employee's contribution to the firm or hospital's product is, in all likelihood, less than the wages paid. This discrepancy between productivity and wages, plus the direct costs of recruitment and training, amount to the stock of employer capital invested in each worker. Through the course of the employee's anticipated work life with the firm, his contribution to production should exceed wage costs. This excess of productivity over cost represents the return on employer investment. In order to ensure that the return is realized, the employer attempts to improve worker productivity throughout the employee's tenure, to establish programs that reward seniority in an effort to keep the employee with the firm, and continually to pay wages high enough to ensure against the highly skilled employee's leaving, which would allow the subsequent employer to "cash in" on the investment already made in the employee.

IS THERE A SHORTAGE OF NURSES?

Armed with the basic concepts of the economics and workings of labor markets, the reader may ask the question of whether there is a shortage of nurses, with some understanding of the complexities of the answer an economist must formulate. While overwhelming evidence of unfilled nursing positions exists, the question may not be whether we have too few nurses but, rather, why nursing vacancies aren't filled by trained persons. Aiken and Blendon have presented data that clearly show that the absolute number of positions for nurses has been declining for 15 yr, and at the same time the number of beds and hospital occupancy rates have been falling.[5] Simultaneously, the number of nurses has doubled.[6] These data suggest that the shortage we are facing is not absolute in the sense that skilled and qualified persons able to fill the positions do not exist. The situation is not akin to that encountered during World War II, when the armed forces had to launch intensive training programs because we were producing more airplanes than there were people who knew how to fly them. Rather, it appears that the question is, Where have all the nurses gone? We know they have been trained and that absolute demand has fallen; nevertheless, budgeted vacancies acutely outweigh the amount of labor the nurse pool is willing to offer.

WHERE HAVE ALL THE NURSES GONE?

As with any problem where facts are few and concern is high, there are many theories offered to explain why nurses are not seeking employment in hospitals, when the demand for their services is so apparent. From the perspective of economics, however, it is important to distinguish between those "theories" that are more in the nature of observations, and the underlying hypotheses that attempt to predict or explain the occurrence or nonoccurrence of these observations.

For example, perhaps the most often encountered explanation of the shortage is that nurses are working in non-nursing-related jobs, or that, while not leaving nursing as a profession, they are simply choosing not to work at all. These phenomena are observable, and if they are in fact observed, can an economic theory be developed that predicts or explains their occurrence?

The answer is yes; the explanation that has been offered by economists is that the perceived shortage is a result of the depression of nurses' wages relative to those of other workers, both within the hospital industry and in other non-health-related occupations. If this theory is sound, then an economic analysis would predict the existence of several observable results. For example, if the wage level of nurses has not kept up with that of other female professional, technical, and kindred workers, then the relatively higher wages offered by these other occupations should induce nurses to leave nursing to work in other jobs, or abandon nursing altogether, perhaps to devote time to childrearing. In economic parlance, this is a shift of the entire supply curve inward (or to the left), and, as shown in Figure 3-4a, there would be a shortage of $Q_0 - Q_1$ until wages for nurses were bid up to W_2.

The truth is, however, that this widely held belief that nurses are either not working, or working in other jobs, does not seem to have a basis in fact. Aiken and associates report that only 3% of nurses are employed in occupations outside nursing, and an examination of the labor force participation rate (the number of nurses working divided by the number licensed and trained) reveals that 75% of all nurses are actively employed, and that this proportion

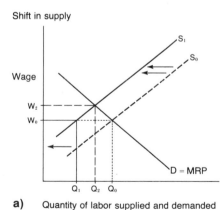

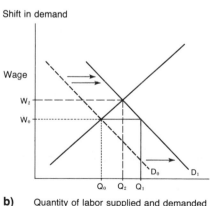

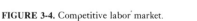

a) Quantity of labor supplied and demanded **b)** Quantity of labor supplied and demanded

FIGURE 3-4. Competitive labor market.

has risen over the last few years.[7, 8] Does this mean that the underlying theory — nurses are underpaid relative to other workers — should be discarded? For several reasons, the answer is no.

First, the nature of nurses' education may be such that it prevents them from moving out of the nursing or health care field and into other occupations, such as teaching or accounting. In addition to restrictions on mobility resulting from the lack of portability of nurses' skills and training, there may also be geographic restrictions on mobility, such as obligations to a spouse or family. While these considerations tend to explain why nurses are not leaving nursing to seek other work, they also seem to argue that the supply curve has not in fact shifted inward, and thus there is not a shortage of supply.

The same underlying theory, however, can still explain why a perceived shortage of nurses exists. If the wage level of nurses has not kept up with that of other, less-skilled workers in the hospital, then employers will have an incentive to substitute higher skilled nurses for those less-skilled workers, as this will increase their revenues proportionately more than it will increase their costs. In short, the demand for nurses will grow. From an economic perspective, this is a shift of the entire demand curve outward (to the right), and, as shown in Figure 3-4b, there would be a shortage of $Q_1 - Q_0$ until wages were bid up to W_2.

If, as a result of this relative wage differential, there is excess employer demand, then nurses may be used to perform less-skilled tasks, thus causing morale problems and exacerbating the apparent shortage. Finally, this proposition reflects the importance of institutional forces within the nursing labor market. The existence of unionism within many of the less-skilled occupations has worked to push up the salaries of non-nurse employees. In order to keep the overall labor costs in the hospital down, nurses' wages are not increased to a level that would create a wage gap sufficient to limit the use of nurses in the hospital to tasks requiring the special degree of skills they possess.

Perhaps the "burnout" phenomenon, another explanation offered for the acute lack of nurses, could also be properly considered as an institutional force. From the economist's perspective, the disenchantment with nursing and the high-level emotional stress of dealing with disease and death usually encompassed by this phrase suggest that from time to time in the work life of the individual nurse, the nonmonetary, or psychic, income connected with nursing becomes negative instead of positive. At such a point the money wage is insufficient when compared to the required tasks or to other opportunities, including not working, and the person drops out of nursing, probably for a finite period. In this respect the burnout phenomenon resembles the declining relative wage explanation immediately above. The professional ethic, and the sense of the work being sufficiently rewarding, which traditionally are seen as motivating the person to offer services without strict regard for corresponding compensation, are eventually overpowered by a sense that the work one does is of marginal importance, requires little skill, and ultimately is useless in fighting back the advance of death and disease.

If in fact the problem is one of insufficient supply or excess demand, it would seem that in a properly functioning, purely competitive market there would be pressure on the wage level to rise. To review, an upward movement in price or wage would attract more nurses to the market, and at the same time reduce the employers' demand. Why has not the market adjusted price upward to a point of equilibrium, thus correcting the shortage?

One answer may be that the market is in the process of adjusting but that it will take additional time before results are seen. Even a properly functioning market cannot be expected to adjust instantaneously to changes in supply and demand. While the length of time required for a market to reach equilibrium is a function of numerous factors, one of the more important is the degree of inelasticity associated with the market's supply and demand curves. The more inelastic these curves are (i.e., the less responsive changes in quantity are to changes in price), the longer it will take before a new equilibrium will be reached. This is important because economists have argued that, in the case of married nurses, there exists a backward-bending supply curve.[9] If this is in fact the case, it suggests that the overall nursing supply curve may be relatively inelastic, with relatively large increases in wages producing only moderate increases in the quantity of labor supplied. If this is true, it will take a significantly longer period of time before a new equilibrium is reached.

The fact that there has been a chronic perceived shortage for at least 15 yr has prompted other economists to argue, however, that this disequilibrium in the market may be of a more permanent nature.[10]

The explanation offered is that the nursing labor market is not a properly functioning, purely competitive market, but is instead a monopsonistic market, which means there exist only a few firms who employ the majority of nurses. The fact that in most communities there are only a handful of hospitals, and the fact that the majority of nurses work in hospitals, is evidence that supports this theory — that the labor market for nurses, from the standpoint of hospital employers, may indeed be a buyer's market. This is especially convincing in light of the occupational and geographic restrictions on the mobility of nurses, and the fact that there is little competition between hospitals elsewhere for nurses.

If the market for nursing labor in hospitals is in fact characterized by monopsony, then vacancies could exist even though the market is technically in equilibrium. Figure 3-5 illustrates this situation — monopsony — in a market where only one purchaser of nursing labor exists, a large hospital, for example.

In this situation, the individual hospital faces an upward sloping labor supply curve, labeled S in Figure 3-5, unlike the horizontal supply curves facing the many individual employers in competitive labor markets. As a result, the monopsonistic employer must pay higher wages to attract more nurses, and moreover, he must also give existing nurses the same wage paid the newly hired nurse. Consequently, the hiring of each additional nurse raises his total labor cost by more than the cost of the nurse's wage alone, and this increase in total labor cost per additional nurse hired is the hospital's marginal factor cost (MFC). The remaining curve is the MRP schedule for nurses in the hospital, representing (as discussed earlier) the number of nurses that could profitably be hired if recruited at the corresponding wage; this curve is in essence the hospital's demand curve for nurses.

According to economic theory, the profit-maximizing firm will hire the quantity of labor at the point where MFC=MRP, that is, at the intersection of these two curves (Q_0). If the hospital employer is a monoposonist, and unworried by the threat of competition from other hospitals bidding up the wage level, he will hire Q_0 units of labor at wage W_0. But if asked how many units he would *like* to hire at wage W_0, he would report X_0. This difference, $X_0 - Q_0$, represents the number of unfilled positions, and these vacancies would exist in a market that is technically in equilibrium.

If the market for nurses has in fact been monopsonized, economic theory would predict the occurrence of one interesting phenomenon that has been observed. Since the hospital would like additional labor at the wage level it sets, but would not be willing to pay the increased wage required for that additional labor to be offered (because of the effect on total labor costs), a compromise might be reached. The hospital might be able to offer a premium for part-time work, or work on unpopular shifts, that it would not have to pay the existing full-time workers on traditional shifts. Our recent experience demonstrates this flexibility being offered nurses in choosing the manner and

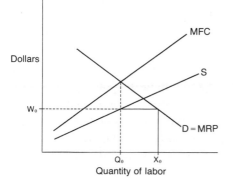

FIGURE 3-5. Monopsony labor market.

units in which they will work. Nurses may, in Chicago or Baltimore, work three 10 hr days per week and be paid for 40 hr. They may work back-to-back shifts on a weekend and be paid for a full week's work. In nearly all communities, many nurses work on a part-time basis. This flexibility being accorded the nurse, uncommon in other professions, may be one symptom of a monopsony market.

WHAT IS TO BE DONE?

Policymakers are inclined to do something about the nursing shortage. With the limited data at hand it is difficult, however, to say exactly what the extent of the problem is and how long it will continue. And, far more important, the preceding section has demonstrated that the existing data can sometimes be read in antagonistic or conflicting ways. For example, while the presence of a problem is irrefutable, whether it is an issue of excess demand or insufficient supply is not altogether clear.

The most common analysis argues that it is a problem of supply — insufficient numbers of nurses exist — and thus efforts must be taken to increase the number of new nurses and induce previously trained but idle nurses to enter the labor market, in order to expand the total supply. Over the past 15 yr, enormous amounts of federal, state, and local funds have gone to subsidize the education of additional nurses. If, however, the monopsony theory of the market is correct, then it would predict that these efforts would be to no avail. In fact, in certain circumstances, it can be shown that an increase in supply will actually lead to an increase in the number of unfilled positions. While an economic explanation of this seemingly unlikely result is beyond the scope of this paper,[11] it does suggest that policymakers should reconsider the appropriateness, from an economic standpoint, of the measures presently being taken to relieve the shortage.

Other authorities, such as Aiken and Blendon, agree that such supply-focused policy may be misdirected, and argue that the problem may be more accurately characterized as one of excessive and inappropriate demand resulting from the depression of nurses' incomes relative to those of other workers.[12] If this in turn is a function of the monopsony power that hospitals apparently exercise in the nursing labor market, then the potential solutions may not be market solutions. In other words, while it would seem that the single best solution to relieving the shortage lies in raising nurses' salaries relative to those of other workers, a monopsony market, lacking in competition between buyers, will not provide this upward adjustment, if left to its own devices.

Consequently, efficacious solutions will be nonmarket ones, such as fix-ing, through government intervention, the wage of nurses at some level above the market price. While this is unlikely, a solution that similarly capitalizes on the government's power to regulate a market might be the use of state rate-setting commissions. For example, these agencies could, in determining hos-pitals' prospective budgets or rates, grant exceptions for increases in the salaries of nurses. Alternatively, the solution may be to somehow "break" the monopsony power hospitals apparently exercise, perhaps by increasing com-petition among hospitals for nurses. For example, inner-city hospitals, which are currently experiencing the most difficulty in attracting nurses and thus are feeling the brunt of the shortage, may need to be given subsidies or simi-lar relief, perhaps from those funds that are being used now to subsidize nurs-ing education. Finally, perhaps the solution will be for nurses to unionize, and exert an upward pressure on wage level through collective bargaining.

Two final considerations, which may serve to reduce the attractiveness of a solution based on raising the salaries of nurses, should be mentioned. The first is that some authorities, as already discussed, have concluded that the presence of backward-bending supply curves for a large proportion of nurses casts serious doubt on the efficacy of wage incentives as a method of increas-ing supply.[13] Second, and more important, a policy of raising nurses' salaries would undoubtably lead to an increase in hospital cost inflation, an ailment that policymakers are trying desperately to correct.

Finally, in light of the fact that many of the potential solutions may in-volve government intervention in the market, one last caution is in order as a closing consideration. When the question is posed as to whether we have enough nurses, or how many should we have, our experience with attempts to correct previously identified perceived shortages must be called to mind. Almost by definition, explicit attempts to rectify manpower shortages will produce errors of great magnitude that prove costly both in terms of dollars and human resources. Two examples of manpower policy resulting in nonin-tended outcomes are the case of engineers in the 1970s and physicians in the 1980s.

In the late 1950s it was determined that the United States was desper-ately short of engineers. As a result, federal policy emerged that stimulated the production of engineers by subsidizing new engineering schools and stimulating the growth of existing training resources. By the 1970s it was ap-parent that too many engineers had been produced. Federal support of engi-neering education was drastically reduced and thousands of engineers were unemployed or subemployed at great social and personal cost.

Likewise, the extraordinary expansion of our medical training apparatus in the 1960s has led to what is universally regarded as an impending surplus of physicians. To employ all of these new doctors will force unneeded expansion of the health care sector, whereas to leave them unemployed or subemployed will involve great waste of the social and personal costs their training represents. Many economists feel that the potential for overreaction to today's manpower shortages, and the immense lag time in changing the production mechanism are such that crash programs aimed at expanding the production of persons with specific and nontransferable skills should be avoided at all costs. In conclusion, then, the reader must consider just what the ultimate ramifications of taking steps to correct the apparent shortage of nurses today will be, in the light of a potentially huge number of nurses in 15 yr who may be unwanted by the health care system and unattractive to everyone else.

REFERENCES

1   See, for example, Pilcher J, Simpson JC: Florence Nightingale wants you. Time: August 24, 1981; Miller S 37,: Programs get support to deliver local nurses. The Evening Sun: C–1, December 29, 1980.

2   See, for example, The Irish Times: August 9, 1981 (offering employment in Arkansas).

3   Link CR, Settle RF: Wage incentives and married and professional nurses: A case of backward-bending supply? Economic Inquiry 19:149–55, 1981.

4   Becker GS. Theory of Human Capital. Chicago, University of Chicago Press, 1974.

5   Aiken LH, Blendon RJ: The national nurse shortage. National Journal: 948–949 May 23, 1981.

6   Ibid.

7   Aiken LH, Blendon RJ, Rogers DE: The hospital nurse shortage: A new perspective. Ann Intern Med 95:365–372, 1981.

8   Ibid.

9   Link CR, Settle RF, op cit, pp 149–55.

10   Yett DE: The chronic shortage of nurses: A public policy dilemma. In Klarman H (ed): Empirical Studies in Health Economics, pp 357–389. Baltimore, Johns Hopkins University Press, 1970.

11   For both a straightforward intuitive explanation and a concise mathematical analysis of this phenomenon, see Altman SH. Present and Future Supply of Registered Nurses, pp 33–34. (DHEW Pub. No. (NIH) 72–134). Bethesda, MD, US Department of Health, Education and Welfare, Public Health Service, National Institutes of Health, Bureau of Health Manpower, Division of Nursing, 1971.

12   Aiken LH, Blendon RJ, op cit, p 950.

13   Link CR, Settle RF, op cit, p 155.

2

FERMENT IN HOSPITAL NURSING

Hospitals are the single most important setting for nursing practice. The public places a high priority on hospitals. In most communities, hospitals remain central institutions enjoying broad public support. Two-thirds of all practicing nurses are employed by hospitals; hence, the public's image of nurses is largely derived from their perceptions of the roles of nurses in hospitals. The excitement and challenge of hospital nursing has been captured in novels and movies over the past 25 years influencing many young people to select nursing as a career. But in recent years, the image of hospital nursing has not been as positive. Although the drama is still here, the picture that emerges is one of stress, underpay, shortages, and high levels of dissatisfaction. As this image becomes more and more commonplace in the news media, enrollments in nursing schools decline. The problems in hospital nursing rapidly become generalized to the entire profession. Hence, resolving those problems is a major priority for nurses in the 1980s.

The current shortage of hospital nurses and the high levels of dissatisfaction among nurses who practice in hospitals have been causes of major concern. Consumers are worried about the effect of the shortage on the quality of care, as is evidenced from extensive press coverage of the shortage. Physicians also fear that care may be compromised, especially in critical care units, or that nurse "burnout" will be increased further exacerbating high staff turnover rates. The shortage has also resulted in delays in scheduling elective surgery and other problems, which directly impact on physicians' practices. Similarly, hospital administrators have been frustrated by disruptions in the day-to-day operation of their institutions, revenue lost from beds closed because of insufficient nurse coverage, and the high costs of recruitment and use of supplemental nursing service agencies.

The chapters in Part II examine both the problems and challenges in hospital nursing. Chapters 4 and 5 provide indepth analyses of the issues in hospital nursing and suggest strategies for change. Chapter 6, written by Clifford, is a case study of a success story, a hospital which has reorganized nursing services to promote professional nursing practice.

Many of the current problems in hospital nursing are attributed to the poor economic rewards for becoming and remaining a nurse. Nurses' salaries did not keep pace in the 1970s with salaries of other professionals with comparable responsibilities. Hospital cost containment efforts have been blamed for holding down nurses' salaries. In Chapter 7, Atkinson and Schramm explore this hypothesis by examining the effects of the Maryland Health Services Cost Review Commission on nurses' salaries. The authors present a convincing case that in Maryland there has not been a direct attempt by the Commission to hold down nurses' salaries. Hospitals have considerable latitude in allocating additional funds allowed each year by the Commission to nurses' salaries or to other areas of concern. Atkinson and Schramm conclude that at least in Maryland nurses have not been adversely affected by state cost containment programs.

However, the editors would like to point out that other labor economists studying national hospital cost containment efforts have reached different conclusions. Frank Sloan at Vanderbilt University, for example, concludes from his studies that hospital cost containment programs have indeed impacted negatively on the growth of nurses' salaries. He further notes that nurses covered by collective bargaining contracts have fared better under cost containment efforts than other nurses. What seems clear from these different analyses is that cost containment programs impose an overall cap on hospital expenditures. In the absence of pressure from nurses, there is a tendency to hold nurses' salaries constant and invest available funds in new equipment, renovation, other salaries, or other areas of need. Hospital cost containment programs are of major concern to the economic welfare of nurses in the 1980s, and should be the topic of continuing study.

Chapter 8, written by Walker, analyzes the actual cost of nursing care in hospitals by separating nursing from the standard daily room charge to patients. Contrary to popular opinion, nurses are not a major operating expense of hospitals; they generate considerable revenue since their services are reimbursed by third party payors or patients. Walker's analysis indicates that nursing care accounts for less than 20 percent of average total hospital charges. This is somewhat surprising since many argue that the need for 24 hour a day nursing care is primary reason for hospitalization.

MARGARET L. McCLURE
M. JANICE NELSON

4

TRENDS IN HOSPITAL NURSING

NURSES' ROLES IN HOSPITALS

An analysis of trends in hospital nursing is probably best begun by examining briefly the role of the nurse in such settings. This will provide a description of the backdrop against which changes are occurring. The role of the nurse can be viewed in two distinct classifications that, for ease of discussion, can be labeled *care-giver* and *integrator*.

The care-giver role is the one that is best understood but, at the same time, most underestimated. It is understood in terms of function, that is, the nurse is responsible for meeting the following patient needs:

1 Dependency needs (bathing, grooming, toileting, feeding, safety).
2 Comfort needs (physical and psychological).
3 Monitoring needs (vigilance to signs and symptoms, including appropriate response based on the data obtained).
4 Therapeutic needs (medications, treatments, dressings).
5 Educational needs (including the fostering of coping mechanisms).

The value of the care-giver role of the nurse is frequently underestimated. Few people comprehend explicitly that nursing is the *raison d'etre* for inpatient facilities. If patients do not need *nursing* care, they have no need to be admitted to a hospital; all health care can be provided on an outpatient basis. For example, the reason that a patient is admitted to a hospital for surgery is because of his perioperative *nursing* care needs, and he is discharged when he no longer has need for the level of nursing care that is provided in that particular setting. Clearly this is what nursing is all about and the reason that most young people choose nursing as a career.

The second component of the hospital nurse's role is that of integrator. This is a term that is derived from the theoretical analysis of organizations provided by Lawrence and Lorsch in which they explicate the ideas of *differentiation* and *integration*.[1] They state that organizations are divided into subsets of people who specialize in particular functions. This they label differentiation. Within these subsets the employees are enmeshed in their own areas of concern and develop their own sets of values, attitudes, and norms that effect their behavior. At some point, however, there is need for the work of the various differentiated groups to come together for the purpose of fulfilling the organization's goals and producing its product, and this process they term integration. Because integration is necessary, the organization must have persons employed who will serve as integrators.

One can readily see the relevance of the Lawrence and Lorsch framework in the analysis of the hospital setting. Our institutions are, in fact, organized into highly specialized departments, for example, medicine, nursing, laboratory, radiology, food service, maintenance. Thus the differentiation aspect exists. Further, it is clear that integration must be performed in order for us to accomplish our goal, which is service to patients. All of these differentiated parts must somehow come into play at the right place and the right time if the patient is to benefit. The person who integrates these various differentiated segments in the hospital is the nurse.

CHANGES IN HOSPITAL NURSING

While the role and responsibilities of the nurse have not changed in recent years, the substance of hospital nursing has changed rather dramatically in several important interrelated ways. First, because the acuity level of hospitalized clients has risen dramatically, there has been a concomitant change in the level of knowledge and sophistication required to carry out the nursing role. Second, there has been a continuous increase in the number of registered nurses hospitals require. And third, there has been a change in the system of delivering nursing care in hospitals. The interplay of these three factors has led to a crisis in supply and demand that will necessitate a great deal of vision and creativity on the part of nursing leadership if the profession is to continue delivering adequate care to the hospitalized American public.

INCREASING ACUITY OF ILLNESS

The steady advance of medical knowledge, coupled with technologic improvements has enabled more seriously ill patients to survive and thus require hospital care. This trend is so pronounced that it led one official of the

Department of Health and Human Services to predict that "hospitals will be huge intensive care units by 1990."[2] Fetal monitoring, hemodialysis, and volume respirators are but a few examples of the kinds of developments that are becoming commonplace, even routine, in many hospitals. Patients who only a few years ago would have been housed in intensive care units are now cared for on "regular" medical–surgical units. The knowledge explosion has been well documented in all fields, but in health care the situation seems to be most severe and the impact on hospital nursing has been great. In addition, an older patient population, more critically ill than ever before, is demanding increased nursing skill and nursing time. Between 1973 and 1978, the number of patient days in hospitals per year dropped for the total national population; however, hospital days for patients aged 65 and older increased 9% during that same period.[3] These older people come into the hospital with multiple-system problems. For example, in addition to the admitting diagnosis, they may have hearing or vision impairment, decreased mental acuity, ambulation problems, loss of skin integrity, and lack of self-care skills such as feeding, toileting, and dressing, all of which may be exacerbated by the primary condition requiring the hospitalization.

The increased acuity of hospitalized patients is also due, in part, to the increased regulation of inpatient facilities that has resulted in reductions in the length of stay for patients. The consequence of the utilization review process has been to force patients out into the community earlier, with the result that they need more care at home or in ambulatory care settings than was required previously, and the hospital beds that they vacate are rapidly filled by more acutely ill patients.

The foregoing has had a direct effect on the numbers of personnel needed to deliver care. An analysis of employment trends, published by the American Hospital Association (AHA), is presented in Table 4-1; this reflects the increased growth of nursing and other services between 1977 and 1980.[4] The greatest increase in employment was in nursing and in therapeutic services, which include respiratory therapy, therapeutic radiology, hemodialysis, intravenous therapy, pharmacy, and social services. It is particularly noteworthy that the rate of increase in nursing service hours almost doubled, from 3.1% to 6.1%, in the period between 1977 and 1980. According to the accompanying report, the largest increase in nurses was in intensive care units (17.6%) and newborn nurseries (16.6%).[5] This latter phenomenon can probably be accounted for, in part, by the fact that increased sophistication in fetal monitoring had a direct effect on the rate of caesarean sections performed; these almost doubled from 5.4 per thousand population in 1973 to 10.2 per thousand in 1978, thus saving those high-risk infants who might not have survived otherwise. Likewise, cardiac catheterizations increased from 3.0 per thousand population in 1973 to 5.7 per thousand in 1978 with a direct

TABLE 4-1 Employment Statistics, 1977-79

Service	Distribution of Total Hospital Employment (1979)	Percentage Change 1977-79	Distribution of 1977-79 Increment
Nursing services	36.3%	6.2%	28.3%
Diagnostic services	9.2	9.9	11.1
Operative services	6.3	4.1	3.3
Therapeutic services	6.2	20.3	14.1
Outpatient services	3.3	11.9	4.7
Patient care support	16.4	4.7	9.9
Professional support	3.9	12.7	5.9
Administrative services	18.3	10.2	22.7

Cohen, Carol F. and Backofer, Henry J.: "A Summary of Trends in Hospital Employment." Hospitals, 54:18:65, September 16, 1980.

Employment Statistics, First Quarter 1980

Service	Average Annual Percentage Change 1977-79	First Quarter Percentage Change 1979-80	First Quarter Distribution of 1979-80 Increment
Nursing services	3.1%	6.1%	40.7%
Diagnostic services	4.8	3.6	6.3
Operative services	2.0	0.9	1.1
Therapeutic services	9.7	11.2	12.8
Outpatient services	5.8	2.1	1.3
Patient care support	2.3	4.3	13.1
Professional support	6.2	6.4	4.5
Administrative services	5.0	5.9	20.2
Overall	4.0%	5.4%	100.0%

Cohen, Carol F. and Backofer, Henry J.: "A Summary of Trends in Hospital Employment." Hospitals, 54:18:65, September 16, 1980.

consequence of increased cardiac surgery.[6] The report points out that in comparing the first quarters of 1979 and 1980, over 40% of the increase in staffing hours in hospitals occurred in nursing. Within that category 38.8% of the increase was in intensive care areas.[7]

TECHNOLOGIC ADVANCES

One important variable inherent in the acuity issue is the specialization phenomenon. Technologic advances have effected increased medical specialization, which in turn has led to increased nursing specialization and, concomitantly, to the specialization or segregation of patient care areas and to the rise of specialized intensive care units (ICUs). While this pattern is generally peculiar to large medical centers, the rate of technologic diffusion to smaller facilities is unquestionably on the rise. In order to remain competitive, provide equitable services for their clientele, and attract well-qualified care providers, smaller hospitals are, in a sense, forced to acquire the necessary electronic equipment. Thus, the technologic impact on hospitals, patients, and personnel is similar regardless of hospital size, differing only in rate and intensity.[8]

Nursing has had to keep pace by greatly expanding its knowledge base. As the ever-present care-giver and integrator of therapeutic services, the nurse becomes the pivotal person who bears primary responsibility and accountability for the patient's well-being. In order to accomplish this, nurses must have a current, working knowledge of laboratory values; of the action, side-effects, and uses of a voluminous number of drugs; of the nutritional needs of patients; of environmental control, including cleanliness, isolation, and reverse isolation techniques, along with other infection control measures; of thermostatic heating and cooling effects; and, not surprisingly, of mechanical engineering. Additionally, in certain specialties nurses must be capable of differentiating such abnormalities as cardiac arrhythmias in order to determine when intervention is required; they must have a working knowledge of chest tubes, various suction apparatus, central venous pressure (CVP) lines and other types of catheters, fluid and electrolyte balance along with intake and output norms, and the interrelatedness of temperature, pulse, respiration, and blood pressure to any or all of the above.

To go a step further, the nurse is expected to address the psychosocial needs of patients, work with anxious families, and cope with other stresses such as death and dying, combative or angry patients, multiple specialty services on a single nursing unit, and the ongoing, never ending introduction of yet newer equipment, newer drugs, and changes in various policies and procedures.

Critical to the responsibility of the nurse is the articulation of nursing and medical intervention. For example, the nurse can monitor a bleeding patient, apply or change dressings if indicated, and determine frequency of blood pressure, temperature, pulse, and respiration checks. However, it is the ability to conceptualize the totality of the process—that is, understand the upper and lower limits of physiologic norms and know when to communicate this information to the physician—that is of the essence. What is required, therefore, is an ability to integrate and synthesize a volume of differentiated knowledge in order to translate that knowledge into coordinated, safe patient care. It is precisely because of this knowledge base requirement that the need for professional nurses has mushroomed while the need for nonprofessional nursing staff has not kept a similar pace. In fact, many institutions have attempted in recent years to move toward a nursing staff almost totally composed of registered nurses, recognizing that the potential contribution of lesser prepared persons is rapidly declining.[9]

INCREASED DEMAND FOR REGISTERED NURSES

The changing demand for nurses in hospitals is clearly reflected in Table 4-2.[10] These data represent a portion of that which is collected annually by the AHA from the more than 7,000 registered hospitals in the United States and associated areas, of which approximately 90% respond. They show that despite a 10.6% decrease in hospital beds between 1973 and 1979, there was a 40.5% increase in registered nurses compared to a 15.5% increase in licensed practical nurses.

It would seem rather evident that few professions would be able to produce enough new practitioners, on an annual basis, to supply this enormous demand. In fact, the vacancy rate that hospitals report reflects, in large degree, the extent to which the supply has not kept pace with the demand. During 1980, surveys of the nation's hospitals revealed 90,000 to 100,000 unfilled registered nurse positions, with 80% of all hospitals indicating such vacancies.[11]

An examination of the supply side of the equation is at once enlightening and discouraging. The American Nurses Association (ANA) has published the findings from their most recent (1977) comprehensive survey of registered nurses in the United States. These show the following: In that year, there were more than 1,400,000 people holding registered nurse licenses, 70% of whom were actively employed in nursing.[12] (It should be noted that this proportion of employed practitioners is considerably larger than that of other predominantly female professions.)[13] Of the 978,234 employed registered nurses, more than 61% (601,011) were working in hospitals; while this figure represented a marked increase from the previous survey conducted in 1972, it is important to note another finding, namely that "more nurses were employed in out-of-institution settings than previously."[14] Thus, hospitals are in competition with community settings in which the demand for nurses has also increased significantly.

A vital part of the supply information, of course, relates to newcomers to the field, graduating from the nation's schools of nursing each year. The National League for Nursing (NLN) collects and publishes data in this regard,

TABLE 4-2 Employment of Nursing Personnel in the United States Registered Hospitals

Year	Number of Hospital beds	Number of RNs (FTE) *	Number of LPNs (FTE) *
1973	1,534,726	446,387	222,599
1975	1,465,828	510,118	239,949
1977	1,407,097	570,117	253,184
1979	1,371,849	627,215	257,209

American Hospital Association. Hospital Statistics, 1974, 1976, 1978 and 1980 editions. Chicago: AHA.
*FTE (Full time equivalent)

the most recent of which reflected the situation in 1979. These showed that we are beginning to lose ground in the numbers of new nurses that we produce, which is reflected in Table 4-3.[15] This table indicates that we avoided a hospital staffing crisis through the mid-1970s because of the marked yearly increase in the number of new nurses entering the field. However, it is plain that we have begun to experience a plateau and will soon see a decline in the preparation of such persons. Since 90% of all new graduates start out their careers in hospital nursing, the impact of this change has been and will continue to be most severe in acute-care settings.[16]

An additional set of findings, when placed in juxtaposition, indicates another area for concern. Johnson, in his analysis of the NLN data, indicates that we have been maintaining our recruitment levels for new nurses as high as they have been in recent years by attracting large numbers of persons who are 21 yr of age or older. For example, he reports that in 1975, 36.9% of all admissions to basic registered nurse programs were in this somewhat older category, as compared with 10.4% in 1962.[17] The older student, then, would appear to be an important source of supply, and could hold promise for solving some of our difficulties.

On the other hand, the data from the 1977 ANA survey reveal that practitioners are retiring from nursing at an earlier age than they ever did before. Moses and Roth, in their description of the data, indicate that there was a significantly lower activity rate for those 55 and older.[18] They suggest that this decline is related to marked changes in retirement benefits in the health care industry. For those involved in hospital nursing, however, this early retirement phenomenon may be more related to the nature of the work itself. Hospital nursing has always been physically taxing. It continues to be as physical as it has been in the past, the only notable change being that the pace has accelerated. In addition, there are added mental and emotional demands that make the work itself difficult, with the result that much of hospital nursing is beyond the capability of the older professional. Hospital nursing may be rapidly becoming, and perhaps in many situations has already become, a young person's job. If this trend continues, the recruitment of older candidates for schools of nursing may not prove as beneficial to hospitals as might be expected initially.

For the future, manpower statistics indicate that supply and demand for hospital nursing are on a collision path. On the one hand, there is every indication that hospitals' requirements for registered nurses will continue to escalate; the Department of Labor has estimated that there will be 240,000 new jobs in nursing by 1985, many of which will be in hospitals.[19] On the other hand, unless recruitment into the field is greatly and suddenly increased (an unlikely occurrence), there is every reason to believe that we will continue the downward trend in the supply of new nurses.[20]

TABLE 4-3 Graduations from Basic RN Programs and Percentage Change from Previous Year, By Type of Program: United States, 1958–59 to 1977–78

Academic Year[1]	All Basic RN Programs[2]		Baccalaureate Programs		Associate Degree Programs		Diploma Programs	
	Number of Graduations	Percent Change	Number of Graduations	Percent Change	Number of Graduations	Percent Change	Number of Graduations	Percent Change
1958–59	30,136	−0.3	3,943	+7.4	462	+8.7	25,731	−1.6
1959–60	29,895	−0.8	4,132	+4.8	789	+70.8	24,974	−2.9
1960–61	30,019	+0.4	4,031	−2.4	917	+16.2	25,071	+0.4
1961–62	31,006	+3.3	4,292	+6.5	1,159	+26.4	25,555	+1.9
1962–63	32,223	+3.9	4,477	+4.3	1,479	+27.6	26,267	+2.8
1963–64	35,050	+8.8	5,053	+12.9	1,962	+32.7	28,035	+6.7
1964–65	34,497	−1.6	5,376	+6.4	2,510	+27.9	26,611	−5.1
1965–66	34,909	+1.2	5,488	+2.1	3,349	+33.4	26,072	−2.0
1966–67	37,931	+8.7	6,122	+11.5	4,639	+38.5	27,170	+4.2
1967–68	41,245	+8.7	7,132	+16.5	6,163	+32.8	27,950	+2.9
1968–69	41,801	+1.3	8,355	+17.1	8,578	+39.2	24,868	−11.0
1969–70	43,103	+3.1	9,069	+8.5	11,483	+33.9	22,551	−9.3
1970–71	46,455	+7.8	9,856	+8.7	14,534	+26.6	22,065	−2.2
1971–72	51,304	+10.4	10,968	+11.3	18,926	+30.2	21,410	−3.0
1972–73	58,881	+14.8	13,055	+19.0	24,497	+29.4	21,329	−0.4
1973–74	67,061	+13.9	16,957	+29.9	28,919	+18.0	21,185	−0.7
1974–75	73,915	+10.2	20,170	+18.9	32,183	+11.3	21,562	+1.8
1975–76	77,065	+4.3	22,579	+11.9	34,625	+7.6	19,861	−7.9
1976–77	77,755	+0.9	23,452	+3.9	36,289	+4.8	18,014	−9.3
1977–78	77,874	+0.1	24,187	+3.1	36,556	+0.7	17,131	−4.9

National League for Nursing. Nursing Data Book 1979. New York: NLN, 1980, p. 29.
[1] Time period is September 1 through August 31 for academic years 1958–59 through 1969–70, and August 1 through July 31 for subsequent years.
[2] Excludes Guam, Puerto Rico, and the Virgin Islands.

SYSTEMS OF NURSING CARE DELIVERY

Comprehensive or total patient care became bywords in the 1950s. There was a distinct shift from functional to team nursing in order to ensure continuity of care, maximize use of professional nursing skills, and, at the same time, provide high-quality care to hospitalized patients.

Over the last decade, additional efforts have been made to increase nursing effectiveness while attending to individualized patient care. From this, a "new" modality of delivery system has emerged, that of primary nursing. Primary nursing gives the nurse direct responsibility and accountability for comprehensive care for a caseload of patients over a period of time. As Zander put it, "Primary nursing puts nurses on the line; their actions can be studied, audited, and evaluated according to priorities."[21] Although the concept of primary nursing appears to be a product of the 1970s, indeed it is not. Its true origins may well be rooted in the case method of yesteryear, although this is a moot point. The modality is, however, traced back generally to the early 1960s when Lydia Hall was instrumental in establishing the Loeb Center for Nursing and Rehabilitation at Montefiore Hospital in the Bronx, New York City. At that time, Mrs. Hall's chief goal was to put nurses back at the bedside and assign nonnursing tasks, such as making unoccupied beds, to ancillary personnel. Out of this evolved the current concept of primary nursing described by Zander:

> Most significantly, the primary nurse assumes first-line accountability for whatever nursing care is done or not completed. Her role includes health-teaching, working with families, and documentation of the patient's physical and emotional responses to treatment. In carrying out her responsibilities, the primary nurse becomes her patient's advocate in the health care system.[22]

While the cost of primary care has been questioned, repeated studies have demonstrated that this system of care delivery results in greater job satisfaction, greater job enrichment, and better use of the professional nurse's judgment, knowledge, and skills. Further, it provides greater professional autonomy and independence at the bedside. Other research demonstrates that primary nursing improves retention, decreases absenteeism, and greatly enhances patient satisfaction with nursing care.[23,24,25,26]

Many tend to believe that primary nursing is synonymous with "good" team nursing, but there is a distinct difference. Team nursing is as the name implies. Nursing personnel of all levels are assigned to a team, which is responsible for a specific group of patients. Patient assignments, designated by the registered nurse team leader, are determined by the level of patient care required. Thus, a licensed practical nurse, for example, may be responsible for the total care of a group of patients whose nursing needs match that person's level of skill. In contrast, the primary nurse bears individual accountability for a small group of patients, often six or fewer. Ancillary personnel are assigned to the primary nurse who then delegates specific tasks to the ancillary person; however, at no time does the licensed practical nurse or nurses' aide assume full responsibility for any one patient.

There is also an important difference in the staff composition required for the two systems. Where team nursing functions with fewer professional staff and more ancillary staff, primary nursing, on the other hand, requires more registered nurses, but fewer ancillary personnel. This development should not be interpreted as adding salary costs to hospital budgets. Most institutions have found that in the conversion to primary nursing they may add registered nurses, but they decrease the total numbers of nursing staff required due to the increased productivity of those providing care.[27]

In an effort to respond to the increased acuity of patients, the increased need for registered nurses, and the introduction of primary nursing, hospitals are experimenting with various approaches to staffing and staffing patterns. For example, earlier in this chapter a staffing pattern was mentioned that was composed almost exclusively of registered nurses. Studies have been conducted on the financial effect of such an effort with results reflecting that this approach is cost effective.[28,29,30,31] While such staffing may not be feasible where professional nurses are in short supply, an all-registered nurse staff has proven to reduce turnover, increase retention, and increase job satisfaction among nurses; it may, therefore, serve to alleviate the shortage for particular insitutions, especially in areas where large numbers of nurses choose to be unemployed.

A great deal of attention has also focussed on flexible hours in an effort to make hospital nursing more attractive. The introduction of the 10-hr day, 4-day work week has proven to be cost effective, particularly in ICUs where it has been demonstrated that a third day off duty is useful in reducing stress and burnout. Other variations offer 7 days on and 7 days off, three 12-hr work days per week, guaranteed long weekends, and combinations of shifts of varying lengths, all designed to accommodate life styles, increase job satisfaction and retention, reduce burnout, and increase the quality of patient care.[32,33,34,35,36]

One of the most controversial staffing issues facing American hospitals today is the proliferation of temporary staffing agencies. Professional nurse registries have been with us for a long time. Until the emergence of ICUs, the registries provided private duty nurses around the clock for those patients desiring or requiring one-to-one care. The nurse independently contracted with the patient or family on a fee-for-service basis; there was no question regarding the usefulness and necessity for such a service. No one perceived these nurses as dropouts from the system, and no one questioned their preference for this type of practice.

The decade of the 1970s, however, witnessed a steady increase in proprietary organizations providing temporary nursing staff to hospitals. The arguments as to their value are diverse. Hospitals claim that these agencies are drawing nurses away and placing added stress on an already overburdened market. On the other hand, the agencies claim that they are recruiting nurses who would not otherwise be working. Hospitals claim that the agencies are adding to the nursing shortage while the agencies assert that they are a *result* of the shortage, not the *cause* of it.[37]

Multiple surveys have revealed that nurses leave hospitals because of inflexible hours, poor salaries, lack of professional recognition, and few opportunities for advanced education.[38,39,40,41] The agencies respond that they can offer flexible time, thus freeing up nurses to raise small children, attend school, or engage in other activities that may provide a respite from burnout.

From another perspective, however, authorities point out that temporary agencies are the result of a need and that hospitals do have the capability of addressing nursing issues. Thus, it is clear that the response of hospitals can determine the survival or demise of what some consider to be an unparalleled and unprecedented competitor for hospital nursing services.[42]

IMPLICATIONS OF CHANGING HOSPITAL TRENDS FOR NURSES

Four major, interrelated trends have been explored in this chapter, namely:

1   The increased knowledge level required of the nurse as a result of the increased acuity of patients.
2   The increased need for nurses in the face of a declining supply.
3   The increased demand for registered nurses.
4   The change to primary nursing as a system of nursing care delivery.

Underlying all of these trends is a common problem that is the source of much of the difficulty facing the profession in the 1980s. It is the problem of powerlessness and it affects both the care-giver and the integrator aspects of the nurse's role.

As far as the care-giver role is concerned, the sense of powerlessness is probably most severe in interprofessional relationships with physicians.

Today's nurses are knowledgeable professionals who have a high degree of self-worth and an understanding of the contribution they can and do make to patient care. In addition they are in a unique position to develop that knowledge because they spend more time with the patient and his family than other members of the health care team. They therefore have an expectation that their input into clinical decisions should be valued. In many situations, however, this is not the case and nurses become frustrated and demoralized by their lack of power. Evidence of this abounds, examples of which commonly include instances when they are unable to convince physicians that pateints need attention or are in need of a particular kind of therapy; these are, of course, most frustrating when the nurse is an experienced practitioner and the physician is not. In any case, such situations are always demoralizing when the nurse perceives the patient's welfare to be in jeopardy.

It was most heartening to see the progress made in solving some of the care-giver problems through the development of demonstration models of collaborative practice under the auspices of the National Joint Practice Commission. The Commission was sponsored by the American Medical Association (AMA) and the ANA for the express purpose of developing more productive and positive practice relationships between the respective professions. While the AMA has decided not to continue participating in this formal organization, a publication was produced by the Commission, before its demise, that is most useful in spelling out the kinds of structure and process that tend to support collaborative practice endeavors in hospitals.[43] These principles can be applied in a variety of settings and have the potential for reducing the sense of powerlessness that nurses experience in their care-giver role.

The powerlessness that surrounds the integrator role is perhaps more diffuse but it is also amenable to change. Without question, the increased intensity of service to hospitalized patients has resulted in more integrator activities for the nurse. These services have increased both in number and in kind. In their analysis Lawrence and Lorsch describe the integrator as a person who has no formal authority over the various specialized departments but rather derives authority from the knowledge that he has of the situation; only under unusual circumstances should the integrator need to resort to the formal chain of command to carry out the role. While it is certainly true that the nurse is the person who possesses the knowledge required of the integrator for patient services, the truth is that this knowledge frequently fails to give the nurse the appropriate authority in the eyes of representatives of the differentiated support services. Coaxing a late tray from the dietary department, convincing an X-ray technician that a film needs to be done immediately, and arguing to obtain urgently needed medications from the pharmacy are commonplace experiences that make up a normal workday for the average nurse. Only rarely are these problems referred to the formal chain of command.

Compounding the difficulty is the fact that these activities take the nurse away from her central care-giver role. It should also be noted that the integrator aspects of the role are most problematic at night, on weekends, and on holidays; during those times services from other departments are often minimal and sometimes nonexistent.

The changes required to reduce the powerlessness for the nurse in relation to the integrator role involves two steps. First, it is necessary that the top levels of administration make it clear to the respective department heads that they expect a high degree of responsiveness to patient needs. This means taking corrective action wherever there are failures in the system.

Second, each hospital should ensure that it is treating registered nurses as the scarce and essential resource that they are. In many cases, this may mean embarking on a careful study in order to be certain that nurses are expending the majority of their efforts on those activities for which they are uniquely prepared. As inpatient care has evolved over the years, many support functions have become the responsibility of nursing departments more by default than design; quite often this has been related to the 24-hr availability of staff. In the evaluation of these functions it is quite likely that a significant number of nursing hours could be identified for redeployment to direct care activities in most institutions. As the nursing shortage worsens, it will become increasingly important to capture those hours for patient care.

It seems quite clear that the increased acuity of hospitalized patients that has resulted in the need for more and better prepared nurses is leading us into a crisis of unprecedented proportion. That crisis can be averted, however, if hospital administrators and physicians, the influentials in the health care delivery system, become convinced of and committed to the need for significant change in the directions noted above. The powerlessness that pervades the care-giver and the integrator aspects of the nurse's role must be mitigated. Only when nurses begin to perceive themselves, and to be perceived by others, as having authority commensurate with their responsibility will the dual problems of recruitment and retention for hospital nursing be solved. The changes required are substantial but they can readily be achieved in most settings. Responsible parties must be willing to expend this necessary effort in order to safeguard the welfare of the hospitalized American public for the future.

REFERENCES

1   Lawrence, Paul R. and Lorsch, Jay W. *Developing Organizations: Diagnosis and Action.* Reading, Mass : Addison-Wesley Publishing Company, 1969.
2   Levine, Eugene. "Hospitals Headlines," *Hospitals*, 54:18:19, September 16, 1980.

3   *Health, United States. 1980.* Hyattsville, Md.: U.S. Department of Health and Human Services, 1980, p. 180–181.

4   Cohen, Carol F. and Backofer, Henry J. "A Summary of Trends in Hospital Employment," *Hospitals,* 54:18:65, September 16, 1980.

5   *Ibid.,* p. 66.

6   *Health. United States. 1980, op. cit.*

7   Cohen and Backofer, *op. cit.,* p. 66.

8   Fagerhaugh, Shizecho, et al. "The Impact of Technology on Patients, Providers and Care Patterns," *Nursing Outlook,* 28:11:668, November, 1980.

9   Alfano, Genrose (ed.). *The All-RN Nursing Staff.* Wakefield, Mass.: Nursing Resources, 1980.

10 American Hospital Association. *Hospital Statistics.* Chicago: 1974, 1976, 1978, 1980.

11 American Hospital Association. *Statement of the AHA Before the Subcommittee on Health and the Environment of the House Committee on Energy and Commerce on Nursing Education and Foreign Medical Graduate Proposals,* March 21, 1981. mimeo, p. 5.

12 Moses, Evelyn & Roth, Aleda. *Nursepower. AJN,* 79:10:1745–1746, October, 1979.

13 Fralic, Maryann. "Nursing Shortage: Coping Today and Planning for Tomorrow," *Hospitals,* 54:9:65, May 1, 1980.

14 Moses & Roth, *op. cit.,* p. 1756.

15 National League for Nursing. *Nursing Data Book 1979.* New York: NLN, 1980, p. 29.

16 *Ibid,* p. 99.

17 Johnson, Walter L. "Supply and Demand for Registered Nurses," *Nursing and Health Care,* 1:2:76, September, 1980.

18 Moses & Roth, *op. cit.,* p. 1748.

19 "Commission Studies Nurse Shortage; Job Satisfaction is Big Issue," *Hospital Management Quarterly,* Winter, 1981, p. 9.

20 Johnson, *op. cit.,* p. 77.

21 Zander, Karen S: *Primary Nursing Development and Management.* Germantown, Maryland: Aspen Systems Corporation, 1980, p. 21.

22 *Ibid.,* p. 53.

23 Cisk, Karen. "Primary Nursing Evaluation," *American Journal of Nursing,* 74:8:1436–1438, August, 1974.

24 Marram, Gwen, et al. *Cost Effectiveness of Primary and Team Nursing.* Wakefield, Mass.: Contemporary Publishing Co., 1976.

25 Carey, Raymond G. "Evaluation of a Primary Nursing Unit," *American Journal of Nursing,* 79:7:1255, July, 1979.

26 Fairbanks, Jane E. "Primary Nursing: More Data," *Nursing Administration Quarterly,* 5:3:51–62, Spring, 1981.

27 Mundinger, Mary O'Neil. *Autonomy in Nursing.* Germantown, Md.: Aspens Systems Corporation, 1980, pp. 74–75.

28 Osinski, Elsie G. and Morrison, William H. "The All-RN Staff," *Supervisor Nurse,* 9:10:68–74, September, 1978.

29 Osinski, Elsie G. and Powals, Jill. "The All-RN Staff Three Years Later," *Supervisor Nurse,* 9:10:25–27, October, 1978.

30 Forster, J.F. "The Dollars and Sense of an All RN Staff," *Nursing Administration Quarterly*, 2:1:41–47, Fall, 1978.

31 Osinski, Elsie G. and Powals, Jill. "The Cost of All RN Staffed Primary Nursing," *Supervisor Nurse*, 11:1:16–21, January, 1980.

32 Cales, Alice D. "A Twelve Hour Schedule Experiment," *Supervisor Nurse*, 7:6:71–76, June, 1976.

33 Shaw, Pearl. "The 10 Hour Day in the 4 Day Week," *Supervisor Nurse*, 9:10:47–56, October, 1978.

34 Simendinger, Earl A. and Gilbert, Vicki. "Flexible Staffing," *Supervisor Nurse*, 10:3:43–46, March, 1979.

35 "The Demise of the Traditional 5–40 Workweek?," *American Journal of Nursing*, 81:6:1138–1141, June, 1981.

36 Price, Elmira. "Seven Days On and Seven Days Off," *American Journal of Nursing*, 81:6:1142–1143, June, 1981.

37 "Nurse Registries. Part of the Problem or Part of the Solution?," *Hospitals*, 55:6:65, March 16, 1981.

38 McCarty, Patricia A. "Nurse Leader Urges Change in Hospital Power Structure," *American Nurse*, 12:10:1+, Nov.-Dec., 1980.

39 Wandelt, Mabel A., et al. "Why Nurses Leave Nursing and What Can Be Done About It," *American Journal of Nursing*, 81:1:72–77, January, 1981.

40 "Many Nurses Leave Hospital – Fewer Return," *Nursing Careers*, 2:1:1+, Jan.-Feb., 1981.

41 McNally, James. "Do National Surveys Reveal Fact or Fiction?," *Hospital Financial Management*, 11:5:16-23, May, 1981.

42 "Nurse Registries. Part of the Problem or Part of the Solution?," *op. cit.*, p. 65.

43 *Guidelines for Establishing Joint or Collaborative Practice in Hospitals.* Chicago: The National Joint Practice Commission, 1981.

ADA JACOX

5

ROLE RESTRUCTURING IN HOSPITAL NURSING

Nursing is the diagnosis and treatment of human responses to actual or potential health problems.[1]
The nurse's place in the division of labor is essentially that of doing in a
responsible way whatever necessary things are in danger of not being done
at all.[2]

The discrepancy between these two conceptions of what a nurse is and
does provides some explanation for the present frustration and anger of
nurses concerning their role in the health care system. How the discrepancy
is resolved will be the major factor in determining who will provide nursing
care for America's sick.

E. C. Hughes noted that what bothers professionals most are differing
notions of what their work is or should be and how it is possible to accomplish that work.[3] Building on Hughes' work in an analysis of the medical profession, Freidson characterized medicine as the dominant profession in the
health occupations and discussed the factors that determine how much functional autonomy other health-related occupations can achieve. He noted that
"the process determining the outcome is essentially political and social rather
than technical in character — a process in which power and persuasive rhetoric are of greater importance than the objective character of knowledge, training, and work."[4]

The discrepancies between the two definitions of nursing clearly are the
result of social and political factors in which an occupation made up almost
totally of women has tried to define its role in relation to medicine, an occupation traditionally composed primarily of men and commonly viewed as near

the top of the occupational hierarchy in social prestige. In more recent decades, nurses have been confronted by hospital administrators, a professionalizing group also largely made up of men, who have assumed it their prerogative to manage and control the practice of hospital nursing. These facts are the foundation for the majority of problems cited today as contributing to the "nursing shortage." From them spring the low economic status of nurses, the still lingering notion that the nurse's primary responsibility is to follow the physician's orders, the expectation that nurses will accept whatever tasks are given to them in the hospital and whatever hours the hospital needs them to work, and the lack of authority in determining policies related to patient care and hospital operation. While these are not the only problems identified in the numerous studies documenting sources of nurses' dissatisfaction, they are the most common ones. Successful attempts to resolve them will have to deal with the occupational overlap between medicine and nursing, with a view toward restructuring both roles.

In this chapter we first consider the nature of nurses' work and the economic and social value placed on it. Definitions and control of professional expertise are considered as the basis for suggesting the kinds of role restructuring that must occur, particularly at the hospital level, if hospital nursing is to emerge as anything other than a low level, poorly reimbursed occupation capable of attracting primarily those persons who have limited options for pursuing more interesting and satisfying work.

THE NATURE OF NURSES' WORK

Educational programs that require students to take the examination to become registered nurses include basic science courses such as chemistry, physiology, psychology, and sociology. Building on this general knowledge are nursing courses that usually focus and on the *nursing process*, which is the assessment of patients' needs, development and implementation of a plan of nursing care, and evaluation of the effectiveness of the care. Understanding both biologic and psychosocial aspects of patient behavior and promoting wellness, in addition to caring for the ill, are emphasized. Faculty generally teach that professional nurses not only carry out the medical orders of physicians, but also have an independent role in areas such as counseling and teaching patients about their illness and health care, providing emotional support for patients and families, and exercising clinical judgment in planning and carrying out nursing care. Students are given very small numbers of patients to care for, and high value is placed on individualized patient care, with the understanding that giving such care is the most important part of the nurse's role.

The "reality shock" encountered by graduates of baccalaureate nursing programs when they enter hospital wards and learn how different the patient care situation is from how it was portrayed in the educational program has been well documented.[5] This phenomenon also occurs to varying degrees for graduates of associate degree and hospital diploma programs, depending on the nature and extent of contact students have had with the clinical situation and how well socialized they have been into the culture of the hospital.

What the new graduates find is more like Hughes' definition of nursing — they are expected to perform in a variety of roles ranging from housekeeper to housestaff. They are responsible for doing bits of care for large numbers of people and for acting as messengers and coordinators for other workers in the hospital. The result is that nurses have little time to give the individualized patient care they have been taught to value as students. Interestingly, the recommended means for dealing with the reality shock has been to teach students more about what they would be encountering in the actual patient care situation and how to adapt and deal with it. Only recently is serious attention beginning to be given to changing the hospital and the way nursing care is delivered to make it more consistent with the value placed on individualized patient care.

The nature of work performed by nurses in today's hospitals requires mental, psychological, and physical abilities to carry out the role in a safe and effective way. A higher proportion of patients in hospitals are seriously ill and have shorter lengths of stay than in years past; the technology related to patient care has become increasingly sophisticated, and the numbers and types of workers in hospitals has vastly increased. Twenty-five or thirty years ago the hospital world was a comparatively simple structure involving nurses. physicians, dietary and maintenance personnel, administrators, and a few other professionals such as social workers and physical therapists; now it is exceedingly complex. There are more medical specialties, an explosion of technicians, technologists, and therapists, and a proliferation of jobs in the administration of the hospital. Where previously one administrator with a few assistants managed the affairs of the hospital, it is not unusual now to have dozens of people in the hospital's administration, each running a piece of the system. Thus, not only has the nature of the work with patients become more complex and demanding, the intensity and complexity of the system in which that work is performed has increased significantly.

It has been estimated that approximately 30% of nurses in acute care hospitals today work in units that provide intensive care to patients. Such units require substantial technical and clinical knowledge, including the ability to interpret accurately the various monitoring devices commonly found in the units, knowing when the monitor is reflecting the true state of a patient's condition and when it is only showing "noise" or machine error. Nurses must be able to diagnose among six or eight different conditions that occur com-

monly in the coronary care unit, for example, and take the appropriate immediate response to alleviate the condition by giving a medication or performing
cardiopulmonary resuscitation or other measures. Assessment and management often must be done even before calling a physician for assistance. Similar activities are normal expectations for nurses working in neonatal intensive
care units, neurologic intensive care units, or any of the other intensive care
units that constitute a major part of the hospital.

It is possible to conceive of a continuum of work-related responsibilities,
at one end of which are complex situations in which the nurse is expected to
handle highly sophisticated technology and difficult physiological problems,
and at the same time be attentive to the personal and social concerns of the
patient and family. At the other end of the continuum are those tasks that
often are not an explicit or intended part of the professional nurse's role but
that no one else may be available at the time to perform. They include
transporting patients from one part of the hospital to another, answering the
telephone in the absence of a ward clerk, passing out nourishments to patients,
delivering mail, providing messenger service between physicians and laboratory, retrieving a patient's chart for a physician, and similar kinds of activities that require little more than the ability to walk, talk, and follow simple
directions.

A study of five Boston hospitals in the mid-1970s classified the activities
carried out by hospital personnel into six categories. The first three categories
were ordered in terms of increasing difficulty, using criteria such as amount
of practical experience and education necessary to perform the task. Class 1
activities included such things as locating and setting up simple equipment
and assisting in moving patients to another floor. Category 2 included giving
routine morning care, and lifting patients on and off litters; category 3
included doing cervical smears, using electrocardiographic (ECG) equipment,
and participating in a cardiac arrest team. Both nursing personnel and house
staff physicians were observed for amount of time spent on tasks of various
levels. There was a great deal of overlap in the performance of various functions regardless of educational preparation, and the most highly skilled persons spent large amounts of time on functions they and others considered
well below their technical capabilities. Considerable overlap was apparent
among levels of nursing personnel in the tasks performed, and there was similar overlap with physicians. Nearly half of the physicians spent approximately 23% of their time in category 1 functions, 77% of the registered
nurses spent 28% of their time on such functions, and 81% of the nurses' aides
spent 57% of their time on these simple activities. The researchers concluded
that "hospital tasks are performed by the medical personnel who happen to
be available, with little regard for the training, certification, or degree of competence of the individuals involved,"[6] They suggested that restructuring the

health occupations should begin with clear delineation and modification of physicians' functions so that the remaining functions could be performed more efficiently by other health occupations.[7]

Aiken and Blendon also addressed the interchangeability among nursing personnel, noting the shift in the proportion of nurses in hospital nursing services during the past 10 yrs. They reported that between 1968 and 1979 the percentage of nurses in hospital nursing service personnel increased from 33% to 46%. The percentage of licensed practical nurses remained at about 19% of the total, while untrained nurses' aides declined from 51% to 35%. The authors concluded that there has been a direct substitution of nurses for nurses' aides. They state that this substitution is possible largely because the salary differential between nurses and nurses' aides is so small that it is advantageous to the hospitals to have nurses perform all jobs rather than only those requiring special training.[8]

Finally, testimony presented by nurse administrators at a series of public hearings sponsored by the American Hospital Association (AHA) in the spring of 1981 provided current evidence of the underutilization of nurses.

> On the patient care unit, professional nurses spend an inordinate amount of time stamping charge slips for Central Supply, reordering medications for pharmacy, explaining TV charges to patients for the Business Office, collecting body fluid specimens for the laboratory, arranging employee vacation schedules for personnel, and settling conflicting department schedules as they occur.[9]

In addition to these tasks requiring little nursing skill or ability, there is another order of activities that falls outside the legal and professional definitions of a nurse's role. Nurses in many hospitals throughout the country assume the functions of other professionals in the hospital when these persons leave at 5:00 PM on weekdays and for the weekend. While some hospital departments keep services open on a scaled-down basis, many expect nursing supervisors on evenings, nights, and weekends to perform functions ordinarily carried out by other professionals and by hospital administrators. In Hughes' words, "The nurse's place in the division of labor is essentially that of doing in a responsible way whatever necessary things are in danger of not being done at all." The nurse has been expected to be and has in fact been a general all-purpose worker who has moved into whatever role the system has demanded.

A significant part of that role, and one that produces a great deal of stress, has been to ensure safe patient care in the hospital. The hospital is a place where mistakes and errors in judgment can have profound consequences. Nurses, in particular those in head nurse and supervisory positions, have long been expected to detect the mistakes of others and to protect patients, physicians, and hospitals against the consequences of such mistakes. Quoting again from Hughes:

> In medicine, the physician, who stands at the top of the hierarchy, takes the great and final risks of decision and action. These risks are delegated to him, and he is given moral and legal protection in taking them. But the pharmacist, who measures out the prescribed doses, and the nurse, who carries out the ordered treatment, are the great observers of ritual in medicine. . . . The ritualistic punctiliousness of nurses and pharmacists is a kind of built-in shock absorber against the possible mistakes of the physician.[10]

The responsibility for completion of accident or incident reports in hospitals has traditionally been the nurse's, even when the act of omission or commission resulting in error was not the nurse's. Because of their constant presence on the patient care units, nurses have been expected to observe and report mistakes made by anyone in the hospital including themselves, dietary aides, housekeepers, house staff, and attending physicians.

A related factor contributing to the frustration associated with hospital nursing is the rigid ritualism and standardization of procedures, accompanied by an absence of decision-making freedom, often extending even to such minor areas as deciding a patient can take a shower or wash his hair. Partly as a way of minimizing risk to patients and protecting physicians and hospitals from malpractice charges, and partly as a means of maintaining the dominance of physicians and hospital administrators, the practice of nursing in hospitals commonly is highly regulated by procedures and policies. In many hospitals nurses may not, except in emergency situations, independently decide that a patient should have his nasogastric tube irrigated, have his visitors limited, be taught before discharge about drugs he will be taking following hospitalization, and similar functions without an explicit order from a physician.

The discussion of the nature of nurse's work has focused on hospital nursing. In other settings as well, nurses perform a wide range of activities that overlap with those of both other health professionals and nursing personnel with considerably less training. While the nurse has little autonomy or decision-making freedom regarding patient care, nurses are frequently assigned the role of ensuring safe patient care.

THE VALUE PLACED ON NURSES' WORK

The value of work can be measured in numerous ways; two common indicators of work value are economic reimbursement and social prestige. The economic value placed on nurses' work is difficult to evaluate for many reasons. One is that in hospitals, the costs of nursing care commonly are included with general costs related to room and board, which include maintenance, house-keeping, and other hotel-like costs as well as nursing department costs. Nursing costs are computed as part of the cost per patient day, making it difficult to identify those costs related specifically to professional nursing care.* A second reason for the difficulty in assigning economic value is that a substantial part of the reimbursement for nurses' work has historically gone to organizations or persons other than nurses.

The late Joann Ashley documented the practice early in this century of hospitals establishing nurse-training programs in order to gain a ready supply of persons to give the nursing care in hospitals.

> Many of the hospitals were small, private "doctors' " hospitals, which were financially remunerative to the physicians who operated them because of the free labor of student nurses. Reliable statistics for the year 1905 indicate that more than half of these private profit-making hospitals had "schools" for women. Though the "hospital" may have been limited to 40 beds, it established a so-called "school" for nurses in order to obtain nursing service at the least possible cost.[11]

A common practice was to send student nurses into patients' homes to deliver patient care, with the hospital receiving reimbursement. At an American Hospital Association (AHA) meeting in 1913, the superintendent of a Minneapolis Hospital encouraged other hospital administrators to require students to have private home nursing during their training. "And of course the hospital should charge for this service. Properly managed, the training school of even a small hospital can contribute a good deal toward the support of the institution, without any abuse of the curriculum."[12]

There are currently a variety of ways in which those other than nurses receive reimbursement for what nurses do. Two of these are physician reimbursement for services performed by nurse practitioners and supplementary nurse agencies.

In an article reviewing the practice of third party payers, in which physicians are reimbursed for the work of nurse practitioners and physician's assistants employed by them, the authors estimate that a 46% reimbursement rate is the point at which physicians will break even in hiring a nurse practitioner or a physician's assistant. If the nurse practitioner is used efficiently to provide the highest level of service possible, the physician can earn up to 54% profit.[13]

Robyn and Hadley note that

> approximately two-thirds of the primary care physician's duties could be delegated to an NP or PA; ... From the standpoint of economic theory, it is irrelevant whether nurse practitioners and physicians' assistants are reim-

---

* This issue is dealt with in detail in Chapter 8.

bursed for their services directly or indirectly through a supervisory physician or facility. Theoretically, as long as the service provided is reimbursable, an NP or PA could receive an equivalent income in the form of a salary paid by the employer. In practice, however, indirect reimbursement has considerable economic, legal, and symbolic importance. Indirect reimbursement permits physicians to realize higher incomes from the development of the NP and PA occupations. More important, indirect reimbursement guarantees that the role of NPs and PAs in health care delivery will be one of dependence on physicians.[14]

A second way in which physicians benefit economically from the work of nurses is when nurse practitioners and other nurses employed by the hospital and paid as part of hospital costs perform work for attending physicians. Such work may include doing admission histories and physicals, making rounds on chronically ill hospitalized patients, ordering routine medications, and carrying out diagnostic and treatment procedures for the physician. These and similar activities are formally delegated to the nurse by the physician with the provision that the physician must "validate" the service by countersigning the admission history and physical examination or the treatment rendered. The physician then collects a fee for validating the work of the nurse, who was paid by the hospital.

A recently developed type of organization benefiting economically from nurses' work is the temporary service agency discussed at length by Prescott in this volume. In this arrangement, the nurse works for and is paid by the temporary service agency, which in turn is paid by the hospital. The agency collects the full costs of the nurses' services as well as an amount, often substantial, for serving as a broker between nurse and hospital.

A somewhat paradoxical issue related to who benefits economically from nurses' work is how the costs of nursing services are treated in hospitals. The primary reasons why patients are hospitalized are (1) to enable the physician to carry out sophisticated diagnostic or treatment procedures unavailable in the physician's office and (2) to receive highly skilled nursing care, also not available in the physician's office. In the first case — diagnostic treatments and procedures — the services are treated as revenue generating, with hospitals highly valuing these as a source of income. In the second case — provision of skilled nursing care — the service is treated as a cost or liability.

A significant dimension of economic value is the salary a nurse actually receives in comparison to salaries received by others doing comparable work. This, of course, is a general contemporary socioeconomic issue, related not only to nursing but to all occupations with high percentages of women and minorities. Aiken and Blendon cite figures indicating that in the past 20 years, the gap between what nurses and nurses' aides are paid has narrowed. In 1960 nurses' aides' incomes were 65% of registered nurses' salaries; today aides receive 71% of registered nurses' salaries. Furthermore, while the salary

TABLE 5-1 Salaries for Male Job Classifications and Nurses in Denver

100% Male Job Classifications	Monthly Starting Salary
Sign painter	$1245.00
Painter	1088.00
Tree trimmer	1040.00
Tire serviceman	1017.00
Parking meter repairman	994.00
Nurse Salaries	
Graduate nurse 1 (Beginning staff nurse—97% women)	929.00
Mean Monthly Starting Salary	
100% Male Classes	1592.81
100% Female Classes	1090.77

range within nursing has narrowed, that between nurses and physicians has widened. Thirty-five years ago nurses received approximately 33% of what physicians received; today the figure has dropped to 20%.[15]

The low salaries of nurses in comparison to other workers is clearly illustrated in a recent lawsuit by a group of nurses in Colorado.[16] Lemons and colleagues complained that they were discriminated against in the salaries they received because nursing is primarily a women's occupation.* At every level in the classification system employed by the city and county of Denver, starting salaries for jobs requiring comparable or lower qualification and responsibility were higher than those for nursing. Table 5-1 demonstrates some of the classifications:

Lemons, the director of nursing, was required to have a master's degree, had 12 yr administrative experience, had administrative responsibility for 575 employees, and administered an annual budget of $3.5 million. The director of nursing was not classed with other equally prepared administrators, but with the graduate nurse 1 class. According to those classifying the positions, the director of nursing was placed in the job cluster with graduate nurse 1 because the two jobs were functionally similar, that is, both were nurses. The director was more an administrator than a nurse in that she administered a large budget, supervised other supervisory personnel, directed

* The case was tried in United States District Court in April 1978. The nurses asserted that the job classification system used by the city and county of Denver discriminated on the basis of sex, and that the standards used were vague and inconsistently applied. Educational equivalence was a common requirement for all jobs within a particular class in 22 out of 27 key class groups. Four of the five groups that were educationally mixed were headed by key classes that were traditionally identified as female. In these predominantly female classes or groups of jobs, the educational standard was ignored. For example, the job of program aide 2 (100% of positions held by females) was in a related class group with the nursing service director, although the program aide 2 was not required to have even a high school education and the nursing service director was required to have a master's degree.

recruitment, supervised policy drafting, shift management, and inservice training, and did not give patient care. Her job was labeled by the city itself as "administrative," rather than "professional," which is the label given the bedside nurse. Nevertheless, she was paid according to the general duty nurses' scale rather than the general administrative series scale. Since the pay of the latter was based upon the prevailing rate of pay given to professionals and administrators within the Denver area and since the director of nursing was tied to the pay of the beginning level staff nurse, she was paid $497 less than other similarly prepared administrators in the same system. The salary discrimination was at all levels in the nursing hierarchy in this hospital and generally applies to pay scales in other hospitals. The judge who heard the case noted that

> we are confronted with a history which I have no hesitency at all in finding discriminated unfairly and improperly against women. . . . I think they (the nurses) have established that by and large, male dominated occupations probably pay more for comparable work than is paid in the occupations dominated by females. . . . I accept that nurses have been discriminated against, but so have other occupational groups. The nurses don't have it as bad as the clergy, for example.[17]

While he was not reluctant to say that nurses had been discriminated against with regard to salary, he ruled against them because he felt it could lead to a disruption of the American economy. The district judge's decision was upheld in the Appellate Court, and the United States Supreme Court would not hear the case upon appeal. The Denver nurses' case illustrates well the economic and social value placed on nurses' work and how these are interrelated.

Another indicator of social value of an occupation is how it is treated in the literature describing various kinds of work. Occupational sociology is a subdiscipline within sociology that studies work and occupations. The titles of two of the more prominent texts, both dealing in some detail with nursing, give a clue to the sociologic perspective: *Men and Their Work* (Hughes), *Medical Men and Their Work* (Freidson). The profession of medicine has been used by sociologists as the contemporary model profession against which other professions are often evaluated. Nursing is viewed as an adjunct to medicine and given such labels as paramedical, semiprofessional, quasiprofessional, and emerging professional. One analysis of three "semiprofessions" — nursing, social work, and teaching — even suggested that none of the three has a clear possibility of becoming a "full profession" because they are comprised primarily of women, and society does not like to grant women the autonomy necessary to become a full professional.[18]

Literature in the health field also reflects the notion that nurses and nurses' work are inferior to the work of physicians. A review of studies comparing nurse practitioner and physician performance was done by Prescott and Driscoll. The reviewers noted that a large number of studies demonstrated differences favoring nurse practitioners. Twenty different variables on which nurses received higher scores than physicians were identified. These included such things as continuity of care, emphasis on preventive medicine, completeness of history and physical examinations, accuracy of disposition, patients' knowledge of appropriate activities and exercises, control of blood pressure and hospitalization rates, symptomatic relief, and similar areas. According to the authors, "Even with this wide array of positive findings for nurse practitioners, the most common interpretation was that no differences existed between physician and nurse practitioner performance. In one instance, nurse practitioner superiority was attributed to a placebo effect."[19]

PROFESSIONAL EXPERTISE

Discussion in the previous section considered the occupational and economic value placed on nursing. Important determinants of the value placed on work are the amount of knowledge required to do the work and who controls how that knowledge will be used.

In his analysis of the medical profession, Freidson emphasized that a profession must have autonomy—a position of legitimate control over its work. To achieve professional autonomy the occupation must control an area of work that can be separated from the dominant profession (in this case medicine) and can be practiced without routine contact with or dependence on the dominant profession.[20] The attempt to differentiate nurses' work from the work of physicians has been pervasive in the nursing literature in recent decades. Physicians have a clear mandate, protected by law, to diagnose and treat illness. How far that mandate extends to other areas of human behavior is a continuing debate between physicians and others. Psychiatrist Thomas Szasz, for example, rejects the idea that psychiatric problems belong in the physician's domain.[21] Psychologists have succeeded to some extent in separating their claim for this area of human behavior from the control of medicine, but their success in achieving autonomy even in this area has been slow.

Nursing has tried to make the dual claims that its focus is primarily on promoting health and wellness and that it contrasts with medicine in its concern with the behavioral as well as the biologic aspects of human behavior. Medicine has been portrayed as oriented to the *cure* of biologically based illness, and nursing as concerned with the *care* of patients. Despite this effort to define an area of work separable from the practice of medicine, nursing in hospitals continues to be dominated by the physician on the one hand and hospital administration on the other. To the extent that nurses have moved away from hospital settings, they have had more success in achieving control over their work separate from that of physician domination and administrative supervision. In most acute care hospitals, however, the physician and administrative control over nurses' work remains firm and pervasive.

The notion of expertise — what composes it and how it can be evaluated — is basic to the control that medicine has achieved over all other health occupations. Freidson suggests that

> expertise is more and more in danger of being used as a mask for privilege and power rather than, as it claims, as a mode of advancing the public interest. . . . Conspicuous in the public eye by providing a personal service, medicine has come to dominate an elaborate division of labor, and its jurisdiction is broad and far ranging, having expanded into areas once dominated by religion and law — i.e., faith and politics.[22]

That physicians dominate the health care field and act to protect that dominance is reflected widely in the literature. Clark Havighurst, for example, observed that

> as the result of their long enjoyment of substantial professional autonomy, physicians now respond almost reflexively to outside interference in "their" affairs by taking collective action through their local, State and national professional associations. Indeed, professional societies are so accustomed to guarding their frontiers against intrusion — by other health professionals, by lay groups representing consumers' interests, or by government — that they will not take kindly to even the suggestion that some of their customary defensive practices may violate the antitrust laws.[23]

In the legal arena, organized medicine repeatedly has made strong and usually successful efforts to restrict the practice of other health professions, including nursing, by successfully persuading state and federal legislators of the dangers that might attend the delegation or sharing of work. The major argument used against delegation of medical tasks to nurses and against acknowledgment of nurses' competence to perform certain areas of work independently is the claim that nurses are inadequately prepared educationally. Accompanying this claim have been strong efforts to limit the educational preparation of nurses.

On the one hand, nurses have been pressured by their own profession to upgrade their educational preparation for the increasingly complex jobs they are expected to do. The emphasis of the nursing profession has been on those aspects of the role that require clinical knowledge and judgment, and strong efforts have been made by organized nursing to move the educational preparation of nurses totally into the system of higher education. On the other hand, organized medicine and hospital administration have tended to deemphasize the importance of formal preparation and to place low value on the knowledge needed by nurses.* The need for increased knowledge has been experienced by all other health professions and by hospital administrators as health and medical care and the systems in which they are delivered have grown more complex. A suggestion seriously proposed for nursing, however, is to return to hospital-based diploma programs to prepare nurses. Such programs traditionally emphasized a limited amount of formal course work and a maximum amount of clinical service. Accompanying the recent call for a return to diploma school education have been attempts in some states to reduce the educational requirements for taking the licensure examination to become a registered nurse. As the increased knowledge needs of other health professionals have been acknowledged, the call for hospital nursing is to decrease or eliminate the formal preparation required to practice.

Concern about nurses being over educated is not new. The president of the Pennsylvania State Board of Medical Examiners noted in an address given in 1909 that "the instruction commonly prevalent in hospital training schools is not only absurdly too comprehensive, but dangerous. It is sufficient to almost entirely result in nurses assuming the right to usurp the functions of physicians."[24] Beates noted that the nurse should "never attempt to appear learned and of great importance . . . she should be able and willing to render intelligent obedience to the instructions of the attending physician, and carry out his orders to the letter."[25]

Organized medicine was not without challenge in its claim for control of nurses and nursing education. The editor of the *National Hospital Record*, the official organ of the AHA, announced in 1908 that "there is only one organization in existence in America that seems fitted to broadly, impartially and effectively deal with this issue of an apprenticeship in the training of nurses. . . . The American Hospital Association."[26]

These earlier committees of physicians, hospital administrators, and others have their counterparts today. At this writing, the Institute of Medicine of the National Academy of Sciences is conducting a study of nursing and nursing education; the AHA in 1980 appointed a National Commission on Nursing to address nursing-related problems in the health care system; and the Health Care Finance Administration, a federal agency, has commissioned a group of health service researchers to study how well nursing education programs are meeting the needs for nursing care. All groups are expected to make recommendations concerning the educational preparation and practice of nurses.

* It should be noted that this statement does not characterize a number of individual physicians, whose efforts to promote the upgrading of nursing and to enable a more effective use of nurses' abilities are reflected most recently in the development of nurse practitioner programs and in efforts to work collaboratively with nurses.

The discussion thus far has been an analysis of nursing as having conflicting role definitions. Nursing has been characterized as comprising a broad spectrum of activities that overlap with other nursing personnel and with other health professionals. The broad and varied set of expectations for nurses has been accompanied by social and economic devaluation of the worth of the nurse's work, attempts by organized medicine and hospital administration to deemphasize the need for formal education of nurses, and the continuing suppression of independent decision making by nurses. The widespread and continuing interest of various groups in studying and making recommendations regarding nursing was noted. The remainder of this chapter will consider changes in the role of nurses (in particular, nurses in hospitals) intended to resolve some of the problems identified in the first part of this chapter.

ROLE RESTRUCTURING

Explicit in parts and implicit in much of the first part of this chapter is the need for major realignment of roles in the health care field to make more efficient and effective use of health care personnel, including both nurses and physicians. Acknowledging the strong resistance to such restructuring by those currently in control of and profiting most from the health care system, there must be sustained effort to match the education and experience required to perform certain activities with the necessary legal and organizational sanctions. Accompanying this must be reimbursement related more directly to who is performing what services for patients. Although the need is for role restructuring throughout the health care system and involving not only nurses, but other nursing personnel, physicians, administrators, and other health professionals and technicians, the remaining comments are directed primarily toward role restructuring of hospital nursing.

Two recent major modifications in the structure of hospital nursing are instructive in understanding the general nature of changes that may be required. These are the introduction of primary nursing and the widespread growth of temporary service agencies. Primary nursing is a form of nursing in which an individual nurse is assigned 24-hr responsibility for planning, evaluating, and carrying out a good part of the nursing care of specific patients. The purpose is to assign responsibility for total nursing care of the patient to an individual nurse rather than assigning patients to nurses collectively, such as to all nurses on a unit or to a team of nursing personnel. Primary nursing, initiated by Marie Manthey approximately 10 yrs ago, has spread quickly to many kinds of hospitals and into many settings. It has been characterized by nurses as providing them with satisfaction from direct patient care they had missed under team nursing and other forms of staff assignment. Other nurses have not been as enthusiastic about primary nursing, commenting that they do not like having to carry out all aspects of patient care, including bed making and similar activities. Comments are beginning to be heard regarding how expensive primary nursing can be and the inappropriateness of it for certain kinds of settings. Nevertheless, its popularity continues in nursing and no new modes of nursing care delivery have been proposed recently as alternatives.

A second change that has occurred that reflects nurses' dissatisfaction with hospital nursing has been the emergence of temporary service agencies, described in detail in Chapter 12. The nurses employed by temporary service agencies frequently comment on the increased flexibility they have in choosing both work settings and hours and days to work. Additionally, they express favorable comments regarding being released from some of the coordinative and administrative activities usually expected of nurses working in hospitals, being able to spend their time instead on direct patient care.

These two recent changes reflect the interest of nurses in having more involvement in direct patient care and in having greater control and flexibility in determining their working conditions. Although the adoption of primary nursing and the introduction of temporary service agencies have been useful in helping some nurses achieve these goals, additional ways must be developed to serve the same ends. Primary nursing may be very useful in some settings but too restrictive and expensive in others. Similarly, while the individual nurse employed by temporary service agencies may experience increased satisfaction as the result of increased flexibility, the cost of delivering nursing services under such a mechanism has increased markedly.

Serious reconstruction of the hospital nurse's role needs to be considered to make more efficient and effective use of nurses' knowledge and abilities and to ensure a continuing supply of nurses. Three main overlapping areas of reconstruction are considered: (1) the work itself; (2) working conditions; and (3) where the role of the nurse is placed in the total organization.

THE WORK ITSELF

The prime consideration in restructuring the work is acknowledging and emphasizing the clinical knowledge and judgment required of the hospital nurse and eliminating to whatever extent possible activities not requiring such knowledge. It is in the clinical knowledge component of the nurse's work that there lies the most potential for developing a more interesting and satisfying role; but it is also this area that is accompanied by great resistance to change, for it is here where overlap with physicians is greatest. It is also here where administrators resist change, since they are not accustomed to viewing nurses as knowledgeable professionals, but as a work force to be managed and controlled.

The introduction of the clinical specialist with a master's degree in the mid-1960s met with acceptance from some physicians but generally great resistance from others, who objected to a nurse being openly identified as having advanced clinical knowledge. This resistance is explained in large part by the traditional nurse–physician relationship. Leonard Stein, in an analysis of the "doctor–nurse game," noted that

> the object of the game is as follows: The nurse is to be bold, have initiative, and be responsible for making significant recommendations, while at the same time she must appear passive. This must be done in such a manner so as to make her recommendations appear to be initiated by the physician. . . . The cardinal rule of the game is that open disagreement between the players must be avoided at all cost. Thus, the nurse must communicate her recommendations without appearing to be making a recommendation statement. The physician, in requesting a recommendation from a nurse, must do so without appearing to be asking for it.[27]

With Stein's analysis as the underlying dynamic of physician–nurse relationships, rejection of the notions that a nurse can have advanced knowledge, be capable of making independent decisions, and provide consultation to physicians as well as to other nurses, is understandable. Nevertheless, it is precisely this lack of acknowledgment of clinical knowledge and ability and the opportunity to apply them in patient care that is a common complaint of the nurse in the hospital and that must form the foundation for any role restructuring.

There are numerous ways in which such emphasis and visibility may be accomplished. Three interrelated ways are the redefinition and expansion of the traditional nursing staff development department, the further development of specialized clinical roles, and closer collaboration between academic and practicing nurses. None of these ideas is new to hospital nursing. Elaine Bellitz, president of the New York State Nurses' Association, presented testimony at The Institute of Medicine's public hearing in Spring 1981, in which she stated that continuous study of the "nursing shortage" and factors related to it, unaccompanied by significant change, was socially irresponsible, since the causes were well known and had been documented repeatedly.[28] This is also the case with regard to suggestions for restructuring the hospital nurse's role. Staff development departments have been primarily responsible for orienting and updating the knowledge of nursing staff. Some nursing administrators have begun to view staff development departments as having research and development functions rather than being limited to orientation of nursing personnel and updating them on changes in hospital procedures. In addition to nurses with advanced clinical knowledge, nurses with knowledge of research and evaluation processes are used to assist the total nursing department to evaluate how care can be structured and delivered most effectively to produce positive patient care outcomes. A major concern is to help transfer new findings from basic and clinical research into practice.

Research and development departments, appropriately staffed and structured, also can assist in the evaluation of the need for and preparation of nurses to serve in various and changing specialist roles. The kinds of expertise required by health professionals change rapidly as new technology is developed. Formal education of professional nurses often prepares them broadly for practice, with acknowledgment that specific practice will vary according to patients and settings and as new knowledge becomes available. Hospital nurses in some settings have developed a multiplicity of specialist roles. These have included nurses with expertise in ostomy nursing, working with families, crisis counseling, pain management, discharge planning, teaching for self-care, health promotion activities such as exercise and control of diet, prevention of substance abuse, and similar areas requiring high levels of clinical knowledge and judgment. Such nurses, in addition to providing direct care themselves, serve as consultants and advisors to other nurses in developing their skills in similar areas.

Another kind of specialist role that has emerged in the hospital in recent years is the nurse practitioner.[29] In the development of this role, there has been significant overlap with physicians, both housestaff and attending. With the addition of nurse practitioners to inpatient settings, particularly those hospitals or services without residency programs, nurse practitioners are carrying out admission histories and physical examinations and providing for the medical supervision of patients between the attending physician's visits.*

It would be possible to develop a role in the hospital that combines these traditional medical functions of histories, physicals, and patient monitoring with some of the more traditional nursing functions valued by nurses. These latter include such activities mentioned above as teaching about the illness, explanations regarding the diagnostic and treatment procedures being carried out, and discharge planning. The combination of nursing and routine physician activities into a single role could both make a major contribution to the safe care of patients in hospitals and provide a more challenging role for nurses.

Consistent with the need to develop specialized roles in that of develop-

---

* A number of hospitals are beginning to employ salaried physicians to do some of this routine medical care, monitoring and responding to emergencies in the absence of the attending physician. With the oversupply of physicians projected in the Graduate Medical Education National Advisory Committee (GMENAC) report, there may be more interest and availability of physicians for employment in such positions, very likely accompanied by expectations for salaries substantially greater than those received by housestaff, nurse practitioners, and physician's assistants, all of whom perform essentially the same functions in this role.[30]

ing career ladders, another mechanism recently introduced that acknowl-
edges clearly that nurses have different levels of clinical expertise, and
rewards this knowledge and ability by promoting people in a clinical rather
than administrative sense.

In developing strong visible programs emphasizing and using nurses' expertise, it will be important that such specialties be integrated into the system and used to help in the development of other nurses—and not seen as
stripping the role of its most interesting aspects, leaving the remainder of the
work to be done by the rest of the nurses. Development of specialized knowledge in the professional nursing staff must be done in a systematic way considering the complementary roles of other nurses, physicians, and others in
the system.

One factor that has contributed significantly to the worsening employment conditions in hospitals has been the gradual separation between nurses
who educate students and those who practice nursing. A large number of
nurses have been prepared in recent years at advanced levels of clinical practice, administration, and research. A large proportion of these, however, have
remained in academic institutions rather than put their increased knowledge
and skills into use in practice settings. As Christman has observed, "Nursing
is the only profession which by willful intent and deliberate design withholds
its best practitioners from the public it is supposed to serve—and that's the
way I see nurse faculty: completely detached from the delivery of care."[31]

The split between academic and practicing nurses is relatively recent.
Before World War II, faculty who taught nursing students also were actively
involved in giving patient care or administering nursing services. The effort
over the last 3 decades to move education of nurses out of hospitals and into
educational settings has been successful in producing graduates with improved educational backgrounds. It has had the negative consequence, however, of separating academic from practicing nurses.

During the period of emerging education–service separation, problems
of nursing care delivery have grown increasingly complex, as have problems
in health care delivery generally. It is unfortunate that the knowledge and
ability of nurses with advanced preparation in clinical practice, administration, biologic and behavioral sciences, and research methods have been essentially unavailable to those in clinical settings trying to deal with increasingly difficult nursing practice and delivery problems.

The movement of the best prepared nurses into academic rather than
practice settings is understandable not only because of the need to educate
students but also because of the conditions commonly existing in hospitals.
As noted above, the clinically well-prepared nurse has been strongly resisted
in practice settings, resulting in discouragement of knowledgeable nurses to
practice there. Most go instead to schools of nursing or to ambulatory prac-

tice settings. The movement of nurses with advanced preparation back into the hospital through the widespread development of joint appointments of nurses to both faculty and hospitals' staffs would greatly strengthen the capability of the department of nursing to ensure a well-prepared staff.

A part of the redefinition of the nature of the work performed by nurses and others in hospitals is to reassign activities so as to minimize the amount of time that skilled professionals spend performing low-skill tasks. Goldstein and Horowitz's data showing that more than 75% of the registered nurses in the Boston hospitals spend about 28% of their time on functions requiring no formal preparation and often very little practical experience suggest that high priority ought to be placed on eliminating a large percentage of that kind of activity from the nurse's role. Similarly, much of the coordination of other peoples' work does not require professional clinical training and could be performed by lesser trained personnel. Some hospitals have redesigned the nurse's role to enable the major focus to be on providing nursing care and coordinating the care-related activities. At Rush University is a prime example of this kind of role redesign. Here a unit manager performs many of the coordinating functions traditionally assigned to the head nurse role, while the "practitioner teacher" assumes responsibility for the clinical supervision of the nursing care of patients.[32]

Emphasizing the clinical knowledge required, further developing roles to enable nurses to use this knowledge effectively and promoting closer collaboration and cooperation between academic and practicing nurses would contribute substantially to restructuring the work of hospital nurses. Such restructuring could simultaneously make more effective and efficient use of a large work force in hospitals toward the end of improved patient care, and could make hospital nursing a more attractive career.

RESTRUCTURING THE WORKING CONDITIONS

Much has been written of nurses' dissatisfaction with the staffing patterns that have characterized hospital nursing. Until very recently it was the widespread expectation in many hospitals that a high percentage of nurses would rotate shifts, sometimes working days, nights, and evenings all within the space of a few weeks. Often only a nominal differentiation is paid for working evenings and nights and after 5 yr the pay scale for nurses on any shift remains essentially flat. Collectively bargained contracts have made some changes in these conditions and nurse administrators have made changes in other situations. It was the advent of temporary service agencies, however, that forced relaxation of the rigid conditions, and nurse administrators generally have moved to develop more flexible staffing patterns. These changes have been discussed in other chapters of this volume and will not be elaborated upon here, except to note that restructuring of the conditions under which nurses work as well as the components of the work itself is necessary.

Again, restructuring the nurse's role means restructuring the roles of other workers in the hospital as well if activities requiring more clinical skill are to be emphasized. Eliminating from the nurse's role those functions commonly assumed by nurses on evenings, nights, weekends, and holidays for other workers will require additional changes. If, for example, the nurse is no longer to be used as a substitute pharmacist or radiology or laboratory technician on the off-hours, those departments will need to provide necessary coverage on the unpopular days and hours. Reassignment of these activities should provide more time for nurses to provide skilled clinical nursing.

In a similar vein, how nurses spend their time on various shifts and days should be carefully analyzed as a basis for a realistic staffing plan. While it is necessary to have 24-hr, 7-days-a-week professional nurse coverage of nursing units, the accompanying need is to ensure that nurses are doing higher level nursing, rather than aide work.

Although team nursing is largely out of favor and being replaced by primary nursing, two points should be considered. One is that having a nurse with 3 or more years of education performing activities not requiring such education is unnecessarily costly, unless doing them is combined with some function requiring higher level of skill such as teaching the patient about his illness and care. One of the reasons why primary nursing has been shown not to cost significantly more than traditional nursing care, which is shared by registered nurses, licensed practical nurses, and nurses' aides, is the relatively small discrepancy among what the three positions are paid. If the restructuring of the work itself were combined with a higher economic value placed on the higher level professional skills of the nurse, team nursing in some settings would be both more effective and less costly. Second, while some nurses apparently enjoy doing total patient care, others do not and resent having to spend substantial amounts of time on lower level tasks.

It may well be that primary nursing is both useful and cost-effective in intensive care situations but not so on some general patient units. On the latter, it may be more appropriate to have some form of team nursing in which the professional nurse in fact is responsible for the coordination of the clinical care, carrying out that part of it that requires higher level skill. Combining the division of labor associated with team nursing and the accountability for patient care associated with primary nursing would take advantage of the strengths of both nursing care delivery models.

Finally, attention should be given to two other conditions associated with hospital nurses' work: the reduction of high levels of stress on the one hand and the boredom associated with many routine and repetitive activities on the other. High-stress conditions generally seem associated with the need to make multiple decisions quickly and repeatedly, such as working in intensive care units or managing a busy patient care unit of any kind. Identifying ways to interrupt the long periods of time spent in intensive care units could reduce the stress to more manageable limits. Rotating nurses across units within the same specialty area is a mechanism used in some hospitals, for example. Nurses who do not tolerate the high stress of a coronary care unit for long periods can spend several weeks on a step-down unit or in a cardiac rehabilitation program, where the stress is generally lower. Periodically changing the set of activities performed can also address the problem of boredom experienced by some nurses. Additionally, giving nurses the opportunity to develop specific areas in intensity and depth would help to alleviate boredom.

Changing the working conditions of nurses, including both when they work and how the work is structured is an important element in the role restructuring needed.

PLACEMENT OF THE NURSE IN THE ORGANIZATION

The final consideration of role restructuring in hospital nursing is the placement of the nurse in the decision-making structure of the hospital. The Hughes' quotation presented at the beginning of this chapter identified the physician as the dominant person in the hospital, and the physician has continued to maintain this dominancy. In recent years, however, the physician's position and authority have been challenged by increasing governmental and voluntary regulation of hospital practice and by increasing strength of hospital administrators. These two groups, physicians and hospital administrators, form an uneasy alliance in the operation of today's hospitals. They are generally in agreement over their opposition to the increasing regulation of the hospital from without, but internally, hospitals are characterized by major authority conflicts between administrators and physicians. Within the hospital, physicians continue to exercise major authority and to resist attempts of others, including hospital administrators, to influence physician practice. Hospital administrators, on the other hand, seek alliance with physicians sympathetic to the need to make organizational decisions on the basis of what is best for the total institution.

In this internal authority conflict between administrators and physicians, nurses are caught between the two groups and expected to be loyal to and protect the interests of both. The director of nursing and the nursing department often function as extensions of both administration and physicians to keep the hospital functioning and the system of care operating.

Nurses have very little formal authority base of their own, however, and are included in the formal decision-making structure of the hospital in very superficial ways. Frequently, the nurse administrator does not occupy the same place in the hospital's power structure as other top level administrators. While some hospitals include the chief administrative nurse as a member of the top administration, others continue to have the director of nursing report to an assistant administrator. To add to the problem, the assistant administrator to whom the director reports frequently has less health experience and sometimes less formal preparation in health administration than the nursing director.

In some instances, chief nurses and their assistants are little more than extensions of hospital administration, acting to carry out the orders of the latter, with little independent authority afforded to the position itself. Many assist in developing and implementing rigid standardization of the nursing staff, with little regard for independent decision making by nurses — or their inclusion in the overall decision-making structure of the hospital.

It is commonplace for hospital committees to omit nurses as members or to appoint a token nurse to comply with regulations. A review of the composition of the administrative and committee structure of most hospitals will indicate that nurses generally are not included significantly in the planning and operational structures that make the major decisions regarding the hospital and its programs.

The total committee structure in hospitals should be analyzed with a view toward incorporating nurses, both administrative and clinical, into whatever committee is concerned with planning, implementing, or evaluating the hospital's programs. This includes long-range planning groups, budget committees, patient care committees, hospital-wide quality assurance committees, and research and evaluation committees. Attempts by hospital nurses to implement programs of nursing research and evaluation have often met with resistance from others in the same way as their attempts to develop programs of care have. Nurses' integration into the full committee structure of the hospital should reflect their ability to contribute significantly to the operation of the hospital. It should simultaneously serve to legitimate such activities as nurses engaging in clinical research and evaluation to improve their practice and to ensure the quality of nursing programs.

The discussion of nurses' authority to this point has focused primarily on authority in decisions affecting the total organization. Equally if not more frustrating to nurses is their inability to exercise much control over how they practice their own profession. The term "autonomy" began appearing in the nursing literature only a decade ago, but discussion of the need for nurses to achieve it is now a dominant theme in the literature and at professional meetings. Studies of nurse dissatisfaction uniformly find lack of autonomy or inability to control how nursing is practiced at or near the top of unsatisfying conditions. The strong move to develop nursing bylaws, often patterned after medical bylaws, is another indication of nurses' rejection of their power-lessness in hospitals.

CONCLUSION

Nurses, in particular, hospital nurses, have increasingly rejected the interpretation of their role in the past few years, and there is little to indicate that they will change unless conditions in hospitals change substantially. Attempts at cosmetic surgery or quick and easy solutions to the problems identified in the beginning of this chapter will not be enough to turn the present situation around.

Continued devaluation of the intellectual component of the nurses' work, accompanied by pressure to lower or eliminate education standards, may result in more licensed bodies on hospital units, but in the long run poorer education of nurses will be detrimental to patient care. Use of temporary service agencies, internal float pools, flextime, and other staffing arrangements should offer temporary alleviation, but serious and massive effort is required to make the hospital a place where nurses are willing and able to do what they are prepared and want to do — provide good nursing care. Nurses at every level — from staff nurse to top administrative nurse — are asking to have the value of their work acknowledged. Yesterday's nurse who accepted long, difficult, and inconvenient working hours, disrespect from those with whom she worked, and low salaries while at the same time remaining loyal to the physician and the hospital is rapidly fading from the scene.

Increasing options for women has taken its toll on nursing as one of the few occupations traditionally open to women. Additionally, increasing options in community health and in private practice, where nurses have better salaries and more control over how they practice, are pulling nurses away from hospitals where conditions are so much less favorable and satisfying.

It has taken many years to arrive at the present critical problems of nurses in hospitals. Numerous factors have contributed to this, including the devalued position of women in society, the disproportionate authority and dominance of physicians, and highly stressful working conditions in hospitals. The judge who heard the Denver case noted that he accepted the fact that nurses have been discriminated against, but ruled against them because he felt it could lead to a disruption of the American economy. If the role of the hospital nurse is acknowledged to be a frustrating and dissatisfying one in which nurses' knowledge and ability are undervalued socially and economically but the organization refuses to undergo major change, the future of hospital nursing is likely to be fraught with increasing conflict and turmoil on the part of everyone involved. If there is public acknowledgment of the need for safe and effective patient care in hospitals and a serious intent on the part of federal and state legislators to provide for that care at a lower cost, major restructuring in hospitals is required.

REFERENCES

1 American Nurses' Association, *Nursing: A Social Policy Statement*, Kansas City, Mo.: ANA, 1980, 9.

2 Hughes, Everett C., *Men and Their Work*, Glencoe, Ill.: The Free Press, 1958, 74.

3 *Ibid.*, 76.

4 Freidson, Eliot. *The Profession of Medicine, A Study of the Sociology of Applied Knowledge*, New York: Dodd, Mead & Co., 1971, 79.

5 Kramer, Marlene, *Reality Shock: Why Nurses Leave Nursing*, St. Louis: C. V. Mosby, 1974.

6 Goldstein, Harold, and Horowitz, Morris A., *Utilization of Health Personnel: A Five Hospital Study*, Germantown, MD.: Aspen Systems Corp., 1978, 80.

7 *Ibid.*, 50.

8 Aiken, Linda H., and Blendon, Robert J., The National Nurse Shortage, *National Journal*, (May 23, 1981) 952.

9 *National Commission on Nursing, Summary of the Public Hearings*, Chicago: American Hospital Association, July 1981, 28.

10 Hughes, *Op. Cit.* 97.

11 Ashley, Joann, *Hospitals, Paternalism and the Role of the Nurse*, New York: Teachers' College, Columbia University Press, 1976, 21.

12 Olson, J. W., "How the Small Hospital May Be Made Self Supporting," Transactions of the American Hospital Association 1913, 434, as quoted in Ashley, *Ibid.*

13 Schweitzer, Stuart O., and Record, Jane C., "Third Party Reimbursement for New Health Professionals in Primary Care, An Alternative to Fractional Reimbursement," Paper presented to a conference sponsored by The National World Center on "Nurse Practitioners/Physician Assistants, A Research Agenda," Airlie, Virginia, June 21-22, 1977, as quoted in Robyn, Dorothy, and Hadley, Jack, National Health Insurance and The New Health Occupations, Nurse Practitioners and Physicians' Assistants, *Journal of Health Politics, Policy and Law*, 5: 4 (Fall, 1980), 457.

14 Robyn and Hadley, *Op. Cit.* 459.

15 Aiken and Blendon, *Op. Cit.* 950.

16 Barnes, Craig S., Denver: *A Case Study*, Unpublished paper, Denver, Colorado, 1978.

17 Lemons vs. City and County of Denver, Civil Action No. 76-1156, Denver Colorado, 1977.

18 Simpson, Richard, and Simpson, Ida Harper, Women and Bureaucracies, in The Semi-Professions, *The Semi-Professions and Their Organization*. Amitai Etzioni (Editor), New York: The Free Press, 1969.

19 Prescott, Patricia A., and Driscoll, Laura, Nurse Practitioner Effectiveness; A Review of Physician — Nurse Comparison Studies, *Evaluation in the Health Professions*, 2:4 (Dec. 1979) 414.

20 Freidson, *Op. Cit.* 67.

21 Szasz, Thomas, *The Myth of Mental Illness*, New York: Hoeber-Harper, 1961.

22 Freidson, *Op. Cit.* 337.

23 Havighurst, Clark, The Role of Competition in Cost Containment, *Competition in the Health Care Sector: Past, Present and Future*, Warren Greenberg (Editor), Germantown, Md., Aspen System Corp., 1978, 299–300.

24 Beates, Henry, *The Status of Nurses: A Sociologic Problem*, Philadelphia: Physicians' National Board of Regents, 1909, 6., as quoted in Ashley, *Op. Cit.*, 80.

25 *Ibid.*, 80.

26 Essentials of a Nursing Education, *National Hospital Record*, II (January 1908), 2-3, as quoted in Ashley, *Op. Cit.*, 23–24.

27 Stein, Leonard I., The Doctor-Nurse Game, *The Archives of General Psychiatry*, XVI, (June 1967), 669–670.

28 Bellitz, Elaine. Oral and written testimony presented at open meeting, Committee of the Institute of Medicine for a Study of Nursing and Nursing Education. May 18, 1981, Washington, D.C.

29 Ford, Loretta C., A Nurse for All Settings. The Nurse Practitioner, *Nursing Outlook*, 27 (August, 1979), 516–521.

30 Graduate Medical Education National Advisory Committee (GMENAC): Report to the Secretary, Department of Health and Human Services (Pub No (HRA) 81-656). Washington, D.C., U.S. Government Printing Office, 1980.

31 Christman, Luther, Luther Christman Anthology, *Nursing Digest*, Summer 1978, 8–9.

32 *Ibid.*

JOYCE C. CLIFFORD

6

PROFESSIONAL NURSING PRACTICE IN A HOSPITAL SETTING

Several years ago, a small group of registered nurses from all levels of the nursing organization at Beth Israel Hospital joined me to improve the quality of nursing care provided to patients through the development of a professional department of nursing services. That was our first stated objective and has remained an overall umbrella objective for all other activities we have pursued. Experiences with primary nursing or a professional practice model were not common at that time, and to some extent we felt the need to pioneer for ourselves what "improved nursing care" could be in our hospital.

The quest for professional status by nurses at Beth Israel Hospital was no different than it has been for other nurses throughout the history of nursing. In recent times nurses have become far more aggressive in their demand for their rightful recognition within the health care delivery system, and they are more willing today to speak out against perceived injustices. Yet full recognition as professionals remains a unfulfilled goal for a majority of nurses, and traditional, sometimes archaic nursing services continue to exist.

Professionalism is described by Pointer as follows:

> The essence of professionalism is control over both the performance of professional tasks and the immediate environment in which tasks are performed.[1]

This statement is consistent with the search in nursing for greater autonomy or self-direciton in our activities as well as for increased participation in decision making in those activities that are relevant to us as professionals. It also points out that the environment in which one practices is as important as the practice itself. This fact is often overlooked by nurses as they attempt to improve the practice of nursing in a health care agency. Traditional delivery systems of nursing and the hierarchical structures supporting these systems have not facilitated achievement of the goals of nursing professionals. Ignoring that these factors are a prime concern for the professional nurse is the downfall of many institutions and departments of nursing. On the other hand, understanding the concepts of autonomy, authority, and accountability as applied to the professional within a bureaucratic organization is perhaps the most relevant knowledge base today's nurse administrator can possess.

The need to integrate professional requirements for practice with organizational requirements was identified early in our pursuit of change at Beth Israel. A few basic statements were initially formulated as guides for our activities. These have remained as part of our statement of philosophy as a nursing service.

> We believe that patients have a right to expect that their care will be personalized and will be planned for and evaluated by a professional registered nurse. Patients have a right to the best care available and care which promotes continuity and incorporates them and their family in decision making.
>
> We believe that nurses have a right to provide care in a manner that maximizes their knowledge and skill and optimizes their own professional practice. These rights include the right to enter into the decision-making process for patient care and services and the right to assume accountability for their own practice.
>
> We believe the hospital, as a health care facility dedicated to the provision of quality care to the community, has a right to expect that care will be provided in an efficient, comprehensive, and cost-effective manner.[2]

With full recognition that the needs of patients, nurses, and the hospital must be mutually satisfied, the development of a professional department of nursing was considered a realistic goal, and in 1974 a change began in the conventional practice system in existence.

LEADERSHIP: AN ESSENTIAL INGREDIENT

One of the most crucial elements affecting the quality of patient care in any health care setting is the nursing leadership. Through nursing leadership, directions for patient care decisions are set and the climate within which nurses practice is established. The quality of nursing leadership cannot be underestimated or overstated as a major factor in the development of a professional department of nursing. Such leadership needs to reach beyond a narrow focus of a few individual positions and encompass an integrated view as a total professional group. Leadership must be accepted as a function of *all* professional roles in nursing and must be perceived as essential for values clarification, standard setting, and program development. The attitude that nurses and nursing are powerless in a hospital organization needs to be changed! Thus, one of the first performance expectations established for all registered nurses at the Beth Israel Hospital is leadership. Since it is our intent that nursing assume a significant leadership role within the hospital, each nurse must view herself as a vital leader in the achievement of overall departmental and nursing practice goals. In an attempt to reinforce this belief, we have carefully avoided job titles such as "clinical leader" or "nurse leader" since we assume this to be a role function for all registered nurses. The title "head nurse" continues to be used by us to describe the unit-based managerial role expected to provide major leadership functions for the staff, the hospital, and the nursing department. A definition of leadership used within our nursing department as a guideline for managers is the following:

> True leadership is not domination: it is a process of mutal stimulation in which the leader not only influences the group, but is, in turn, influenced by it and is thus able to assemble the various wills into one, unified, driving force.[3]

DECENTRALIZATION

Significant change has occurred in our nursing service since 1974. For one thing, we have changed from a traditionally organized, highly centralized nursing department to a very decentralized nursing organization. While organizational structure has been flattened, decentralization in our system is viewed in the context of decision making. When decentralization is not implemented from this frame of reference, it often leads to fragmented departments, areas, or staff members—none of which promotes the components necessary for a full professional department of nursing. Thus, at Beth Israel nursing is viewed as a total professional department rather than the sum of many fragmented parts.

One simple but tangible example of this is our hospital policy, which is circulated each year when new physicians arrive on staff. It indicates that *any* nurse hired to function in a position using her nursing capabilities, regardless of whether that position is budgeted in the nursing division, is accountable for nursing practice to the vice president for nursing or her delegate. The hiring process, salary quoted, and subsequent performance review is through the nursing department. As a result of this policy, nurses throughout the hospital have reestablished their identity with nursing. The fact that their salary comes from a non-nursing cost center is considered more of an accounting convenience than an accountability process.

Decentralized decision making has required a number of changes in our organizational structure. The long, hierarchical structure of the past has been replaced by a flattened organizational structure rather than multiple supervisory layers. Within the hierarchy, there is now a four-tier organizational design from staff nurse to vice president for nursing. This structure has been developed to facilitate decentralized decision making. It is our belief that administrative roles exist to support other professional roles — not to supervise other professionals.

These changes in the organizational structure occurred following the articulation of professional practice expectations and the role clarification of the head nurse and the primary nurse. In other words, professional role development dictated the organizational structure, not the other way around.

Clarification of decision-making authority for each layer in the line organization consumed extensive time and continues to be a significant factor in our ongoing development of professional roles. Distinct areas of responsibility have been identified, promoting more effective communication, efficiency in decision making, and tighter accountability systems. Other roles, not in the line organization, include program directors for each of the areas of education, research, and quality assurance and other educational and clinical consultants to the staff. Concentrating on the direct care provider, that is, the staff nurse, as the professional who is ultimately accountable for the care delivered helps formulate the basis of role clarification and decision-making authority among clinical experts. This area of role clarification is the most troublesome to apply consistently, yet is perhaps the most critical element ensuring appropriate decision making and accountability by those providing direct care.

The status of nursing within an organization relates ultimately to the position and status of the chief executive officer in the nursing department. It is essential that this nurse administrator be a member of the executive management team of the hospital and, in the case of a teaching hospital such as the Beth Israel, be accorded organizational status commensurate to the chiefs of other professional services. The hospital organizational chart of Beth Israel (Fig. 6-1) depicts this dual relationship of the vice president for nursing. The position is parallel with the medical chiefs and, like them, responsible in a colleague relationship to the executive vice president and director of the hospital for the overall operational activities of the department of nursing. Control of nursing practice for the institution is the domain of the vice president for nursing. Through this organizational design, nursing maintains professional accountability for nursing and is able to influence future policy direction of the institution. Such influence requires that the chief nurse administrator spend much of her time in planning and policy activities with other members of administration, the medical staff, the board of directors, and the community. Such activity leaves little time for direct observation and intervention in

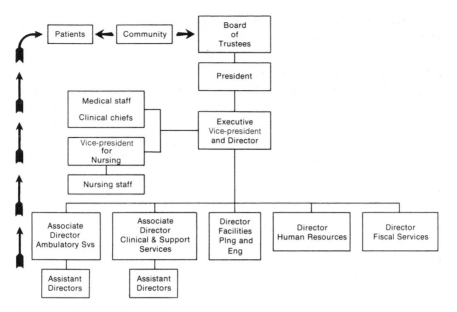

FIGURE 6-1. Beth Israel Hospital, Boston, Administrative Organization.

the daily operations of the nursing department, a fact that leaves many nurse administrators in a dilemma.

A critical element in organizational reorganization is the development of systems of accountability that allow the chief nurse administrator a mechanism for remaining fully aware of those aspects of the organization relevant to her area of decision making. Not all activities are relevant—some certainly not as relevant as some others. Just as the decision-making authority of the primary care provider must be made explicit, the role of the chief nurse administrator within the organization must also be clarified explicitly. The nurse administrator who involves herself with daily operational activities best accomplished elsewhere in the organization will deter the total professional group from its pursuit of professional activities and objectives. A hard lesson to learn, but nevertheless an important one, is that role development must occur at the top of the organizational hierarchy as well as at every other level.

THE PRACTICE SYSTEM

Three basic characteristics of a professional system were identified as essential components for our nursing department. They are as follows:

- *Continuity of care* planning with interdisciplinary and intradisciplinary communication from care-giver to care-giver.

- A sense of *accountability* for nursing practice, with practice defined by the individual practitioner rather than directed by routinized tasks and tight supervisory controls.
- *Decentralization* of the organizational structure with authority and accountability for decision-making functions invested in those closest to the point of delivery of services.

As part of the change toward decentralization, the traditional team-functional method of care delivery was replaced by a system that now provides continuity for patient care and accountability of the practitioner for that care. These two concepts are considered essential in order to maximize the professional role of nursing. This system, identified by Manthey as primary nursing, could just as easily be called professional nursing practice.[4] Primary nursing is, however, a term the public as well as the profession has been able to identify with easily. In our situation, it served the purpose of helping to change the image of nursing generally held by our patients. Primary nursing is now identified by our patients as a quality of nursing practice that is superior to that experienced previously. It has been a vehicle through which the lay public and our medical colleagues have been able to learn and understand more about professional nursing.

The traditional delivery system employed at the Beth Israel had the usual pitfalls in terms of both patient outcomes and nurse satisfaction. Responsibility for care planning was widely distributed and lacked any identifiable nurse professional as being accountable for that care. Such a system alluded to the head nurse as the accountable professional for all patient care, but it also usually acknowledged, in one way or another, the inability of a single person, no matter how competent, to assume full accountability for the outcomes of so many individual patient care plans.

Such a system in place at the Beth Israel in 1974 brought strong reaction from both the provider of that care, the nurse, and the consumer, the patient and family. Both groups expressed great dissatisfaction with nursing services that were depersonalized, fragmented, and lacking continuity in either planning or delivery. It was the expression of this dissatisfaction that led us to look for alternatives in the organization of our nursing department. It became evident that we needed to examine closely the environment within which we were asking bright men and women to practice nursing. Nurses expressed the need to have more fulfilling work responsibilities and sought participation in decision-making activities. The challenge was to develop opportunities for nurses to think and act independently within the boundaries of appropriate standards of practice.

Primary nursing is the delivery system now used throughout the nursing department at Beth Israel to facilitate the practice of professional nursing.

The role of the primary nurse, which is analogous to that of the primary physician, requires the ability to form therapeutic relationships with individual persons, to make decisions, and to assume accountability for these decisions. Inherent to the practice of professional nursing is the use of the nursing process, which focuses on the patient and his family and is initiated through a comprehensive assessment that results in the identification of needs. These patient needs are analyzed and arranged according to logical priorities and in terms of nursing goals, representative of the patient's aspirations. The primary nurse must be able to conduct interviews, obtain and assess pertinent data, as well as communicate effectively with peers and other members of the health team. Collaborative relationships become critical in order to fulfill the responsibilities inherent in the professional role.

The primary nurse directs nursing care 24 hr a day through the use of the written nursing care plan and other forms of communication. The nurse is held accountable for planning comprehensive patient care and formulating clear-cut nursing directions for other nurses to continue in her absence. Coordination of activity with the patient, physicians, and other personnel is within the realm of the primary nurse's responsibility, and the individual competency level of each nurse is manifested in respect to performance as a nurse rather than as a manager of people. Professional nursing allows for comprehensive, coordinated patient-centered care. It encourages the nurse to use all intellectual and creative resources and skills to formulate and implement the most appropriate and personalized nursing care plan for a particular patient. When care plans are formulated from the individual patient's needs, professional information can be shared with other members of the health team, and the nurse is in a position to better articulate her own practice. The primary relationship between the nurse and patient inevitably increases the amount of information nurses have about patients. This not only improves communication because there is more relevant patient information to share, but it also supports the nurse's position of leadership and responsibility for patient care.

Before the implementation of primary nursing at our hospital, nursing as a professional group received little respect and recognition. Nursing responded in fragmented ways to needs, issues, concerns, or problems. There was little real control or influence over our own nursing practice. At best, negative communication existed between nursing and other health disciplines such as medicine and social service.

The response of these professional groups to nursing was clearly understandable. Nurses had little to offer that enhanced patient care planning and evaluation and indeed had little time to become involved in such activities. Our concerns had to be related to efficiency of time, for certainly the task-oriented practice system then in existence provided little opportunity for accomplishing more than the basic essentials. When the system did provide opportunities, they were looked upon as luxuries for the day rather than considered appropriate expectations for both patient and practitioner. Today nursing at Beth Israel is considered an important component of *all* planning activities, whether they are activities that involve a single patient and family or activities of an institution planning future patient care facilities and programs. Such involvement is at all levels of the organization and in all issues relevant to us as professionals.

Participatory activities are valued in our setting as a way of ensuring the full development of a professional nursing department. Senior staff members are selected for activities and are encouraged to participate in broader nursing service responsibilities. Committee activities form the basis for most of these activities and have become a popular form of involvement. Our committee structure is established primarily to use the talent and resources of the nursing staff in determining standards of care, policy, and procedures for clinical practice and evaluation, to ensure compliance with overall standards. Staff form the major membership on committees and have proved to be committed to the committee objectives and issues to be resolved. Expectations for committee membership have been developed and the chairperson evaluates each staff person's performance as a committee member. These committee members are vocal, influential nurses who earn respect from their peers as well as their managers for the level of commitment they exhibit in their participation.

As these activities have become incorporated within our routine at Beth Israel, an increase in professional colleagueship is demonstrated. Consultation among staff increases the respect staff provide to each other as peers and to colleagues in other disciplines. Staff now seek consultation and validation of decisions rather than mere assistance in accomplishing a task. Collaboration with each other is a basic expectation of professional practice and is demonstrated in this practice setting. Nurses call upon each other as consultants, and an active sharing of information as peers is promoted and recognized as appropriate professional behavior.

THE NURSING PRACTITIONER

Soon after implementing primary nursing, we recognized the increased learning needs of our staff as they carried out the role responsibilities of a professional direct care provider. Initially, four areas were identified as essential practice requirements as follows:

- *Clinical competency.* Competency beyond the basic knowledge of nursing process, patient teaching, and psychological factors is considered necessary for effective clinical practice in a primary nursing system.

- *Decision-making ability.* The professional nurse is required to gather data about individual patient problems, draw conclusions from these data, and use these conclusions as a basis for nursing actions.

- *Management skills.* The ability to plan, organize, establish priorities, and evaluate one's performance is a critical element for practice. Reliance on routine schedules or tasks to be accomplished at precise times is no longer a part of the system, and individual practitioners are now accountable for determining their own priorities of time and activities.

- *Accountability.* A willingness to assume responsibility for one's own actions and the outcomes of one's own decisions in a reasonable fashion becomes an essential practice requirement in a professional environment.

As primary nursing developed, it became clear that these practice expectations were essential and required further expansion by our nursing practitioner. As a consequence, expectations became explicitly identified through a performance evaluation tool that uses the nursing process as an overall framework for practice.

It also became evident that the graduate of the baccalaureate program seemed best suited in our setting to meet these requirements. As with other aspects of our practice system, the change to a predominately baccalaureate-prepared staff has been evolutionary in nature. For a number of years, we have employed new graduates with baccalaureate degrees while we continue to seek demonstrated performance as the highest priority in the selection of experienced nurses (Table 6-1). Over time, many of our experienced nurses not prepared at the baccalaureate level of nursing have chosen to return to school, either full time or part time, a decision we support philosophically and whenever possible through mechanisms such as tuition reimbursement and scheduling flexibility.

Slightly more than 80% of our total registered nurse staff are prepared minimally at the baccalaureate level (Table 6-2). A number of our staff nurses hold a master's degree in nursing, and now more than 50% of our head nurses do so. All of our clinical specialists and educational resource roles are prepared at the graduate level.

TABLE 6-1 Educational Preparation of All Registered Nurse New Hires

	1974	1975	1976	1980
Diploma	26%	11%	0	5.8%
AD	23%	13%	4.3%	2.0%
BSN	50%	76%	95.7%	92.2%

TABLE 6-2 Educational Preparation of Total Registered Nurse Staff

	1975	1977	1981
Diploma	45%	32%	16%
AD	12%	6%	3%
BSN	39%	55%	73%
Master's	4%	7%	8%

Our experience at Beth Israel led us to conclude that today's nursing practitioner is generally self-reliant, self-confident, and self-directed. We have obviously found the graduates of baccalaureate programs to be successful in their practice in our setting. These nurses come to us with a good sense of professionalism. They consider themselves professionals, and they expect to be recognized as professionals. They expect to be considered equal members of the health care team and desire collaborative relationships with others. At the same time, we value these behaviors and consider them essential in order to effect meaningful change and to meet the holistic needs of patients in an acute care setting such as the Beth Israel Hospital. There are numerous examples of increasing technologic demands coupled with a need for nurses to bridge the gap and ensure personalization of care, all requiring well-prepared nursing practitioners. Consider, for example, the increase in the elderly patient population who often have limited family and financial resources, or the increase in the promotion of life-sustaining supports. These societal concerns translate further into issues of informed consent and skilled monitoring of patient repsonses, each with its accompanying ethical considerations. Additionally, the complexity of problems presented by patients and the challenge of attaining and maintaining wellness requires the collaboration of an interdisciplinary team.

Many of the interactions nurses experience at the Beth Israel are, we believe, a result of the educational preparation of our practitioners. Collaboration, confrontation, and, of course, accountability are terms and behaviors specific to a professional role, and are increasingly more important to nurses who view themselves as professionals with equal rights to participate in decision-making processes. Collegial relationships with peers as well as with other professionals must be fostered and developed as an expectation of practice, not as an accident of that practice. In our view, the nature of the expectations for interdisciplinary and intradisciplinary collaboration, the questions raised around patient care intervention, the judgments to be made, and the decisions to be reached all require nurses who have as their minimal level of preparation a baccalaureate degree in nursing.

Other aspects of professional role development appear to occur more effectively in our system with staff prepared at the baccalaureate level. Interest in educational and research activities directed towards improved nursing care is evident throughout the nursing department. Nurses are highly motivated and often extend themselves beyond the normal working hours to participate in nursing grand rounds, research seminars, or a patient care conference planned by a colleague. A willingness to share their nursing experiences with others extends beyond a small circle of professionals as more and more staff nurses are publishing articles or accepting invitations to speak at programs outside the hospital.

THE HEAD NURSE ROLE

As previously noted, the quality of leadership within an organization cannot be emphasized enough. It is our belief that the single most critical factor in determining success or failure relates to the quality of management and leadership at the unit level. At Beth Israel we believe the head nurse position is one of the most important management positions *within the hospital*, not only within the nursing department. Through this role, the philosophy, standards, and policies of the total organization are translated into action. It is the head nurse who actually controls the implementation of change. Thus, it was the head nurse role that became the initial focus of our change process at the Beth Israel, and it is the role that continues to be identified as most crucial in the development of professional practice at the unit level.

One of the first changes we were able to effect was to identify, by hospital policy, the head nurse as the full manager of the patient care unit. All areas of activity are included and are described in the head nurse position description as *patient care management*, *personnel management*, and *unit management*. It must be understood that patient care management relates to the overall standards of care for the unit's patient population, and the general evaluation of care provided. In no way does this component of the head nurse role interfere with the individual decision-making rights of the primary nurse.

For head nurses, this represented a significant change, because they assumed 24-hr accountability for the unit and were supported in their right to exercise authority over a variety of activities formerly considered only marginally within their area of responsibility. One of the major changes was the right to select and "de-select" their own staff. This is not after consultation with a person in higher authority but is in actual practice the head nurse's total responsibility. Once this practice is implemented, a different level of commitment to the staff member appears to be demonstrated by the head nurse. Head nurses now have a personal, vested interest in the development of their staff. The failure of staff to succeed is considered by many head nurses to be a reflection of their own ability to select and then develop appropriate candidates. No longer can head nurses excuse themselves with "What do you expect me to accomplish with the staff *you* send me?"

Interviewing by the head nurse is also an excellent recruitment tool. Potential staff are able to identify more readily with the practice area and with the person who will provide them daily direction, coaching, and, for new graduates in particular, the development of their practice skills. The candidate meets with the staff with whom they will work and has an on-site view of the work area, which is different from merely a quick tour of the unit. Through this process, the commitment made by the head nurse becomes shared by the staff member after employment. As well as with other factors, retention of staff becomes associated with the relationship established by the staff with the head nurse.

While the change in the head nurse role is very significant to nursing, decentralized decision making and increased authority in all professional nursing roles has considerable impact on the institution as a whole. The traditional role of the head nurse as the central focus of all communication on a patient care unit is eliminated in a primary nursing setting. All professional nurses are accorded status as the primary care providers and assumes responsibility for their own direct communication with other health-providers. In order for change of this magnitude to succeed, the total institution must be educated to the role of nursing in patient care. The executive nurse administrator must assume responsibility for this institutional educational process. Administrators, physicians, and members of other health disciplines and other departments must be reoriented as to how communication and problem solving takes place in a professional practice setting. Nurse administrative roles such as the vicepresident for nursing or the directors of nursing in our organization must be consistent in their responses and their redirection of others to the appropriate managerial or staff level for resolution of a problem or issue. Leadership of the staff nurse must be promoted if improved practice at the unit level is to be achieved.

The role of the head nurse in this setting is to teach staff how to deal with issues often formerly considered only the prerogative of the head nurse or supervisor. For example, direct communication with the physician or family member without seeking permission from another professional is now an inherent part of the professional nurse role at the Beth Israel Hospital. Staff nurses frequently assert themselves as leaders around issues of patient advocacy. It is perfectly acceptable for a primary nurse to initiate a patient care team conference requesting the private physician, personnel from other health disciplines, and the house staff to meet at a particular time to evaluate or determine a patient's plan of care. While support for this activity is given and consultation is provided as requested by the primary nurse, the authority for initiating and carrying out such communication is the primary nurse's. Indeed, it is *expected* that primary nurses will facilitate such a planning process on behalf of their patients.

As noted previously, we believe that the nurse prepared at the baccalaureate level is best prepared to meet the challenges of such interdisciplinary team collaboration. These activities encourage self-appraisal and generate differing points of view and a professional exchange that ultimately benefits the patient. Nurses prepared with a well-rounded knowledge of the humanities and basic science have demonstrated effectiveness in meeting these expectations and a professional orientation that enables nurses to assume accountability for their own practice.

COSTS

Concern for costs is often expressed when discussing primary nursing and the use of baccalaureate-prepared nurses as primary care providers within a practice setting. Studies however, do not necessarily support these concerns. Marram, in a comparison of team and primary nursing, shows that primary nursing was no more costly than team nursing.[5] Both Burt and Forster independently report a reduction in salary and wage costs following implemen tation of an all–registered nurse staff and a change in the organizational structure to support a professional practice model.[6, 7] Others such as Brown and Christman provide strong arguments in favor of the cost-effectiveness of primary nursing and an all–registered nurse staff.[8-11]

A discussion of costs is most relevant when examined within the context of one's own institutional setting. Multiple variables must be considered, and certainly the expectations for patient care outcomes must be incorporated into this analysis. Inadequate staffing patterns are unacceptable no matter what delivery system is used. Changes that improve such patterns generally increase costs. Thus, a nursing service must first examine its staffing patterns from a basic standard of patient safety and minimum expectations for care and make staffing decisions in light of these staffing standards.

Once satisfied that the numbers of staff will provide a reasonable level of staffing around the clock, thorough examination of staffing to provide professional services to patients can begin. An objective of this examination should be to determine ways to increase the use of the registered nurse in the provision of direct care to patients with a concurrent diminishing use of nonprofessionals in direct care. The fulfillment of this objective usually will lead to a reorganization of unit-based activities and eventually to a total system change.

At the Beth Israel our basic staffing complement was developed in early 1974, before the implementation of, or even the planning for, primary nursing began. The staffing methodology and budget accepted by the board of direc-

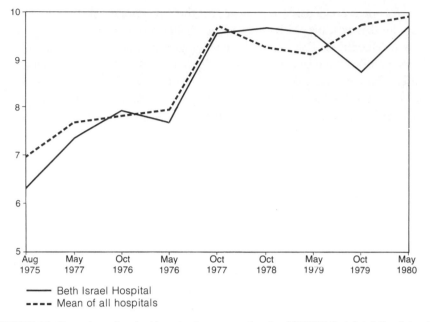

FIGURE 6-2. Comparison of total paid nursing hours per patient day (NHPPD), Beth Israel Hospital and Conference of Boston Teaching Hospitals.

tors at that time has continued until the present to provide the overall framework for our staffing and personnel budget. A building program with the addition of hospital beds, some programmatic changes and hospital organizational changes have resulted in an increase in the number of budgeted (FTEs) within the nursing department. None of these changes, however, was a specific result of primary nursing.

Surveys of nurse utilization conducted by the Conference of Boston Teaching Hospitals' Nursing Group show that even after hospital-wide implementation of primary nursing the relative position of nursing hours per patient day (NHPPD) paid at the Beth Israel Hospital did not significantly change in comparison to other hospitals in the survey (Fig. 6–2). In other words, when compared with area hospitals of a similar nature who do not employ primary nursing throughout their total system. Beth Israel's costs as measured through NHPPD remained constant.

Other findings in these surveys include a decrease in nursing administration as a percent of the total NHPPD worked (Table 6-3). This change represents the reorganization of the nursing services, particularly at the unit level, placing registered nurses in positions of direct care delivery rather than in supervisory positions. We do not use "charge" positions nor do we have layers of supervision between the head nurse and the directors of nursing. We consider this organization change to be one way costs have been contained.

TABLE 6-3 Nursing Administration as Percent Of Total NHPPD Worked. Beth Israel Hospital vs Mean of Conference of Boston Teaching Hospitals (COBTH)

	Beth Israel	All COBTH Hospitals
August 1975	7.41	6.81
October 1976	4.96	5.00
October 1977	4.63	4.30
October 1978	1.07	4.47
October 1979	1.24	4.26
May 1980	1.05	4.39

A major difference in the staffing complement in this system is the change in the mix of personnel we now employ since the implementation of a professional practice system. Nonprofessional positions (licensed practical nurses and nursing assistants) were systematically converted to registered nurse positions on a dollar-for-dollar basis, eventually yielding a higher mix of registered nurse staff to all others.

Data from a 1979 to 1980 Nursing Intensity Study at Beth Israel Hospital reveals that productive work time varies by type of personnel. In this study, head nurses used the least amount of personal time, averaging only 5% of total time worked. Personal time for staff nurses totaled 7% while nursing assistants and co-workers used the greatest amount of personal time, 13% of total time worked. When these data are examined by shift, opposite trends are apparent for registered nurses and nursing assistants or co-workers with respect to personal time. Staff nurses on the evening and night shifts showed decreasing use of personal time while the personal time of nursing assistants increased on each of these shifts respectively (Table 6-4). These data support the idea that registered nurse staff are economical and their use supports cost containment efforts within a hospital.

A major change in our staffing costs occurred with the elimination of private duty nurses to supplement staffing. This practice was in fact analogous to the current practice in some hospitals to use temporary staffing agencies. We have not used private duty nurses to supplement staff for a number of years and have never used temporary agencies to supplement staff. The use of such agencies is contrary to all of the goals of a professional department of

TABLE 6-4 Personal Time By Shift as Percent of Total Time Worked On Medical and Surgical Units

	Head Nurse	Staff RNs	Nursing Assistants/ Co-Workers
Total Personal Time	5%	7%	13%
Days		7.5%	10.5%
Evenings		6.5%	12.0%
Nights		4.5%	16.5%

TABLE 6-5 Private Duty Nurse (PDN) Expense Overview

Year	Total PDN Payroll	Approximate Number of Shifts	FTE
1972	650,135	18,575	71.4
1973	525,344	14,136	54.4
1974	647,128	16,152	62.1
1975	591,236	13,373	51.4
1976	380,420	8,454	32.5
1977	39,000	866	3.3
1978	0	0	0

nursing, and is counterproductive in the development of a practice environment that supports the professional nurse as the primary care provider and in the provision of continuity of care.

Approximately 10% of the total nursing budget was allocated for private duty nurses supplementing staff during the peak years of usage. For 1975 the last full year of our use of private duty nurses in this manner, this represented 51.4 FTE and more than a half million dollars (Table 6-5). As staffing improved and our practice expectations were integrated into the system, this component of the budget was eliminated. Only a few private duty nurses are ever used now, and they are always contracted for by the patient or family. Our policy, however, requires the private duty nurse to work in an associate nurse role to the primary nurse. The patient and family remains as part of the primary nurse's case load and communication continues with the primary nurse assessing with the family the continued need for private nursing services.

While accurate turnover statistics are not available for the first few years of this change process, turnover in our general medical–surgical areas was well over 80% with the hospital totals for the nursing department averaging better than 50%. The total nursing turnover rate for 1980 at Beth Israel was 23%, slightly higher than the 1979 rate of 21.1%. In 1974, the most frequent time for nurses to leave our nursing service was after 3 mo to 6 mo of employment. Today, nurses tend to leave Beth Israel after completing 2.5 yr to 5 yr of employment. Approximately 8% of the staff transfer from general care units to specialty units, while there is virtually no transfer of staff between the general medical and general surgical units. These data substantiate our belief that following a few years of practice nurses seek changes not only in work schedules but even more significantly in responsibilities they consider increasingly challenging to them, a fact that supports the development of clinical promotions or levels of practice within a hospital.

Since a single standard of professional performance is identified for all registered nurses, salary differentials between baccalaureate and non-baccalaureate graduates no longer exist in our hospital. A small differential similar to that of all other area hospitals was part of the salary program in 1974. Because we believed there should be one level of professional practice, this differential was built into the base salary rate for all nurses, avoiding a potentially discriminatory practice of lower wages for the same performance. Salaries at our hospital are within the same relative range of all other area hospitals, and the employment of baccalaureate graduates has not increased the salary and wage budget in our institution.

Attempts to quantify the costs of a professional practice system are usually limited because of the multiple variables present within a dynamic human service organization such as a hospital. We believe our continued ability to recruit nurses prepared at the baccalaureate level, the nonuse of supplemental agencies, our ability to maintain staffing levels that support professional practice, and our ability to remain nonunionized in a unionized climate all must be considered in the examination of costs.

QUALITY ASSURANCE

An evaluative component was incorporated into the early stages of planning for change in this setting. The results of these studies coupled with many anecdotal reports of the staff indicate a high level of satisfaction on the part of the care-giver as well as for patients and families.[12, 13]

Of particular interest were the results of Volicer's Hospital Stress Rating Scale.[14] This scale, based upon Holmes and Rahe's Social Readjustment Rating Scale, asks hospitalized patients to rank 49 stress-producing events related to hospitalization. This study was carried out on four general medical units, of which two had implemented primary nursing and two were still using a team-functional delivery system at the time of data collection. The significant finding was that following the implementation of primary nursing, the stress scores of patients on the primary nursing units were significantly lower than on the units with a conventional practice system (Table 6-6).

This outcome supports to some extent the change in the patients' descriptions of their hospitalization experiences since the implementation of primary nursing. Patients and families express continued satisfaction with their care and when readmitted frequently request a return to their original primary nurse. Letters commending the nursing care received are common, and it is extremely gratifying that primary nurses are now identified by name and often referred to as the major component in the patient's recovery.

It is not uncommon for primary nurses to maintain a relationship with patients and families following discharge from the hospital. Patients referred to nursing homes are often visited by their primary nurse. It is also not un-

TABLE 6-6 Volicer's Hospital Stress Rating Scale In Preimplementation and Postimplementation Phases

	Mean	Standard deviation	Standard error	Test for significance
Time 1	313.06	189.51	29.96	0.71
Exp/Control	343.76	197.24	31.19	
Time 2	236.84	138.21	21.85	1.98*
Exp/Control	311.17	193.11	30.53	
Time 1/2	343.76	197.24	31.19	0.75
Control	311.17	193.11	30.53	
Time 1/2	313.06	189.51	29.96	2.06*
Exp	236.84	138.21	21.85	

*$p = .05$

common for family members of a deceased patient to be maintained by the primary nurse as a primary family throughout their bereavement. These activities have been integrated into the practice of many primary nurses and represent a level of professional commitment not experienced by us in the previous delivery system.

SUMMARY

The intent of this chapter is to describe the nursing services of Boston's Beth Israel Hospital as a demonstration of a professional nursing department using a registered nurse staff prepared predominately at the baccalaureate level. In the years since a professional practice model has been implemented, we have experienced a variety of changes in nursing practice. The development of a professional practice system is not an overnight accomplishment but rather is the result of a great deal of deliberate planning, and at the Beth Israel it represents an evolutionary process in our nursing department since 1974. The intent of our activities was purposeful and was directed not only toward the improvement of care to patients, but also toward the development of a system within an active teaching–research environment that would promote nursing as a major force in the provision of health services.

   The success of Beth Israel relates to the combination of many factors, but clearly is a beginning representation of what professional nurses are capable of providing to society when they are given the opportunity to grow and develop within their sphere of practice. The discussion of Beth Israel's nursing service is of necessity a selective highlighting of the system and the activities that have taken place over a number of years. We are proud of what has been accomplished, yet we recognize that our success is only in relation to where we have been, not in relation to where we believe we need to be. We continue to have great hope for what we have yet to accomplish as professionals now that a strong foundation has been developed.

REFERENCES

1   Pointer, Dennis, D., Ph.D. Hospitals and Professionals – A Changing Relationship, *Hospitals JAHA* 50 (October 16, 1976), 117–121.

2   Beth Israel Hospital, Boston, Statement of Philsoophy, Department of Nursing.

3   Goddard, H.A. *Principles of Administration Applied to Nursing Service*. Geneva: World Health Organization, 1958, 71.

4   Manthey, Marie. *The Practice of Primary Nursing*. Boston, London: Blackwell Scientific Publications, Inc., 1980.

5   Marram, Gwen. The Comparative Costs of Operating a Team and Primary Nursing Unit, *JONA* VI:4 (May 1976), 21–24.

6   Burt, Marguerite L. The Cost of All-RN Staffing, in *All-RN Nursing Staff*, Genrose Alfano (ed). Wakefield, Massachusetts: Nursing Resources, 1980, 87–90.

7   Forster, John F. The Dollars and Sense of an All-RN Staff, *Nursing Administration Quarterly* 3:1 (Fall 1978), 41–47.

8   Brown, Barbara J. Experiences of Setting Up an All-RN Staff, in *All-RN Nursing Staff*. Genrose Alfano (ed). Wakefield, Massachusetts: Nursing Resources, 1980, 13–17.

9   Brown, Barbara J. Reorganizing Hospital-Based Nursing Practice: An Analysis of Patient Outcomes, Provider Satisfaction, and Costs, in *Health Policy and Nursing Practice*. Linda H. Aiken (ed). American Academy of Nursing, New York: McGraw Hill Co., 1981, 119–139.

10 Christman, Luther. Accountability With an All-RN Nursing Staff, in *All-RN Nursing Staff*, Genrose Alfano (ed). Wakefield, Massachusetts: 1980, 19–23.

11 Christman, Luther. Cost Effectiveness in Patient Care, *NAQ* 3:1 (Fall 1978), 51–53.

12 Hegedus, Kathryn S., and Sharon M. Bourdon. Evaluation Research: A Quality Assurance Program, *NAQ* 5:3 (Spring 1981), 26–30.

13 Hegedus, Kathryn S. Primary Nursing: Evaluation of Professional Nursing Practice, *Nursing Dimensions* 7 (Winter 1980), 85–89.

14 Hegedus, Kathryn S. A Patient Outcome Criterion Measure, *Supervisor Nurse* 10 (January 1979), 40–45.

15 *Ibid.*, 44.

J. GRAHAM ATKINSON
CARL J. SCHRAMM

7

HOSPITAL COST CONTAINMENT AND NURSING

When faced with the issue of hospital cost containment programs, two primary questions arise for those interested in nursing in the 1980s. The first is what effect such programs have on the nursing labor force, and the second, and more immediate from the perspective of the practicing nurse, is whether such programs hurt the economic position of nurses.

The nursing labor force issue involves how many nurses are demanded by hospitals subject to cost containment programs and how this has changed through time as a result of these programs. It also involves the mix of nonphysician professional personnel that emerges in hospitals where concern over cost containment is formalized because of government initiative. If the mix of personnel has changed such that lower cost, lesser skilled personnel have been substituted for nurses, those concerned over issues such as nursing shortages or the preservation of the role of nursing in the delivery of hospital care will make different judgments as to the desirability of cost containment. These judgments will depend on the interests they represent or on the values they espouse with respect to the importance of the traditional nursing role. Concerning the second question, we believe that nurses have been "hurt" if the cost containment program has had the effect of reducing their wages.

This chapter is divided into five sections. In Section 1 some background is provided on the way in which the Medicare and Medicaid programs reimburse hospitals, since this has had a profound impact on hospital costs in general and on nursing costs in particular. Section 2 consists of a comparison of regulatory systems in New York, Washington, and Maryland, and looks at the different ways in which they are likely to affect nurses. The following two sections deal with cost containment in Maryland, where the experience of such state-operated programs is most developed and where quality data on the nursing labor force exists. Section 3 provides some general arguments why hospital rate regulation has not hurt nurses, and Section 4 consists of an analysis of empirical data on numbers and wage levels of nurses in Maryland as well as an interpretation of the results. In Section 5 we consider the converse question of whether cost containment has helped nursing by expanding the absolute demand for nurses (which yields more opportunity to the individual), expanding their role or producing higher wage levels.

SECTION 1: MEDICARE COST-BASED REIMBURSEMENT

When Medicare was being debated before its enactment, there was considerable concern that adequate controls be established to ensure the federal government not be overcharged for the services it would be purchasing on behalf of Medicare beneficiaries. At that same time, concern was expressed that the federal government should not interfere with the manner in which those services were provided. In view of these concerns, it was decided that Medicare would pay for services on the basis of a cost reimbursement formula. The fact that it is almost impossible to be a major purchaser of services without affecting the way in which those services are provided was unfortunately ignored by policymakers at the time.

Instead of paying for the care of Medicare patients on the basis of the price or charge established by the hospital for cash-paying patients, the Medicare program — and in some states the Medicaid program — pays what is considered to be an appropriate share of the hospital's costs of producing the care. While this created an immensely complicated financing system, the important point to note is that no matter how much the hospital spends (within certain limits), Medicare, and sometimes Medicaid, will pay its share of those expenditures. In many states, the Blue Cross plans also pay on the basis of a share of the hospital's cost of producing care, regardless of the hospital's decisions in purchasing the necessities for producing care.

There is very little incentive to control costs under a payment system of this type. Indeed, there is a consensus in the literature that the *cost* reimbursement approach has been a principal cause of burgeoning hospital inflation since the enactment of Medicare.

How has this financing system influenced the compensation of nurses? The first observation is that the managers of our nation's hospitals, under this system, have had very little incentive to control the salary level of nurses. As a result, the salary levels have increased more rapidly than salaries and wages in the economy as a whole. An analysis by Feldstein strongly supports this contention.[1] His conclusions are that hospital wages went from being below comparable wages in the nonhospital field in 1957 to a level above comparable wages by 1969. This conclusion was particularly apparent when considering wages for nurses: Those for professional nurses were among the fastest growing for all hospital employees in the period 1963 to 1969. At this point it is interesting to note that the wage and price controls introduced in late 1971 appear to have had the opposite effect.[2]

The observation that cost-based reimbursement created the climate for improvement in the relative wage levels of nurses is further supported by the large difference between the rates of pay for nurses in hospitals and for those in nursing homes. Nursing homes receive a very small proportion of their revenues from Medicare, and many are proprietary, suggesting more tightly controlled wage structures. The pay scales for nurses in nursing homes are generally dramatically lower than the corresponding pay scales in hospitals for nurses of similar background, training, and experience.

In sum, the Medicare program has a financing feature, namely cost-based reimbursement, that, while originally intended to protect the federal government from paying the full price of hospital care, has had the opposite effect. By paying for whatever the hospital may wish to build into the cost of producing hospital care, the cost-based reimbursement system has stimulated high levels of spending. The key to this boomerang is that the system does not significantly impair the discretion of the hospital to build whatever costs it sees fit into the production of hospital care. It is partly this perversity in federal financing, which has had the effect of greatly embellishing the normal hospital "product," that has led several state governments to take direct action to dampen the inflation of hospital prices in their jursidictions.

SECTION 2: STATE EFFORTS IN MARYLAND, NEW YORK, AND WASHINGTON

The impact of state-level cost containment programs would be expected to have different impacts on nurses depending on how the program operates. For example, in a budget review state, where each line item of the hospital's total budget is approved, the impact on nursing would be dependent on the agency's approach to controlling the mix of labor costs. If, on the other hand, the state were guided by a normative policy such as reducing the percentage of hospital costs connected with laboratory testing, the demand for laboratory technicians would probably decrease. While the regulatory philosophy does not set out to injure the position of such groups, it does hurt them as a secondary effect. In non–budget review states, such as Maryland, other cost-controlling approaches are used that may not produce a uniform impact on any one occupation, since each hospital operates within a global budget and determines how resources are allocated within the institution.

This section outlines the cost containment program in three stages. Maryland's program, the subject of detailed scrutiny in the next section, is described in skeletal fashion here, as are the programs of New York and Washington. All three of the programs are discussed with special attention to the regulatory program's policy with regard to wages and employment.

MARYLAND

The hospital cost containment program in Maryland is run by the Maryland Health Services Cost Review Commission. The Commission has the authority to set the rates of all the general acute care hospitals in the state, and all payers, including Medicare and Medicaid, pay on the basis of the rates set by the Commission. The Maryland program sets rates by establishing external incentives for better performance. The Commission does not try to instruct the management of hospitals in how they should run their institutions, how many employees they should have, or what wages they should pay. It concentrates on ensuring that the overall rates charged to the public are reasonable. As part of the process of ensuring reasonable rates, the Commission gives each hospital an annual inflation adjustment. This adjustment is intended to allow for the impact of price changes on the costs of the hospital — both the costs of supplies and contracted services and the cost of personnel. Each year the Commission publishes the inflation factor by which it will routinely allow the total wage, salary, and fringe benefit expenses of the hospital to rise. What the hospital does with the increase is at the management's discretion.

NEW YORK

The regulatory program in New York covers the rates or costs paid by Blue Cross and Medicaid. The prices paid by charge-paying consumers are constrained by a separate charge control law that limits the rate of increase. The New York regulatory system is penalty oriented rather than incentive oriented, and many of the hospitals in the state have experienced financial difficulties. If a hospital has suffered penalties because its average cost per day is above the allowable level for such costs, then the hospital can be expected to respond by giving small wage increases and by laying off the staff. Conversely, hospitals that do not incur such penalties would not be expected to behave in such a manner.

WASHINGTON

The Washington Hospital Commission sets the rates that can be charged by hospitals in the state. At present, this rate does not apply to Medicare and Medicaid. The Washington Commission has taken a different attitude towards wage increases from that adopted by the Maryland and New York programs. The Washington Commission adopted a policy that union-negotiated wage increases should not be interfered with by the Commission, and so they are allowed as pass-through costs. Thus, while the Commission may have some impact on staffing levels, it does not have an effect on the wage rates paid.

SECTION 3: COST CONTAINMENT IN MARYLAND — GENERAL DISCUSSION

This section examines the activities of the Maryland Health Services Cost Review Commission in more detail and provides some general arguments that rate regulation in Maryland would not be expected to diminish the economic position of nurses. The arguments center around the idea that the Commission does not direct the hospitals concerning how they should spend their money or what staffing patterns and levels they should have. The Commission simply ensures that global rates for the hospitals are reasonable in relation to the costs of providing services.

The rate-setting process in Maryland has two main components: the rate review system and the inflation adjustment system. The inflation adjustment system is a more or less automatic system under which a hospital can receive an adjustment to its rates on an approximately annual basis to adjust for the reasonable impact of inflation, as estimated by the Commission. Included in the inflation adjustment is a factor for wage, salary, and fringe benefits increases. The Commission decides in advance on the factor that is to be included in the subsequent year's inflation adjustments for these increases. This factor is then applied to the total amount of such costs that are included in the hospital's rates. During the years 1975 to 1977, the allowance relied exclusively on the increase in the consumer price index; for 1978 and 1979, President Carter's wage and salary guidelines were used as the standard. Currently, the Bureau of Labor Statistics' index for service workers is in use. The allowance is given to each hospital annually whether the hospital actually gives an increase in wages or not.

The indices used were decided upon after much discussion, including public hearings and comment, and are considered fair by most of the parties. The hospitals are free to give increases to more or less than the allowance.

The other component of the rate-setting process is the rate review system. This is the mechanism by which hospitals obtain rate increases if they require more than is provided by the inflation adjustment system. In the course of a rate review, the hospital has the opportunity to justify the level of wages and salaries it considers appropriate for its particular circumstances. The allowance in rates for personnel cost increases may be more or less than the factor included in the inflation adjustment system.

The Maryland rate-setting process had several attributes that indirectly touch on the economic status of nursing. During the period in which hospital rates have been set by the Commission, all hospitals have experienced improvements in their financial positions. Almost all of the hospitals are making profits, and the annual net position (the "bottom line") has improved in each year. What this means with regard to nursing is that the hospitals have discretionary funds that they could, if they felt it necessary, expend in any way they saw fit. One such way would be to pay higher wages to nurses.

The existence of the rate-setting process also has encouraged some innovative experiments. The Commission has been concerned with the shortage of nurses, and has been trying to devise ways in which it could help alleviate the problem. One of the ways it is trying is a nurse scholarship program. The Commission has asked for proposals from hospitals for demonstration projects that would offer retraining for inactive nurses, reopen nursing schools, upgrade the skills of nurses' aides, and so forth in order to increase the number of nurses in the state. Several such projects are already underway, and more are under consideration. Because of the existence of the rate-setting process, it is possible for the hospitals to be given the opportunity to take a longer range approach to solving the nursing shortage than would otherwise be the case.

A point worth mentioning here is that the literature is unclear as to whether increasing the wage rates for nurses will increase the supply of nurses. Some of the literature in the field indicates that there is some relatively small wage elasticity.[3-5] One recent paper on the subject suggests that increasing nurses' wages may even reduce the supply of nurses.[6] Conversely, Aiken, Blendon, and Rogers draw the opposite conclusion from an analysis of data for the period following the enactment of Medicare, and then for the duration of the wage and price controls that were started in 1971.[7]

SECTION 4: DATA ANALYSIS—MARYLAND

The aim of this section is to present and interpret empirical data on the effect of the Health Services Cost Review Comission's activities on nurses. Each year the Commission requires all general acute care hospitals in the state to

TABLE 7-1 Change in Nursing Wage Rates 1978–1979, 1979–1980. Data from the Maryland Health Services Cost Review Commission's Wage and Salary Survey

	% Change 1978–1979	% Change 1979–1980	% Change 1978–1980
Baltimore metropolitan area			
Nurses' aide	4.53	8.55	13.47
LPN	4.97	7.19	12.51
General duty nurse	3.68	12.01	16.12
Supervisor of nurses	3.73	9.93	14.03
Washington metropolitan area			
Nurses' aide	5.98	9.57	16.16
LPN	8.55	11.66	21.21
General duty nurse	6.76	12.50	20.11
Supervisor of nurses	9.26	13.40	24.33
Nonmetropolitan area I			
Nurses' aide	9.91	9.27	20.10
LPN	7.81	9.60	18.16
General duty nurse	0.87	15.91	16.91
Supervisor of nurses	9.77	7.08	17.06
Nonmetropolitan area II			
Nurses' aide	7.60	8.71	16.97
LPN	5.95	10.04	16.59
General duty nurse	6.27	10.13	17.03
Supervisor of nurses	4.57	11.70	16.81

complete a wage and salary survey. This survey includes, among other data elements, the number of employees in the different job categories included in the survey, and the cost per hour for these employees, including the cost of fringe benefits. It is these particular data elements from the surveys done in 1978, 1979, and 1980 that were used in the analysis presented in this section. For the purpose of the analysis the state was split into four regions: the Baltimore metropolitan area, the Washington metropolitan area, and two nonmetropolitan areas.

Table 7-1 presents the results of the analysis of the change in wage costs (including fringe benefits). The number of employees in individual job categories in the nonmetropolitan areas is sometimes so small that the results are not significant. In the period 1978 to 1979, the factor allowed in the inflation adjustment system was 7% for employees earning over $4.00 per hour, and the percentage increase in the Consumer Price Index (CPI) for employees earning under $4.00 per hour. The reader will observe that the increases received by the various nursing personnel were less than this amount. For the period 1979 to 1980, the allowance was 8% for employees earning over $5.00 per hour, and the percentage increase in the CPI for the remaining portion. However, during that period the increases received by nursing personnel were almost uniformly above that allowance. This suggests that the hospital takes factors into account other than merely the allowance in the inflation adjustment system in determining the increases to be given to its nursing personnel.

TABLE 7-2 Change in Number of Nursing Employees (FTEs), 1978–1979, 1979–1980, 1978–1980. Data from the Maryland Health Services Cost Review Commission's Wage and Salary Survey

	% Change 1978–1979	% Change 1979–1980	% Change 1978–1980
Baltimore metropolitan area			
Nurses' aide	− 7.02	10.02	2.30
LPN	10.07	2.19	12.48
General duty nurse	8.41	5.54	14.42
Supervisor of nurses	9.16	11.86	29.77
Washington metropolitan area			
Nurses' aide	− 9.57	− 7.35	−16.22
LPN	20.45	− 8.31	10.43
General duty nurse	12..71	− .46	12.19
Supervisor or nurses	− 4.35	−42.61	−45.00
Nonmetropolitan area I			
Nurses' aide	6.72	− 2.48	4.07
LPN	−0−	− 2.94	− 2.94
General duty nurse	−13.09	31.95	14.68
Supervisor of nurses	− 3.57	1.82	− 1.75
Nonmetropolitan area II			
Nurses' aide	−13.80	2.81	−11.38
LPN	5.32	4.18	9.72
General duty nurse	− 7.81	5.50	− 2.47
Supervisor of nurses	−15.08	− 4.67	−19.05

In addition to examining wage rates, one must also analyze the mix of personnel used in order to determine the full impact of cost containment on the interests of nurses. Table 7-2 shows changes in the composition of the nursing labor force in Maryland hospitals from 1978 to 1980. It appears that, during this period, the wage policy was linked to a strategy intended to increase the skill level of nursing, thus reversing a previously observed trend to substitute lesser skilled for higher skilled nursing personnel. It appears that the general duty nurse category (registered nurse, baccalaureate-prepared nurses) has experienced the greatest growth through the period, with a significant decline in the number of nurses' aides.

SECTION 5: HOW COST CONTAINMENT CAN HELP NURSES

Cost containment has the possibility of being a positive force for the interests of nurses. Two ways in which cost containment may improve the economic status of nurses will be discussed in this section.

The first is improvement in the use of nurse personnel. Presumably nurses enter nursing because they want to care for patients. In practice, much of a nurse's time is spent in performing duties that are not directly related to patient care, or which could be performed by someone with a lower level of training. As hospitals become more cost conscious, they are likely to use nurses to provide the services they were trained to provide, and to use lesser skilled, less expensive personnel to do the jobs that do not require the level of training received by registered nurses. Most nurses would consider this to be a change for the better.

The second is increased flexibility in the use of nurse practitioners. There are a number of different services that specially trained nurses can provide economically. Nurse anesthetists and nurse midwives come immediately to mind. Unfortunately, the ability of nurses to provide and be reimbursed for such services has been severely constrained, mainly at the instigation of the medical profession. If cost containment becomes sufficiently forceful, which it has not done to date, these less expensive providers of medical services may be given the freedom they need to practice their skills to the fullest extent possible. This would benefit nurses greatly, since it would expand the range of services they could provide and would provide opportunities for upward mobility while allowing them to remain in the business of providing patient care. It is significant that nurses are allowed to provide services that are traditionally provided by physicians only in those isolated rural areas in which physicians have little desire to practice. Elsewhere, cost containment pressures have not been sufficiently powerful to overcome the resistance of the medical establishment.

CONCLUSIONS AND SUMMARY

In this chapter we have discussed several state regulatory systems designed to contain overall hospital cost inflation. In some instances it is possible they may have hurt nurses, but in general they do not appear to have done so. In particular, according to data on both salaries and growth rates for various nursing personnel in Maryland, it appears that higher skilled professional nurses have fared well under a comprehensive and rather aggressive cost containment system. While other state systems, particularly those that force many hospitals into a deficit situation, may affect hospitals' decisions both to compensate and use nurses differently than in Maryland, it cannot be concluded that attention to holding down resource consumption in our hospitals will have adverse effects on the nursing profession. On the contrary, continued pressure for cost containment may hold great promise for improved and creative uses of nurses both in the hospital and in other settings.

REFERENCES

1   Feldstein, M.S. *The rising cost of hospital care.* Washington, D.C.: Information Resources Press, 1971.

2   Aiken, L.H., Blendon, R.J., Rogers, D.E. The shortage of hospital nurses: A new perspective. Published simultaneously in *Annals of Internal Medicine*, September 1981, *95*(3):365–371, and *American Journal of Nursing*, September 1981 *81* (9):1612–1618.

3   Bognanno, M., Hixson, J. and Jeffers, J. The Short Run Supply of Nurses' Time, *Journal of Human Resources* (Winter 1974), 80–93.

4   Sloan, F., *The Geographic Distribution of Nurses and Public Policy.* U.S. Department of Health, Education, and Welfare: DHEW Publication No. (DHRA) 73–53, 1975

5   Link, C. and Settle, R. *The Supply of Married Professional Nurses,* Report to the U.S. Department of Labor, 1977.

6   Link, C. and Settle, R. Wage Incentives and Married Professional Nurses: A Case of Backward-Bending Supply? *Economic Inquiry* XIX: (January 1981), 144–156.

7   Aiken, L.H., Blendon, R.J., Rogers, D.E., *op cit.*

DUANE D. WALKER

8

THE COST OF NURSING CARE IN HOSPITALS

There is a widespread concern about the rapidly escalating costs of hospital care. A national effort has been launched to reduce unnecessary hospitalizations by having physicians perform as many diagnostic and therapeutic procedures as possible on an ambulatory basis. Presumably, more patients are hospitalized because they require continuing nursing care and ready access to physician services.

Acute care hospitals have been under scrutiny and attack for over a decade in regard to their part in the exorbitant and ever-increasing costs of health care. A report of the National Council on Wage and Price Stability recently concluded that during the 1965 to 1975 period, hospital costs and physicians' fees rose more than 50% faster than the overall costs of living.[1]

Beginning in 1971 with federal wage and price controls, followed by state rate commissions and voluntary hospital cost-containment efforts, hospitals have been under considerable pressure to control their costs. Nursing service is the hospital's largest department, and therefore has been particularly vulnerable to cost-containment policies.

The nursing service department has been singled out as a major cost in hospital's operating expenditures.[2-4] Yet the actual cost of nursing care is unknown because it is embedded in the daily hospital room charge. The cost of nursing care has been synonymous with the room rate, which is very high by any standard. It is not surprising, therefore, that many assume that the rapidly rising costs of hospital care are due to increased nurses' salaries.

SEPARATING NURSING CARE COSTS FROM NON-NURSING COSTS

This paper proposes to examine the question, How much does nursing care in hospitals really cost?

To answer the question, we need to probe hidden costs and to find answers to the following interrelated questions:

- How should the relative cost of nursing care be determined?
- Are *all* expenditures in the nursing service operating budget specifically related to direct or indirect nursing care services?

Since these questions, relative to the high costs of nursing care, have been critically analyzed and a preliminary study conducted at a leading university teaching hospital, some background information and initial findings from the study will be presented in order to sort out costs of *nursing care* services from *non-nursing* hospital services.

THE SETTING

Stanford University Hospital (SUH) is a 668-bed private, nonprofit, teaching hospital, owned and operated by Stanford University. Its income is derived primarily from patient revenues (97%). SUH serves as a community hospital for patients from adjacent areas and as a regional medical center for patients with advanced and difficult medical problems.

The primary goals of the Nursing Service Department at SUH are to provide patients with quality nursing care and educational services, and to foster a nursing practice environment that will provide nurses with challenges, satisfaction, and rewards. Some of the programs the department of nursing offers are the following:

- Four-level clinical nursing career ladder.
- Department of nursing research.
- Continuing education opportunities.
- Primary nursing practice.
- Distinguished lecture series.
- Administrative residency program in nursing management.

The Nursing Service Department is composed of seven major clinical regions, each headed by an assistant director of nursing. Each unit within a clinical region is managed by a clinical nursing coordinator (head nurse). In addition, there is an assistant director of nursing for administrative services and one for educational services; these administrative services provide support to the clinical regions. Overall direction of the department is provided by the associate administrator/director of nursing along with an associate director of nursing. At present, the department employs 1,200 registered nurses, 20 licensed practical nurses, 225 nursing assistants, seven unit managers, and 110 unit clerks. The modality of nursing practice consists of primary nursing and team nursing.

Each nursing unit is structured as a separate cost center, and each clinical nursing coordinator, with assistance from a unit manager, prepares the nursing unit's budget. The budgets are based on the projected acuity of illness of the patients to be served. Assistant directors of nursing, assisted by the unit manager, defend their budgets at hospital budget hearings.

It should be noted that the Nursing Service Department at SUH supports the proposition that nursing care is limited only to direct and indirect activities required for the management and delivery of nursing care *per se*. These direct and indirect nursing activities include the following:

DIRECT NURSING CARE. Those nursing care activities (including the "laying on of hands" in performing nursing functions at the unit level), unit nursing management, and only those recordkeeping, clerical, and management tasks that are required specifically for the provision of nursing care.

INDIRECT NURSING CARE. Activities performed at the nursing department administrative level, including general administration of the department; nursing supervision (general supervision on evenings, nights, weekends); environmental management; classification of patients; nursing quality assurance programs; nursing staffing and recruitment; nursing educational services (orientation, inservice, and continuing education, patient education programs, other special programs); and nursing research. (*See* Table 8-1 for a complete list of direct and indirect nursing activities.)

THE METHOD

As a first step, the cost of nursing care must be separated from the plethora of non-nursing tasks and services frequently lumped with nursing under the misleading title "room rate."[5-8] However, as a prerequisite to this step, the nursing service director needs to take steps to ensure that nursing staff members are indeed performing *nursing* tasks rather than a myriad of other non-nursing tasks. Primary components of nursing care are the direct care requirements of patients and families, which depend upon the acuity of the patient's condition, the necessary related nursing tasks, and the time needed to perform these tasks. These components (acuity, nursing tasks, and nursing

TABLE 8-1 Hospital Services Included in the Daily Room Rate

Direct	Indirect
Direct Nursing	**Indirect Nursing**
Clinical nursing coordinator, Clinical assistant director of nursing, bedside nursing staff Unit manager, clerks, and equipment technician	Nursing administration Nursing orientation Education and development
Direct Medical	**Indirect Medical**
Medical supplies Interns and residents	Medical school contracts Anatomic pathology Medical staff office Utilization review and quality assurance
Other Direct	**Financial Affairs**
Dietary Housekeeping Laundry and linen Messenger and mail service Central supply items Minor equipment and pharmacy stock Social services Telephone Admitting Patient placement Infection control Chaplain	Financial adjustments (Medicare/ Medicaid disallowances, bed debts, discounts and allowances, provision of capital) Depreciation (buildings and equipment) Patient accounting Finance and data processing Insurance Interest Purchasing
	Other Indirect
	General administration Maintenance and repairs (plant, grounds, equipment) Personnel Utilities Medical records Office supplies Communications Facilities protection Community relations

time) were identified and quantified at SUH as the basis for a computerized patient classification system that reflects levels of nursing care. This system enables the prediction of staffing needs, and provides a data base for validation of budet requirements and the setting of differential charges for direct nursing care to the patient.

As will be discussed later, this classification system is similar to others that have been developed, and it has some of the same shortcomings. It has the potential, however, of allowing one to put a more realistic price tag on levels of nursing care throughout the hospital. In order to understand how the patient classification system can be used as a tool to determine the cost of nursing care on a particular unit, the following description of nursing care costs on an adult intensive care unit is presented.

NURSING CARE COSTS OF INTENSIVE CARE UNITS. On the adult intensive care units (ICUs) at SUH, the patient classification system consists of five levels of direct nursing care that range from the least nursing care required (level I) to the most nursing care required (level V). Each patient's acuity is assessed and classified three times a day by a nurse caring for the patient. The nurse makes this assessment 4 h before the next shift, which enables adjustments to be made in staffing patterns for that shift. To record each assessment, the nurse completes a form by darkening appropriate squares with a pencil. This form is then read by an optical scanner, and the information goes directly into a computer.

At present, the *per diem* room charge in the ICUs is based on the five levels of nursing care. Payments for charges are determined on this basis, and were negotiated with third party payers. Although the level of nursing care is identified on the patient's bill, the actual dollar figures for a particular level do not appear on the bill distinct from the room charge.

In the ICUs all *non-nursing* tasks have been reallocated to the appropriate departments through negotiation. Therefore, nurses on these units do *not* perform non-nursing tasks, ensuring that the nursing care charge represents the actual cost of providing nursing care.

Two methods are useful in examining the relative costs of nursing care in hospitals. The first is to examine the components included in daily room charges. To determine the cost of nursing care *versus* the room rate, data were collected for level III nursing care over a 1 month period. The average daily census of patients requiring this care level was 20.

Figure 8–1 illustrates the proportionate daily cost of nursing care *versus* other non-nursing charges included in the average *per diem* rate for level III care. The categories used, other than nursing, were selected to show expenses related to providing services directly to patients ("direct" categories) *versus* overhead costs ("indirect" categories).

The nurse–patient ratio for level III ICU care is 1:1. Patients who are classified as level III have the following nursing care requirements:

- Continuous observation and hourly intervention (nursing activities directed toward evaluating and correcting patient problems or complications).
- Increased number and frequency of vital sign determinations and treatments.
- Vital signs determinations every 15 min to 30 min: temperature, pulse, respiration, blood pressure, apical and radial pulses, central venous pressure, electrocardiogram monitoring, and other determinations as indicated.
- Continuous ventilatory support.

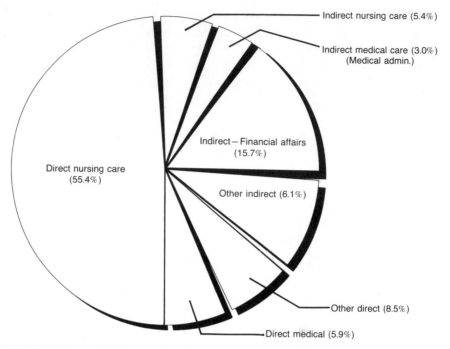

Indirect nursing care (5.4%)

Indirect medical care (3.0%)
(Medical admin.)

Indirect—Financial affairs
(15.7%)

Direct nursing care
(55.4%)

Other indirect (6.1%)

Other direct (8.5%)

Direct medical (5.9%)

FIGURE 8-1. Percent of daily room charges for intensive care attributable to nursing care and non-nursing services.

- Pulmonary therapy every 30 min to 60 min: intermittent positive pressure breathing treatments, percussion, postural drainage, and other procedures done by registered nurses.

- Continuous drug infusions (vasopressors, vasodilators, and antiarrhythmics.

- Increased monitoring of other parameters with appropriate therapy.

- Blood gases.

- Fluid and electrolyte management.

- Increased monitoring for life-threatening complications.

- Increased care due to total dependency (inability to participate in own care).

- Isolation.

COMPARATIVE COSTS OF NURSING CARE VERSUS NON-NURSING CARE COSTS

A second way to examine the relative cost of nursing is to ascertain the share of total hospital charges attributable to nursing. Data were collected and analyzed from a sample of five patients with similar lengths of stay in each of

TABLE 8-2 Percent Distribution of Charges in Average Total Cost of Hospitalization by Diagnosis*

Diagnosis	Room charge (excluding nursing)	Nursing Care	Clinical Professional's Fee†	OR, ER PT OT	Inhalation Therapy	Anesthesia	X-ray and Radiation Therapy	Laboratory	Surgical Supplies	Central Supplies	Drugs	Blood	Total
Coronary artery bypass graft	14.8	14.8	13.9	11.4	2.5	1.3	2.5	19.0	13.2	1.8	4.6	0.1	100.0
Aortic valve repair; mitral valve repair	12.4	12.4	12.6	9.0	2.1	1.0	2.0	13.9	29.5	1.2	4.0	—	100.0
Chronic obstructive pulmonary disease	20.7	20.7	5.7	5.1	9.0	—	6.9	16.8	0.9	5.3	8.7	0.1	100.0
Hodgkins' disease; lymphoma; leukemia	21.0	21.0	5.1	1.6	4.0	0.1	6.6	26.9	0.3	4.5	8.9	—	100.0
Craniotomy	20.5	20.5	22.1	12.4	3.3	1.2	4.1	8.4	1.7	1.5	4.1	0.1	100.0
Thoracotomy; aortic-femoral bypass	17.1	17.1	15.9	14.1	5.8	2.4	6.8	11.5	3.0	1.7	4.5	—	100.0

* Sample of 5 patients in each diagnosis category.
† Includes surgeon's fee. where applicable.

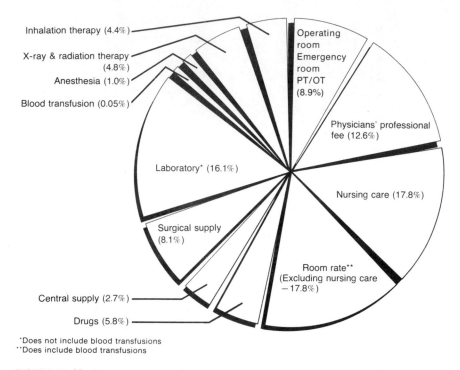

Inhalation therapy (4.4%)

X-ray & radiation therapy (4.8%)

Anesthesia (1.0%)

Blood transfusion (0.05%)

Operating room Emergency room PT/OT (8.9%)

Physicians' professional fee (12.6%)

Laboratory* (16.1%)

Nursing care (17.8%)

Surgical supply (8.1%)

Room rate** (Excluding nursing care −17.8%)

Central supply (2.7%)

Drugs (5.8%)

*Does not include blood transfusions
**Does include blood transfusions

FIGURE 8-2. Nursing costs as percent of average total hospital charges for 6 diagnoses.

six disease categories ($N = 30$). Since the sample size is small generalizability is limited. However, the data are presented as an exploratory approach in determining and comparing the cost of nursing care with other hospital services.

Charges that make up the average total cost of hospitalization for the sample of 30 patients are presented in Table 8-2. The total nursing care cost was approximately 50% of the room charge. The percentage may be somewhat high since these patients received intensive care during part of their hospital stay. It should be noted that the table shows mean figures only and does not reflect variations within categories.

Examination of Table 8-2 reveals that the cost of nursing care accounts for a relatively small proportion of total hospitalization charges (approximately 12% to 20%). In four of the six diagnostic categories, the nursing care cost is similar to the cost of physicians' services. Figure 8-2 represents the proportionate costs of hospitalization when data from Table 8-2 are combined and the six diagnostic categories are considered as a group. Laboratory charges account for almost the same proportion of the total cost as nursing care.

Although a more comprehensive study is needed to determine the costs of nursing care, the preliminary findings suggest that *actual* nursing care is not as costly as many hospital administrators and physicians would lead us to believe. For example, when 24-hr one-to-one care is provided by an all-registered nurse staff, as in level III ICU care, the high level of nursing care accounts for approximately 55% of the *per diem* charge. When the cost of professional nursing is compared to that of charges for other hospital services, somewhat less than 20% of the total charges appears to be for nursing care.

DISCUSSION

The general misconception that the cost of hospital nursing care is synonymous with the room rate needs to be corrected. This notion has probably arisen because of the long-standing fiscal practice of combining overhead and other miscellaneous costs with nursing costs, as well as the practice of charging the nursing budget for non-nursing services.

Why has nursing's monetary value and professional identity been buried in this way? Undoubtedly, a large part of the responsibility belongs to nurses themselves. The historical view of nurses as handmaidens has been difficult to change. The subservient attitude that accompanies this view has prompted many nurses to assume responsibility for non-nursing activities that other hospital members have failed to complete.

Nursing administrators need to take more responsibility for fostering the autonomy and decision-making ability of nurses. The nursing budget is a management tool for achieving this end. Not only do nursing directors need to become proficient in budget procedures, but head nurses at the unit level need to increase their knowledge and skills, and play a vital role in fiscal management.

Many nursing directors either do not prepare a budget or do not understand its uses and value.[9] Schmied notes that many directors are remiss in allocating time and energy to fiscal management, even though, as Swansburg points out, "the control of a budget determines who controls nursing service."[10,11] Furthermore, Stevens proposes that nursing administrators work toward realistic representation on both the expense and revenue sides of the ledger, and recommends that nursing service directors take steps to establish the concept of nursing as a revenue-producing department.[8]

To reflect nursing care costs as accurately as possible, levels of care should represent *actual* nursing care, that is, the cost of care when nursing staff are performing only nursing functions. The use of a patient classification system, such as that employed at SUH, is a suitable approach to arriving at a dollar value for various levels of nursing care. This notion has been supported by a number of authors.[12–15] The idea of classifying patients by nursing requirements is not new, and numerous systems have been developed. Although some of the components of the patient classification system are difficult to identify and quantify, soundly developed patient classification systems have proved useful for determining staffing and the nursing budget and setting differential charges for patient care.

Almost a decade ago, Holbrook proposed that nursing care charges be separated from room charges and that they be determined by level of nursing care provided.[6] Recently, a few institutions, such as Massachusetts Eye and Ear Infirmary, and St. Luke's Hospital and Medical Center in Phoenix, Arizona, have initiated charges for nursing care by levels of care, and reflected these charges on the patients' bills.[16] As noted earlier, the actual dollar figures for these charges do not yet appear on the patients' bills at SUH, but it is the appropriate next step in accord with the American Nurses' Association's (ANA) 1977 resolution recommending that "all billing and reimbursement procedures clearly identify both the nature and cost of the nursing care services rendered."[17]

Swansburg recommends that the system of reimbursement for health care costs should not pay for "frills," such as additional food and drinks, daily changes of bed linens, and personal services that patients could perform, provided they are physically and mentally able.[3] Giving patients the option to purchase extra services might be one way of meeting the needs of patients while containing overall costs. Stevens' proposal is similar, and suggests that "it should be possible to set price schedules related to both patient needs and standards of care."[8] This could be accomplished by combining quality control and patient classification systems, and would be useful in nursing and institutional decision making regarding levels of care that could or could not be offered. Either the institution might choose to offer a certain level of care, based on a realistic assessment of its resources, or it might offer a variety of levels and prices, with clients deciding on the price they want to pay.

This concept is analogous to shopping for any item in a free enterprise system. It requires that the seller of the item or service be prepared to deliver that which is purchased. Thus charging for various levels of nursing care requires that the specified level of care will be provided. Nurses may be reluctant to accept the concept that a certain level of nursing care and hospital hotel services will be provided in accordance with choices of the patient. In addition, nurses may have difficulty in accepting the high degree of accountability that goes with identifying and publicizing the monetary value of nursing care. Education of all concerned groups to these changes is essential. Nursing administration needs to work toward changing attitudes of nurses, hospital administrators, other health providers, and perhaps more importantly the consumers.

All groups would benefit from implementation of these fiscal changes. For consumers, benefits will include eliminating the inequitable practice of paying for services not received. Although operating expenditures such as utilities, maintenance, and housekeeping would probably be apportioned equally, a patient who requires and receives minimal nursing care would pay only for minimal care. This patient would not subsidize other patients who receive substantially more hours of nursing care. Consumers would also benefit from the offering of options as to the amount and sources of care or hospital amenities they desire. Such options would not only assist in cost containment, but would also increase the accessibility and scope of services for consumers. An accompanying benefit might be the fostering of self-determination and responsibility, with a lessening of the dependency that hospitals now generally impose on patients and families.

For nurses the anticipated benefits are considerable. Nurses are perceived as an economic drain, rather than as a financial asset. Determining the cost of and charging for nursing care – thereby establishing and validating nurses as income producers – should greatly improve nurses' ability to influence important decisions concerning nursing resources and practice. In addition, the opportunity to demonstrate and establish the relationship between nursing actions and cost-benefits should pave the way for nurses to use their special knowledge and skills more fully.

Finally, the current shortage of nurses may be partly due to frustration brought about through the inability to practice nursing as professional clinicians and teachers, to be valued as important members of the health care team, and to be duly rewarded for the care and comfort they provide their patients. When nurses gain the power and status that goes with recognition of their economic worth, and when their role is more clearly defined through establishment of care levels, they may very well feel more committed to and satisfied with nursing. A satisfied, committed professional nurse is the key to high productivity and quality nursing care.

CONCLUSION

Despite the central importance of nursing care to hospitalized patients, nursing services have traditionally been included under the hospital's daily room charge instead of as a professional service rendered. As a result, many have come to believe that the cost of nursing care is almost synonymous with daily room charges.

Contrary to popular opinion, nursing care accounts for only about half of the daily room charge for ICUs and may be significantly less in other areas of the hospital. Moreover, for the six diagnostic categories examined here, nursing accounted for only 20% or less of total hospital charges.

Nurses are the largest single group of health professionals employed by hospitals. It is not surprising, therefore, that nursing service budgets have been a target of cost containment programs. Despite a widespread shortage of hospital nurses, there is great reluctance to invest additional resources in nursing. However, if the results of this preliminary analysis are sustained by subsequent studies, it would appear that nursing care is one of the hospital's most economical services. It has also been suggested that the cost–benefit ratio could be significantly improved by breaking the costs of nursing care out of the daily room charge and billing patients for professional services rendered. Nurses would be more accountable for their services, and hospitals would have greater incentives to improve the fiscal management of hotel, maintenance, and other institutional operating costs.

The question of how to determine nursing care costs will remain without a definitive answer until unsound fiscal practices such as hiding nursing care costs and revenues are abandoned. It is obvious from a preliminary study that nursing care costs need to be separated from non-nursing hospital costs and that the real problem is presenting costs in their room rate disguise. Indeed, the time is long overdue for a more extensive study of the costs of nursing care. One thing appears certain — if nursing in acute care hospitals and other health care facilities is ever to be recognized and reimbursed as an essential professional service, the time for working toward these goals is *now*.

REFERENCES

1   Council on Wage and Price Stability, Executive Office of the President: The Program of Rising Health Care Costs, p 3. (Staff Report). Washington, DC, April 1976

2   Mullane MK: Foreword. In Donovan H: Nursing Service Administration: Managing the Enterprise, p 3. St Louis, CV Mosby, 1975

3   Swansburg RC: Cost control in nursing. Supervisor Nurse 9, No. 51:3: 12, 1978

4   Porter-O'Grady T: Financial planning: Budgeting for nursing. Part I. Supervisor Nurse 10, No. 35: 3, 1979

5   Baker N: Reimbursement for nursing services: Issues and trends. Nursing Law and Ethics 1, No. 1: 6, 1980

6   Holbrook FK: Charging by level of nursing care. Hospitals 46, No. 80: 6; 11; 12; 1972

7   Jennings CP, Jennings TF: Containing costs through prospective reimbursement. Am J Nurs 77, p 1155: 6, 1977

8   Stevens BJ: What is the executive's role in budgeting for her department? Hospitals 50, No. 83: 6, 11, 12, 1976

9   Goertzen I: Cost effectiveness for nursing: Regulation of hospital rates and its implications for nursing. Nursing Administration Quarterly. 3, No. 59: 11, 1978

10 Schmied E: Allocation of resources: Preparation of the nursing department budget. Journal of Nursing Administration 7, No. 31: 11, 1977

11 Swansburg, RC: The nursing budget. Supervisor Nurse 9, No. 40: 11, 1978

12 Brown B: Editorial. Nursing Administration Quarterly 3, No. V: 11, 1978

13 Evans SK: Laundon R, Yamamato WG: Projecting staffing requirements for intensive care units. Journal of Nursing Administration 10, No. 34: 11, 1980

14 Marriner A: Variables affecting staffing. Supervisor Nurse 10, No. 62: 11, 1979

15 Porter-O'Grady T: Financial planning: Budgeting for nursing. Part II. Supervisor Nurse 10, No. 25: 11, 1979

16 A Patient Classification System for Staffing and Charging for Nursing Services, p. 12. Phoenix, AZ, St. Luke's Hospital Medical Center

17 Commission on Economic and General Welfare: Reimbursement for Nursing Services (Position statement), p. 12. Kansas City, MO, American Nurses' Association, 1977

3

THE CHALLENGES OF LONG-TERM CARE

Long-term care is the most rapidly growing component in American health care, and nursing is the central service required by the health-impaired elderly. Therefore the potential for nurses to assume important roles in long-term care is immense.

The papers in Part III explore the possibilities for nurses in long-term care and identify critical areas requiring nursing leadership in the 1980s. Chapter 9, written by Reif and Estes, is an overview of long-term care policy that provides the context for the remaining papers. Special attention is given to the financing of long-term care, which has become a major constraint in the development of services for the elderly. Although the national resources spent on health care for the elderly are immense, there is an imbalance in the distribution of resources that favors expensive institutional care and mitigates against the development of less expensive and more appropriate alternative services. An understanding of financing issues is essential to nurses as they chart their efforts to improve long-term care services.

Nursing homes have been cause for escalating public concern over the past 20 years. News media reports, public opinion polls, and national commission reports reveal a national uneasiness about the quality of health care and the quality of life of nursing home residents. Unfortunately, nursing homes have become isolated from the mainstream of American health care. Neither nurses nor physicians are much in evidence. On average, there are only 1.5 licensed nursing providers (registered nurses and licensed practical nurses) for each 100 nursing home residents. Even in skilled nursing facilities, only 40% of the homes have at least one nurse present around-the-clock. Physician coverage is even more of a problem. Only 17% of American physicians make nursing home visits at all, and most who do spent only a fraction of their time there.

Chapter 10 is based upon an extensive national inquiry into nursing homes conducted by political scientist Bruce Vladcek who accurately depicts the difficulties of developing appropriate professional care in our current nursing homes. In Chapter 11, two gerontological nurse specialists, with extensive experience in nursing homes, acknowledge the constraints but offer strategies to bring about change. And in Chapter 12, Alfano shares the success of the Loeb Center, a hospital-based extended care facility, where the importance of nursing care in returning long-term care patients to independent living arrangements has been demonstrated.

These papers together present a picture of nursing's potential leadership in long-term care that is both exciting and challenging. If nurses can successfully surmount some of the current problems in the organization and financing of long-term care services, new vistas for autonomous professional practice will emerge, and nurses could provide an invaluable public service by ensuring that elderly Americans receive appropriate health services.

LAURA REIF
CARROLL L. ESTES

9

LONG-TERM CARE: NEW OPPORTUNITIES FOR PROFESSIONAL NURSING

Long-term care encompasses a wide range of services — health maintenance, rehabilitation, medical treatment, personal care, housekeeping, and various kinds of assistance with activities of daily living. These services are delivered both within and outside of institutions, to persons suffering from chronic physical or mental conditions that have significantly impaired their ability to function independently. How best to provide long-term care, and for which groups of patients, has become a major health policy issue in the United States.[22, 28, 48, 50, 51, 54]

A number of factors have given rise to the current concern about long-term care. First, the population in need of long-term care has grown to substantial proportions and is increasing rapidly. Recent estimates suggest over 9 million Americans suffer from severe functional impairments.[54] That number is expected to increase dramatically in the next 50 yr, due to the rapid increase of the elderly population and particularly those groups among the elderly that have the highest risk of disability — those over 85, the poor, ethnic minorities, women, and those lacking social support from family and friends.[54, 17]

Second, the cost of long-term care is very large and escalating at an

The authors would like to express their appreciation to Linda Aiken, Charlene Harrington, Philip R. Lee, Paul Newacheck, and Brahna Trager for their suggestions, criticisms, and comments on an earlier draft of this chapter. We also thank Hank Foley, Lenore Gerard, Susan Gortner, Lauren LeRoy, and Virginia Saba for supplying relevant material on issues related to the employment of nurses and nurse training in gerontology and long-term care.

147

alarming rate. Nursing homes account for the largest amount of expenditures on long-term care, costing about $18 billion in 1979. The cost of publicly financed noninstitutional long-term services amounted to about $1.2 billion in 1978.[54] Expenditures for both nursing home care and home health services grew rapidly over a 6-yr period: 1979 nursing home expenditures were two and one-half times what they were in 1973; spending on medically oriented home care in 1978 was over six times what it was in 1972.[52] Of particular note is the large amount of *public* monies spent on long-term care. Government programs presently pay for 57% of the costs of all nursing home care in the United States. Over 80% of the costs of home health services are paid for by public funds.[52]

A third factor leading to increased concern about long-term care is the widespread belief that current approaches to the problem are ineffective. There has been mounting evidence of the glaring deficiencies and inequities of a system that relies almost exclusively on end-stage intervention, institutional care, medically oriented treatment models, and eligibility criteria that restrict services largely to the aged and very poor.[39, 48, 54, 66, 67, 78, 86, 91] Conservative estimates indicate that over 1 million disabled persons living outside of institutions fail to receive the long-term care they require.[54] The number of persons with unmet needs is expected to grow as changing family structures and a decrease in the ratio of caretakers to dependents erodes the currently high levels of informal support services.[19, 51, 54, 64, 83]

The above mentioned social and demographic trends will likely result in long-term care assuming increasing importance within the spectrum of health and human services, both during the present decade and in the foreseeable future. Policies and programs pertaining to long-term care will have a very significant impact on professional nursing. In 1979 long-term care, particularly nursing home care, was the fastest growing segment of the health services industry in the United States.[54] In that same year over 100,000 nurses* were employed in organizations that delivered long-term care.[5, 32] While 80% of these nurses worked in nursing homes and extended care facilities, the *greatest increase* in employment of nurses between 1972 and 1979 was among those providing long-term care to persons *outside* of institutions. During that 7 yr period, the numbers of nurses caring for people at home tripled.[30, 32]

Registered nurses represent the largest number and percentage of professional workers involved in long-term care.[92] Recent projections indicate that there will be a great shortage of nurses in the specialty areas of long-term care and gerontology. These estimates suggest that by the year 2030 there will be a shortfall of 75,000 nurses, based solely on personnel needed in nursing homes.[92] Given the recent emphasis on noninstitutional long-term care,

---

* Throughout this chapter, the word "nurses" will refer to *registered nurses*, not licensed vocational nurses, practical nurses, or nurses' aides.

and the anticipated decrease in the amount of care provided by the family to its elderly, ill, or disabled members, nurses are likely to become increasingly involved in long-term care. Indeed, in the future, long-term care is very likely to become a key growth area for professional nursing.

In this chapter we present an overview of the current status of long-term care in the United States. We will also attempt to identify some of the key factors that have in the past and are likely in the future to significantly affect policies and programs concerned with long-term care. A major purpose of this chapter is to spell out how developments in long-term care are likely to influence the profession of nursing.

MAJOR DIMENSIONS OF THE PROBLEM OF LONG-TERM CARE

Before describing the characteristics of long-term care in the United States, we would like to describe the nature of the population that is at risk, and contrast that group with those persons who currently use the range of services generally referred to as long-term care. Persons need long-term care when they have a chronic condition that results in functional impairment and causes physical dependence on others.

DISCREPANCY BETWEEN POPULATIONS WHO NEED AND RECEIVE LONG-TERM CARE

While no thoroughly reliable data exist on the number of Americans who require long-term care, the best available information suggests that 7.66 million persons — 3.6% of the United States population — suffer from a functional deficit serious enough to prevent them from carrying out their major activity. Of particular interest is the fact that this population consists of as many persons *under 65* as it does elderly persons.[54] In addition to this population, which resides *outside* of institutions, there are over 1.5 million Americans, 90% of them elderly, who currently live in nursing homes.[54]

In contrast with the large number of persons potentially in need of long-term care, a relatively small proportion actually use formal services. Recent statistics on the use of noninstitutional long-term care indicate that about 2.4 million persons presently receive services.[28] This suggests that as little as 31% of the noninstitutional population who requires care are served by the health and social service system. The problem may be even more severe for the elderly. Recent studies suggest that as few as 20% of elderly persons in need of noninstitutional long-term care presently use home health services.[20, 54]

Even conservative estimates indicate that over 1 million noninstitutionalized disabled fail to receive needed long-term care.[54] However, need likely exceeds use by much more than that, given information available in a recent analysis of the deficiencies of current methods for determining populations at risk.[79] In addition, there is evidence that 60% to 80% of the long-term care of persons at home is provided by family members, and that the percentage of informal care increases with the severity of the functional impairment of the person being cared for.[50, 51, 54]

LIMITED EFFORTS TO REDUCE THE RISK OF DISEASE AND DISABILITY ·

Approaches to long-term care in the United States rely almost exclusively on service strategies designed to provide assistance only when a health-related problem has progressed to the point where it results in substantial functional impairment.[54, 64] Very little attention is paid to the social and economic factors that are associated with disease and disability. Current approaches emphasize dealing with consequences rather than reducing risks, despite the mounting evidence that persons who have a low income, poor nutrition and housing, and a limited support network stand an increased chance of being chronically ill and impaired, and are at much greater risk of being institutionalized in extended care facilities.[10, 11, 12, 17, 27, 85]

Recent reports provide rather convincing evidence for the association between poverty and poor health.[26, 74] Particularly relevant for this discussion are findings showing the relationship between low income and chronic illness or disability. The percentage of persons reporting functional impairments is twice as high among the poor as among those with higher incomes.[26] Moreover, 34 million Americans in the poorest families (below $6,000 income per year) spent twice as many days in bed and twice as many days unable to carry out normal activities.[74]

In addition, there seems to be a striking relationship between use of formal long-term care and certain economic and social factors. A recent paper by Butler and Newacheck presents evidence of higher use of nursing home care among elderly who lack necessary social support.[17] These researchers found that widows and widowers were up to five times more likely to be institutionalized than were married persons. Further, those elderly who were never married, or who were divorced or separated were found to have up to ten times the rate of institutionalization of married persons. Those with low incomes also seem to have an increased risk of institutionalized long-term care.[9, 25, 33] A number of studies show that the availability of informal sources of social support also significantly affects the use of noninstitutional long-term services.[12, 51, 86] There is increasing evidence that only patients who have substantial assistance from family or friends can get along with the limited services most home health agencies supply.[20, 50, 51]

The above findings suggest that an exclusively service-oriented strategy for dealing with the problem of long-term care may not be the most effective or least costly approach. While it is necessary to provide long-term care to those persons who suffer from substantial functional impairment, it may also be prudent to supplement this approach with efforts to reduce the risk of disability and institutionalization by improving income levels, nutrition, and housing for vulnerable populations.[35, 66, 67] In addition, it is apparent that public programs such as Medicaid have not been effective in improving the health of the poor. Recent evidence indicates that chronic diseases among the poor are just as prevalent as they were before Medicaid, and the gap between low-income and high-income groups disabled by illnesses has not narrowed.[74] These findings suggest the need for expanded efforts in preventive health care, prompt intervention in acute illness, and rehabilitation to prevent long-term disability.

THE ESSENTIAL ELEMENTS OF LONG-TERM CARE

The phrase "long-term care" is generally used to describe a range of services that address the health, social, and personal care needs of persons who are unable to care for themselves because of a physical or mental impairment caused by a chronic condition.[54, 64] Long-term care can be used to accomplish one or more of the following goals: (1) maximal possible functional independence, given existing physical or mental impairments; (2) rehabilitation to restore the person to the highest level of functioning that can be sustained; (3) humane care in the least restrictive environment, when incapacity prevents independent activity; and (4) death with dignity for the terminally ill.[18] Services may be continuous or intermittent, but usually are delivered over extended periods of time to persons presumed to have a continuing need for assistance with health problems, mobility, or activities of daily living. Long-term care can be provided in a variety of settings, both inside and outside of institutions. Noninstitutional long-term care is most effective when combined with other forms of support, such as financial supplements to ensure an adequate minimum income, and the provision of adequate housing, including architectural modifications to facilitate independent functioning despite physical impairment.

Leading exponents in the field have argued that the essential elements of long term care include the following:

- *Access for all persons with enduring functional impairments*, with eligibility for services based on incapacity rather than age, income, or other criteria.[71]

- *Linkages with other forms of assistance*, such as income maintenance and help with housing.[66, 67]

- *Availability of a broad range of services*, including health care as well as various types of assistance with essential activities of daily living.[86]

- *Services provided in a variety of settings*, such as in the home, in congregate living situations, outpatient clinics, residential treatment units, day hospitals, and extended care facilities.[18]

- *Case management as a part of care*, in order to ensure proper assessment of need, linkages with resources, periodic monitoring of care, adjustment in service mix and intensity, and coordination. While these may be responsibilities assumed by clients or families, many sick persons cannot manage care and supervise providers unassisted.[18, 71]

- *High-quality services*, which are *delivered on the basis of client need* rather than solely dependent on the availability of funding or the resources and discretion of providers of care.[78, 86]

INADEQUACIES OF LONG-TERM CARE IN THE UNITED STATES

Unfortunately, long-term care in the United States falls far short of the recommended features outlined above. Instead, long-term care currently has the following deficiencies:

- *Funding determines services.* The pattern of long-term care in the United States has largely been dictated by available funding. Federal and state programs provide the major funding for long-term care. Private insurance for this type of care is virtually unavailable.[54] Long-term care is paid for largely from three government programs: Title XVIII (Medicare), Title XIX (Medicaid), and Title XX (Social Services) of the Social Security Act. Medicare, which is available to the elderly and selected groups of persons with severe and permanent disabilities, is basically a medical insurance program. As a result, it funds only a limited amount of care in a skilled nursing facility, and pays for home health services for those in need of short periods of acute, intermittent care. Only 2% of nursing home costs were covered by Medicare in 1979; approximately 2% of the total Medicare expenditures currently are used to pay for home care.[54]

  Medicaid, which funds services for the very poor, and in some states for the medically indigent, currently pays for about 50% of the costs of nursing home care.[54] Medicaid also pays for home health services, and depending on state discretion, may be used to pay for in-home personal care and medically oriented adult day health services. Less than 1% of Medicaid expenditures are used to fund noninstitutional long-term care.[54]

  Title XX of the Social Security Act is used in some states to subsidize homemaker–chore services and social day care. Present expenditures for noninstitutional social–supportive services under Title XX are approximately equal to expenditures for home health services under Medicare. However, Title XX services are only available to the very poor and, depending on state resources and discretion, to the medically indigent. In addition, Title XX home care, while longer in duration, is usually strictly limited to nonmedical types of help.[54]

The major government programs that fund long-term care have had such a substantial impact that services are now defined by what is reimbursable under the benefit structures spelled out by these government programs.[86] As a result, long-term care does not encompass the broad range of services potentially useful to the chronically ill and severely disabled. Rather, services are biased toward institutional care and toward end-stage intervention in situations of acute medical need and severe disability.[54]

- *Dominance of institutional care.* In the United States, long-term care has virtually come to mean nursing home care. This is the result of current funding policies, which reimburse institutional services but fail to adequately cover noninstitutional long-term care. In 1979 88% of all expenditures for long-term care went for care of persons in nursing homes.[54] In that year $18 billion was spent on nursing home care. The extent to which institutional expenditures are disproportionate is apparent when one considers that only about 14% of all persons with severe functional impairments are cared for in nursing homes.[17, 54]

- *Underdevelopment and fragmentation of noninstitutional services.* Noninstitutional long-term care is very poorly developed in the United States.[86] Such care encompasses a narrow range of services. There are very few providers, staffed with limited numbers of personnel. While there are about 3,000 home health agencies in the United States, over half employ fewer than five service staff.[28] There are currently about 700 adult day care programs in this country. However, the majority serve a very limited number of clients.[54] The fact that between 60% and 80% of long-term care in the community is provided by family and friends further testifies to the underdevelopment of noninstitutional resources.[50, 51]

In addition, services tend to be fragmented.[78] Home care agencies usually specialize either in medically oriented care or in supportive services (such as assistance with housekeeping and personal care). This is also true of adult day care programs, which are geared to one of three types of clients — those requiring rehabilitation, those needing medical care, or those coming for social services.[7]

The underdevelopment and fragmentation of noninstitutional services is largely attributable to the limitations imposed by service definitions, eligibility requirements, and reimbursement policies emanating from federal and state programs that fund long-term care.[78, 86] Funding for this range of services is extremely limited. In fiscal year 1978–79, Medicare home health expenditures totaled $520 million — only 2% of all

Medicare expenditures.[54] In that same year, federal and state Medicaid expenditures on home health care were $211 million, representing 1% of all Medicaid expenditures. About $481 million was spent during this same period on homemaker services under Title XX. This amounts to a total of about $1.2 billion in public expenditures on home care. It is important to note that this represents only about 7% of the amount spent on *institutional* long-term care during that year. In fact, over the course of that period, the cost of nursing home care increased by $2.7 billion — an amount that exceeded that year's total expenditures on noninstitutional long-term care.[54]

- *Eligibility determined by age and income.* Access to long-term care is largely determined by a person's age and income. Institutional long-term care is available mainly to those who qualify for Medicaid and for those wealthy enough to afford the out-of-pocket expense. In 1979 public payments covered 57% of the cost of nursing home care, with Medicaid paying almost 90% of this amount. Private payments covered 43% of institutional long-term care, with consumers paying directly for 97% of those costs.[54]

  Eligibility for noninstitutional services is also very restricted. Those eligible for Medicare (largely the elderly) can obtain medically oriented in-home services for very brief periods of time. Persons who are poor enough to qualify for assistance under Medicaid and Title XX can obtain adult day care and various types of in-home supportive services, including some personal care and home maintenance. However, both eligibility and availability of services varies widely from state to state, since states are allowed a great deal of discretion in determining which services shall be provided and for whom.[39, 75]

  Noninstitutional services, when required over long periods of time, are sufficiently costly that they cannot be purchased privately, except by the very wealthy. Insurance policies cover an exceedingly limited range of medically oriented home services, so private insurance does not really cover assistance that might be considered long-term care.

- *High cost of care.* The cost of long-term care in the United States is very high and rising at an alarming rate. Increases in nursing home expenditures have been particularly great, rising from $7.5 billion in 1973 to almost $18 billion in 1979.[52] This represents an increase of 148%, and far exceeded increases in either the consumer price index, which increased 64%, or the gross national product, which increased 81% during the same period.[54] The increased cost of nursing home care is largely due to price increases, not increases in use. In homes certified for Medicare and Medicaid reimbursement, *per diem* costs rose 55.2% between 1973 and 1977 — an increase 50% above the increase in the consumer price index.[46] It is clear from the above figures that our current approach to long-term care — to provide services only when illness results in grave incapacity, and then to deliver that care primarily in institutional settings — is excessively costly.[48]

- *Poor quality of care.* Problems relating to the quality of long-term care have been a continuing concern of the public, health professionals, and legislators. There have been recurrent scandals in the nursing home industry, and more recently similar sorts of problems have surfaced with providers of in-home services.[70, 89, 91] With both institutional and noninstitutional long-term care, quality of services is impaired for a number of reasons, the most important of which are the following: (1) inadequately trained service staff, particularly paraprofessionals; (2) shortages of nurses and aides; (3) high turnover in personnel, particularly in nursing homes; (4) very limited involvement of physicians; (5) lack of uniformity in standards of care, and absence of effective enforcement of even minimally adequate standards; and (6) lack of adequate planning and coordination of care.[62, 78, 86, 91] Recent concerns about the high cost of long-term care, coupled with the increasing fiscal constraints faced by the federal and state governments, have already led to cost containment efforts. Cuts in funding for long-term care will likely exacerbate the problems that presently contribute to poor quality services.

- *Inadequate integration of various forms of assistance.* Long-term care encompasses a variety of services, delivered by multiple, often specialized providers, in diverse settings, employing a wide range of personnel. Efforts to ensure coordination are limited and quite often ineffective, especially in noninstitutional long-term care.[86] Concern about this deficiency has provided some of the impetus for recent efforts to establish case management or brokerage agencies, such as those currently being developed under the federal channeling demonstration.[42] Providing better coordination of services will not resolve the most critical problems, which are caused by the institutional bias of care and the gross underdevelopment of noninstitutional services. However, mechanisms need to be developed to provide better communication between providers and more complete integration of the various care components. In addition, the relationship of long-term care to other types of assistance needs to be closely examined. The provision of long-term care needs to be coupled with efforts to ensure adequate housing, nutrition, income, and medical services during episodes of acute illness. At present, insufficient attention has been given to coordinating these diverse forms of assistance.[35, 48, 66, 67]

In summary, long-term care in the United States is currently very costly, and rather ineffective in meeting the needs of the majority of those who have chronic illnesses and disabilities that substantially impair daily functioning. Delivery of services is heavily biased toward nursing home care. Noninstitutional services, such as home care and adult day care, are underdeveloped and fragmented. Available funding largely determines which services will be provided and which populations can obtain long-term care. Because of restrictions in reimbursable benefits, only a limited range of services is available, and these are available largely to the very poor, the aged, or the very wealthy, who must pay out of pocket for the cost of care. The quality of care is highly variable and often exceedingly poor, particularly in institutional settings. Coordination of services within the same setting as well as across different settings, is very limited and often completely absent.

We would now like to turn to a discussion of the political, social, and economic factors that shape long-term care in the United States.

POLITICAL, SOCIAL, AND ECONOMIC FACTORS AFFECTING LONG-TERM CARE IN THE UNITED STATES

THE ACUTE CARE AND INSTITUTIONAL FOCUS OF PROGRAMS FUNDING LONG-TERM CARE

Long-term care is currently defined by public policy as a health service in the technical sense that it is incorporated in, and paid for through, programs that fund medical care. The enactment of Medicare and Medicaid in 1965 firmly established long-term care as a health policy predominantly of nursing home institutionalization, to be financed either privately or through the public pay mechanisms of Medicaid. This has profoundly affected the scope, character, and cost of long-term care services.[65]

Medicine has placed primary emphasis on disease, acute care, modern hospitals, and advanced technology, and on financial rewards for specialists and subspecialists who treat disease. A wide range of health policies, including those governing the Medicare and Medicaid programs, as well as policies for biomedical research, health manpower, and health facilities construction have reinforced this bias.

The bias toward acute medical care in the allocation of public resources has resulted in a low priority for long-term care. Nursing homes have been required to perform multiple functions — custodial care, treatment of acute illness, rehabilitation, chronic care, and terminal care — without the resources to perform these tasks.[91] Only a small percentage of health care funding has been allocated for noninstitutional approaches to long-term care.[86] Alternative policies for income maintenance and housing have not been adequately considered.[66] Acute care and institutional services, funded under Medicare and Medicaid, have been dominant, and have consumed resources that otherwise could have supported such policies.[67]

PUBLIC PERCEPTIONS: INCREASING CONCERN ABOUT HEALTH CARE COSTS

Public perceptions of the role of government have a major impact on health policies for the elderly and for other groups in need of long-term care. These perceptions are changing.

In the 1960s the problem was defined as lack of access to good medical care and the threat of financial catastrophe for those who became seriously ill. The answer was reflected in Medicare, Medicaid, a variety of outreach programs, and the development of medical resources — each with a large federal contribution.

The health issues of the 1980s are no longer defined in terms of access to services. The major concern with health care is largely with its high and rapidly rising cost and how to contain those costs. Proposed policy solutions do not address the hospital and physician reimbursement policies that have contributed significantly to increasing costs. Instead, policymakers are suggesting that costs can be reduced through stimulation of competition in the private sector, and the removal of government regulation.[34, 41, 91] The mood is one of mistrust of government and its officials, skepticism about the ability of government to deal effectively with complex social problems, and a desire to cut taxes; it is against government regulation and spending.

ECONOMIC CONSTRAINTS

In the 1980s, the issues of long-term care policy in the United States will increasingly be affected by resource limitations, and by the highly politicized decision making that characterizes eras of fluctuating economic realities. The state of the economy affects the manner in which social problems are defined. When the economy is growing at a rapid rate, optimism abounds and generous resources are more likely to become available to deal with social problems of all types.[72] But when economic growth slows, policies tend to favor less costly, more limited social programs, particularly for those populations that are assessed as low in productivity (*e.g.*, the poor and aged).

Fiscal crisis is a term applied to the financial difficulties of a variety of governments in the United States. Fiscal crisis occurs as a consequence of the tendency for government expenditures to rise faster than revenues. Popular and corporate resistance to taxation has been one factor preventing revenues from rising as rapidly as expenditures. The current fiscal crisis and taxpayer reform movements, taking various forms including Proposition 13-style tax revolts, have contributed to severe financial problems for local and state governments. Inflation and budget cuts at the federal level are exacerbating these problems.

While costs are escalating, there are definite limits on funding for health and social services. From above, there are federal limits such as the federal ceiling on Title XX funds and the cap on Medicaid and an attempt to shift costs to the states. From below, there are fiscal crises and tax revolts at local and state levels. Caught in the squeeze, health and social services are involved in a fiscal crisis of their own. During the 1980s, all levels of government will increasingly seek to cut costs and shift expenditures to other jurisdictions.

These conditions have created pressures to redefine the funding relationships among all levels of government. This is a particular problem for Medicaid-funded services. The rapid increase in Medicaid expenditures is outrunning the capacities of state governments to raise the necessary revenues. State Medicaid expenditures are rising rapidly (1) because federal policy requires states to meet their percentage share of total Medicaid expenditures, (2) because of the rapid increase in the cost of medical care, and (3) because of the political risks that have restrained provider and hospital cost-containment strategies. As a result, Medicaid expenditures have risen far more rapidly than revenue increases, creating serious fiscal difficulties for states (as well as for local governments where they share in states' costs).

In response, some states have reduced the number of beneficiaries by lowering the level of income allowed for eligibility, reduced the scope of optional services, reduced the duration of mandated and optional benefits; they have held rates of reimbursement for hospitals, physicians, and nursing homes constant, or increased them more slowly than costs have risen.

As fiscal pressures are spread throughout all levels of government, the major issues are the following: (1) How dramatically will efforts to limit or reduce spending alter current priorities and benefits? (2) What are the consequences of the resultant shifting configurations of long-term care priorities, service foci, target populations, and benefits?

With increasing economic constraints, we can expect intensified power struggles among powerful and vested interests that wish to forward their perspectives of particular problems. Of relevance to long-term care will be the shifting definitions and power struggles that will emerge from the differing ideas and interpretations of what the long-term care needs are, of who the needy are, of the rights (if any) of the population in need of such services, of their blame for current economic problems, and of the extent to which the poor, old, and disabled should be required to sacrifice as program cutbacks ensue.

DECENTRALIZATION

Compounding the increased difficulty of making decisions in the face of economic constraints, is the decentralization of major health and social programs. Decentralization, which reached full swing under Nixon in the 1970s, has now resurged under the Reagan administration. While Nixon employed decentralization in the 1970s as a mechanism for curtailing the growth of federal programs, the result was to transfer the pressures for underwriting program expansion from the federal to state and local governments.[35, 36] Decentralization has also exacerbated fiscal and tax pressures at both levels of government, creating a hospitable environment for taxpayer revolts.

The decentralization policy trend of the 1970s has been accompanied by the fragmentation and diversification of policy in many social problem areas (*e.g.*, Title XX homemaker services), as national policy goals give way to more autonomous and *variable* state and local policy choices across multiple programs, and political and geographic jurisdictions. Further, with a myriad of decision-makers, authorities, and subgovernments that may act at their own discretion, it is extremely difficult to focus with assurance on particular targets of intervention.

Under the broadly defined and decentralized block-grant type enactments in which Congress only vaguely specifies its intention, there is increased potential for the politicization of state and local policymaking and program implementation. The resultant ambiguity provides opportunities for political actors, vested interests, and active health professions organizations to "create" and shape large segments of health and social policies *outside* of the public legislative process—through the less visible implementation and administrative processes.[69] An important issue for long-term care policy is the degree to which increasing decentralization of programs for the poor, aged, and disabled fosters politically motivated, rather than need-based, priorities and allocations. Certainly in the past, decentralization has created wide variations in income, health, and social service eligibility and benefits for the poor, the elderly, blind, and disabled across the states.[39]

A major question that must be asked is whether particular long-term policy goals and priorities should be determined nationally or pushed down on the states and localities—thereby becoming subject to their varying fiscal pressures, resources, and politics. Given the current structure of programs relevant to long-term care, the "national" policy is composed of multiple, variable, noncomparable policies and programs, each of which is different in different states.

Even more important, because the benefits provided by the federal–state programs that now underwrite long-term care are heavily influenced by a state's willingness to continue underwriting the costs, there are mounting pressures for state level policies of retrenchment (cutbacks) as fiscal constraints on state government are rising. Because the most disadvantaged are heavily dependent on state-determined benefits, they are extremely vulnerable in this period of economic flux.

Of particular significance is the Reagan administration's intent to build upon and augment the decentralization and block-grant strategies that are Nixon's "new federalism" legacy of the 1970s. Most crucial in terms of long-term care policy is the administration's federal cap on Medicaid spending, for it will further engender fiscal strain in the states and localities—simultaneously augmenting both the need for alternatives to institutionalization, and the economic conditions that are likely to preclude the possibility of the development of anything more than the most symbolic community-based long-term care policies.[38]

STATE-LEVEL GOVERNMENT: INCREASED RESPONSIBILITY FOR LONG-TERM CARE POLICY AND FINANCING

The decentralization of fiscal and political responsibility from the federal to the state level for major health and social services programs for the poor, disabled, and aged has had a major impact on the availability of various forms of assistance to persons who require long-term care. Such assistance is provided from many different sources—not only Title XIX (Medicaid), but also Title XVIII (Medicare), Title XVI (Supplementary Security Income—SSI), and Title XX (Social Services) of the Social Security Act, as well as the Older Americans Act.[39, 65, 91] All of these federal programs, with the exception of Medicare, provide significant policy and program discretion for the states.

The wide discretion permitted states by federal policies affecting long-term care creates great inequities among states and also creates a variety of problems in determining eligibility, ensuring availability of services across program jurisdictions, coordinating benefits and services, reimbursing services, setting and enforcing standards, and evaluating the effect of alternative policies.

These discretionary policies also create problems relating to accountability and cost control. The major federal programs now funding long-term care were created independently of each other with little or no consideration of provision of long-term care services. There are separate authorizations and appropriations for each of the programs, and each is administered by a different agency at the federal and state levels.

Efforts to assess the impact of long-term care programs are difficult because of the general problems of accountability inherent in federal programs, which are complicated by multiple state policies and accounting systems used for the different decentralized programs.[35, 40] Thus, the increased policy discretion given to states and localities in the 1970s decreased federal capacity to assess the impact of federal funds, particularly in terms of specific population groups served, such as the elderly.[8, 88, 90]

THE FEDERAL STRATEGY: RESEARCH AND DEMONSTRATION IN LONG-TERM CARE

Current federal policy for new initiatives in long-term care is largely limited to research and demonstration efforts. An important dimension of current federal demonstration efforts is their affinity for management–administrative strategies. As an essentially bureaucratic reform measure, the focus is on the screening, functional assessment, and case management of older persons, as well as the integration of funding streams to achieve the desired community-based continuum of care.[4]

Such long-term care policy strategies are consistent with our prior observations that "government-financed service strategies are largely based upon the theory that direct services are not as necessary as the more indirect services that link and provide access for the client to the (theoretically) already available services."[35]

Many of the most popular long-term care policy options now under consideration continue this trend toward indirect services. Based on the assumption that unnecessary institutionalization results from the fragmentation of services (thus necessitating a planning–coordination–management strategy), such policies do little to address the accumulated stresses of low income and loss of social support that dramatically accelerate the risk of institutionalization.

Such bureaucratic reform efforts in long-term care are consonant with the growing national concern over economic scarcity that has made it imperative to find intervention strategies that will not add to either costs or the expectations of the public.

PROJECTED INCREASES IN THE ELDERLY POPULATION

Demographic projections indicate that by the year 2000, the total United States population will be 260.4 million, with almost 32 million (12.2%) being 65 or older, and the number of those who are 85 or older is expected to double — to 3.8 million.[13] Of most significance for long-term care policies in the short term, are the predictions that "between now and 2025 the oldest part of the older population will grow most rapidly, then be reversed between 2000 and 2025 and return to the current trend after 2025 when all rates of growth are much slower, especially in the younger aged."[13]

The projections of an increasing elderly population, coupled with projections of the growth of the total number of disabled as they too have longer life expectancies, have led to predictions of an alarming increase in the need for long-term care.

Based on these and other reports, the White House Conference on Aging Technical Committee on Health Services has projected that by 2010 "we will require half again as many health care providers . . . as we have today just to keep pace" with the older population. Estimates are that by 2030, 2.6 million older persons will be in nursing homes (more than doubling of the total nursing home population) and the number of physician visits is estimated to more than double for elderly — from 187 million visits in 1977 to more than 443 million in 2030.[92] The White House Conference on Aging report predicts a serious shortfall of trained academic geriatric physicians and nurses unless traditional disciplinary educational approaches and policies are changed. This report also predicts a shortage of at least 75,000 nurses in nursing homes alone.

Many of these straight line projections tend to anticipate only incremental variances from current trends in both health status of the population and public policies. Thus, most projections are predicated on an assumption of the continued dominance of the role of medicine in the health of the aged and disabled — and of physician visits, acute care hospitalization, and nursing homes as the major arsenal of services for the long-term care needs of the population.

In contrast, we would argue that many of these projections tend to be of limited and short-range utility, for they largely ignore the post-2025 and post-2050 demographic population trends, as well as potential dramatic improvements in health status.

Any effort to predict future trends for long-term care must take into account more than current population projections. To improve the accuracy of such predictions, other important variables to consider would include projected changes in the health of the population (and particularly of old people); the anticipated economic conditions and political climate; the likely configuration of health and other public policies for the aged, disabled, and poor; and the prospective roles of nursing *vis-a-vis* the long-term care population and the organization of care around the nursing profession and long-term care. Obviously, the policies needed and the role and opportunities for nursing in long-term care are contingent on all of these factors.

One of the most significant of the potential alternate futures would be the realization of the Fries and Crapo projections, with the older population experiencing dramatically improved health as a result of a major delay in the onset of chronic disease.[47] Older persons would then live out (in a healthy state) a biologically determined natural life span of approximately 85 yr.* If, as Fries and Crapo argue, the advent of chronic illness is postponed through life-style changes, the period of a vigorous life will be extended. Thus, the implications of what they call "the rectangular curve" is the improvement of physical, mental, and social functioning "within very broad biological limits."[47]

---

* Fries and Crapo suggest that the maximum life span can be fixed at about 100 yr and the median life span at about 85. A conflicting view expressed by Schatzkin is that major gains in life expectancy are possible through life-style changes, such as reduction in animal fat intake and cigarette smoking and through such medical measures as the effective control of hypertension with drugs. In Schatzkin's view, "The precise biological upper limit to life will remain elusive, but prolongation of life is statistically and biologically possible."[82]

The rectangular curve projection would call for dramatically different long-term care policies and health personnel, aimed largely at prevention and life style changes — in contrast to policies and personnel required by the simple straight line projections that hold constant all but the demographic variables. In all cases, however, a growing elderly population is projected.

ANTICIPATED DECREASE IN THE CARE PROVIDED BY FAMILY AND FRIENDS

Currently, most of the long-term care given to persons who reside outside of institutions is provided by family and friends.[51, 21] However, population projections suggest there will be fewer resources to provide such care in the future. Currently, spouses are the major source of support for about 50% of all elderly and impaired individuals. However, the availability of a spouse will decrease in the future as a result of differential mortality rates between older men and women. The projected increase in the elderly population will be mainly among widowed and single persons.[54]

Furthermore, there will, in the future, be fewer family members available to provide assistance to the elderly and disabled. This is likely for two reasons: (1) The numbers of dependents is increasing faster than the number of caretakers; and (2) the number of adult women available to serve as care agents is decreasing because of increases in the percentage of working women. First, the numbers of persons over age 75 is increasing. Four-generational families are now commonplace. Moreover, the number of persons over age 65 is increasing in proportion to the numbers of adults of working age. In 1980 there were about 18 elderly persons for every 100 working-age adults. Projections indicate that 50 yr from now, there will be nearly twice as many elderly who might potentially be dependent upon that same number of working adults.[83] In addition, there will be fewer women who are able to care for elderly and disabled family members. Employment among women is expected to increase from 48% in 1977 to 57% in 1985 and to exceed 60% by 1990.[16] The above statistics suggest that in the future persons who require long-term care may have to rely more on the formal care system to provide needed assistance.

We would like to conclude this chapter by discussing the ways in which the profession of nursing is likely to be affected by developments in the field of long-term care. We will begin by describing the significant role nurses currently play in the delivery of long-term care in the United States. Next, we present evidence that shows there is presently a shortage of nurses working in long-term care, and why this undersupply is likely to continue in the future. In a final section, we will explore the ways in which nursing practice, training, and research are likely to change as a result of the challenges and opportunities presented by the increased involvement of nurses in long-term care.

CHALLENGE FOR NURSING: THE GROWING IMPORTANCE OF LONG-TERM CARE AND GERONTOLOGY IN NURSING PRACTICE, TRAINING, AND RESEARCH

More than 100,000 registered nurses are working in the field of long-term care. More nurses are employed in long-term care than any other professional group. Registered nurses represent about 68% of all professionals delivering services in nursing homes.[55] Nurses account for the majority of the total staff employed by home health agencies.[20] Moreover, the number of nurses working in long-term care is increasing rapidly. During the period from 1972 to 1979, there was a 42% increase in the number of nurses working in long-term care facilities, and a 200% increase in the number of nurses employed by home health agencies.[5, 30, 32]

SHORTAGE OF NURSES IN LONG-TERM CARE

There is some disagreement about whether the supply of nurses expected to work in long-term care will keep up with future demands.[23] A number of projections indicate that supply and demand for nurses will be in balance over the next 10 yr.[15, 23, 56] However, a careful analysis of factors affecting supply and demand suggests that these projections may seriously underestimate the potential for nurse shortages.[68] Recent evidence indicates that there may be serious shortages of nurses, particularly in the fields of long-term care and gerontology.[55, 59, 92] Factors that contribute to the undersupply of nurses in long-term care include the following: (1) growth of the elderly population, particularly those persons over 75, and a concomitant significant increase in the population that requires long-term services, particularly nursing home care;[92] (2) noncompetitive salaries, limited opportunities for career advancement, and unfavorable work conditions for nurses working in nursing homes and other settings that provide long-term care;[55] (3) anticipated expansion of nursing roles and functions, especially in care of the elderly and persons requiring outpatient and long-term care;[55, 92] (4) expansion of agencies and programs providing noninstitutional long-term services;[24, 57] (5) decreases in applicants to and graduates produced by nurse training programs;[58] (6) the limited numbers of nurses prepared to work in long-term care;[15, 55] (7) the relatively small number of programs that provide training in gerontologic nursing and long-term care;[29, 31, 55, 61] and (8) limitations in the amount of funding available for nurse training in these specialty areas.[6, 55, 87]

Based on projections of increases in the elderly population and, in particular, in the numbers of elderly in nursing homes, a technical paper developed for the 1981 White House Conference on Aging predicts a shortfall of about 75,000 nurses in institutional long-term care alone.[92] Conservative estimates indicate that 101,000 registered nurses will be needed in nursing homes by 1985, and that there will be an average of 6,200 nursing positions opening up every year in nursing homes.[1]

A number of experts both within and outside of nursing have argued that more nurses are needed to provide long-term care *today*, given current shortages of professionals in nursing homes and the limited amount of long-term care delivered by registered nurses to very ill, disabled, and elderly patients.[3, 44, 59, 60, 62] Statistics from a recent study indicate there may be fewer than 9 nurses per 100 patients in skilled nursing facilities (SNF) and only about 3 nurses per 100 patients in intermediate care facilities (ICF).[44] This same study reveals that the average nursing home patient receives direct care by a registered nurse a total of 12 min per day in a SNF, and only 7 min per day in a ICF.[44] The problems related to the absence of adequate nursing care in nursing homes have been thoroughly documented by Kayser-Jones and Vladeck.[62, 91]

LOW STATUS, SALARIES, AND BENEFITS FOR NURSES IN LONG-TERM CARE

Shortages of nurses in long-term care are likely to continue for some time in the future as a result of the low status given nurses employed in long-term care, and because of the low salaries, limited career opportunities, and largely unfavorable work conditions for nurses working in this field.[55] Over 80% of those nurses who provide long-term care are employed in nursing homes. Long-term care facilities presently pay lower salaries and give substantially fewer benefits to nurses than do hospitals and other employers.[55] For example, among nurses working in nursing homes in 1977, only 9.2% had paid vacations and sick leave, only 11% had retirement programs, and only 10.8% had health or life insurance. This contrasts with hospital nurses surveyed during the same period, all of whom had higher salaries with paid vacations and holidays, most of whom had shift differential pay and paid overtime, and virtually all of whom had health insurance and retirement plans.[55] This situation is markedly different from other countries, such as Scotland and the Scandinavian nations, where salary *bonuses* are provided to staff who work in geriatrics and long-term care.[60, 62] Problems faced by nurses working in American nursing homes are compounded by chronic shortages of personnel, lack of administrative support and leadership, and limited opportunities for staff development and career advancement.[55, 62, 91] Given these conditions, it is not surprising that nursing homes have an astonishingly high rate of transition in personnel. A recent survey in California reports that the average turnover of service staff in long-term care facilities was 240% during 1978.[84] This research shows that 90% of the facilities surveyed had a turnover rate of 147% or greater.[84]

EXPANDED ROLES AND JOB OPPORTUNITIES FOR NURSES IN LONG-TERM CARE

The need for nurses is likely to outstrip supply for yet another reason: nursing roles and functions are likely to expand, particularly in settings where nurses care for the elderly and persons with medically stable chronic illnesses and disabilities. One recent report suggests that in the future nurses are likely to assume up to 50% of the outpatient care now provided by physicians.[92] A number of nurse leaders are currently advocating an expanded role for nurses in long-term care institutions.[3, 60] A pioneering study by Kane and colleagues, which describes the need for increased physician involvement in geriatrics, foresees an expanded role for nurses and estimates that as many as 20,000 geriatric nurse practitioners will be required, depending on the amount of responsibility delegated by physicians.[59] These projections are predicated upon the physician's assuming the primary role in directing care of the elderly. If physicians in the future do not play a greater role in geriatrics and in long-term care than they have in the past, nurses will continue to assume major responsibility for delivering, managing, and coordinating services for the elderly and disabled.[3]

The number of agencies that provide noninstitutional long-term services is relatively small at the present time. However, the growth of these programs, and in particular the number of nurses they employ, is quite impressive.[24, 57] The number of nurses who work in home health agencies has tripled over the past 7 yr. While only slightly over 6,600 nurses were working in home care agencies in 1972, this number has grown to exceed 20,000 by 1979.[30, 32] This trend is likely to continue in the future because of government and public concern about the high costs of institutional long-term care. Expansion of community-based services becomes a politically attractive solution because it is easier to divert the population in need into less costly noninstitutional alternatives than to attempt to contain hospital costs or control physicians' fees. The National League for Nursing (NLN) reports that over one-third of all community health agencies surveyed in 1978 showed they had vacancies in registered nurse positions.[73] This shortage of nurses is likely to become more severe because of the growth of noninstitutional services and increases in the population requiring long-term care.

PROBLEMS WITH RECRUITMENT AND TRAINING OF NURSES

Current shortages of nurses in long-term care are likely to be affected by still another trend. There appears to be a significant decrease in applicants to and graduates from programs that train nurses.[58] This is a significant development, since maintenance and development of new nurses is crucial to the supply–demand balance; the pool of inactive nurses cannot be counted on to correct shortages. The supply of new nurses has not increased significantly since 1974. In 1978 a decline in admissions was recorded, the first since the 1960s.[58] If this trend continues–and there is no reason to expect it will not–it could result in a serious shortage of nurses, and particularly affect the availability of nurses for such traditionally low-status areas as gerontologic nursing and long-term care.

In addition to the above factors, which portend an undersupply of nurses for long-term care, there are relatively few nurses who are currently prepared to work effectively in organizations that provide services for the elderly and disabled. Nurses who work in nursing homes generally have limited training in the special problems of long-term or geriatric patients. This is partly due to nursing homes' inability to attract and retain highly qualified personnel because of lower pay scales and poor working conditions, but also contributory is the relatively recent development of specialty training in long-term care and gerontologic nursing.[15, 55] Despite the fact that the American Nurses' Association (ANA) is the only professional organization with a formal recognition program for geriatric practitioners, by 1979 certification had been given to only 217 gerontologic nurses.[77] Moreover, to date only about 1,000 nurse practitioners have been prepared in geriatrics and related fields, such as adult health care and family medicine.[55] The potentially severe shortages of nurses prepared to work as geriatric nurse practitioners becomes very apparent when one considers that Kane and colleagues predict a need for 12,000 geriatric nurse practitioners by the year 2010, assuming moderate delegation of responsibilities from physicians to nurses. That projection swells to 20,000 should nurses assume what Kane and colleagues view as a maximal level of responsibility for the care of the elderly.[59]

THE SLOW DEVELOPMENT OF SPECIALTY TRAINING IN GERONTOLOGIC NURSING AND LONG-TERM CARE

The short supply of nurses with specific training and expertise in long-term care and gerontology is largely due to the very recent development of nursing programs that offer specialized education in these fields. There has been an effort to build geriatric nursing content into programs preparing persons for initial registered nurse licensure. However, the majority of entry-level programs include little, if any, theoretical or clinical content in geriatrics or long-term care.[61] More substantial educational preparation is available in nurse practitioner and graduate-level nursing programs.[55] However, this sort of advanced nurse training in gerontology and long-term care has only been available for a short period of time. As recently as 1977 there were only eight schools of nursing in the United States that had graduate programs in gerontologic nursing; many of these programs were in a rather embryonic stage of development.[14] By 1980 the number of schools offering specialty training had increased to over 20.[61] Currently, of the 70 federally supported advanced nurse training and nurse practitioner training programs, 47 have substantial geriatric content and 23 are specifically designed to prepare gerontologic specialists.[55] There is, however, a great deal of variation in the quality and content of gerontologic nurse training throughout the United States, in large part due to constraints such as inadequate numbers of trained faculty, insufficient development of clinical geriatric training sites, funding constraints, and lack of educational background of students accepted for training.[55, 61]

The relative underdevelopment of nurse training in long-term care and gerontology is closely related to limitations in the amount of funding available to develop and maintain programs in these specialty areas.[55] Much of the impetus for the establishment of geriatric training programs has been provided by the allocation of federal funding, through grants and contracts awarded to schools of nursing under such provisions as the Nursing Training Act of 1975 (Public Law 94-364) and Titles VII and VIII of the Public Health Service Act (Nurse Training Act, 1979), including Section 822 of the Public Health Service Act (which funds training of geriatric nurse practitioners), Section 821 (which funds advanced nurse training) and Section 820 (which funds continuing education).[29, 45, 55] In fiscal year 1980 the federal government provided over $2 million for geriatric nurse practitioner programs.[55] A comparable amount was spent on Advanced Nurse Training grants for the preparation of gerontologic nurses at the graduate level.[87] Another $1.4 million was allocated for curriculum revision and continuing education to upgrade skills of entry-level students and practicing nurses.[29, 87]

It is clear that many of the current training efforts would not have been possible without the influx of federal funding directed at improving nursing education in long-term care and gerontology. Nevertheless, federal support for this sort of specialty training has been quite limited, considering the magnitude of current and projected shortages of nurses prepared to work in long-term care. A significant concern in the future will be the increasing limitations in funding that supports specialty training. The proposed federal budget for fiscal years 1981 and 1982 calls for drastic cuts in funding for nurse training programs and assistance to nursing students. If the proposed recissions are approved, by 1982 funds for advanced nurse training will be only one-tenth of the 1980 level, and nurse practitioner program monies will be cut in half.[6]

Two new initiatives were proposed for fiscal year 1982. One of these initiatives would have funded the establishment of demonstration nursing home centers that would have emphasized nurse training and the development of client care models, at a projected funding level of $2.7 million. The other initiative would have provided money for the development of short-term, work–study programs designed to increase the knowledge and skills of nurses employed in both nursing homes and community agencies that provide long-term care.[55] Given the current move to keep federal spending to a minimum, it is unlikely that new initiatives such as these will be funded.

In summary, although nurses represent the largest group of professionals currently providing long-term care in the United States, there is a shortage of nursing personnel, and this short supply is likely to continue in the future unless there is substantial progress made in improving (1) the status, role, salaries, benefits, and work conditions of nurses working in long-term care; and (2) the availability and quality of nurse training in the specialty areas of gerontology and long-term care. Given the growth of the number of persons — particularly the elderly — who need long-term care, and given the decreasing availability of family and friends to care for these persons, there will likely be an increasing need for specially trained nurses in the future.[54, 92] We would now like to outline how nursing practice, training, research, and professional activities are likely to change as a result of future developments in long-term care.

LONG-TERM CARE: IMPACT ON THE PRACTICE OF CLINICAL NURSING

Increasing numbers of persons suffer functional impairments and physical disability as a result of chronic illness. Indeed, it is chronic disease, rather than acute illness, that presents the major health problem in the United States today. Chronic diseases are the leading causes of morbidity, mortality, and physical impairment, substantially reducing the number of years of vigorous, functionally independent life — especially for older Americans and the very poor.[47, 74] Nursing practice is increasingly being affected by the preponderance of persons who require assistance in preventing, postponing, recovering from, and managing chronic illnesses and the functional impairments that accompany disease or disability. We anticipate that nursing practice will undergo some profound changes, among them the following:

- *Increased emphasis on prevention, health education, primary care, and long-term services.* Given the dominant health problems in this country (*i.e.*, chronic illnesses) and the aging of the population, in the future nurses are likely to become more involved in primary care, prevention, health education, and long-term care for the impaired elderly and disabled. Acute medical care is likely to be required mainly at the onset and for exacerbations of chronic disease. Moreover, acute medical intervention will probably be oriented toward preventing or postponing disability or death that might result from an acute episode of chronic illness. There is likely to be considerably more emphasis on primary care and keeping people healthy through modification of life-styles and early detection of potentially chronic problems. Moreover, since chronic illness, once it develops, is by definition not resolvable by medical intervention, nurses will be involved in providing health education, temporary assistance, and, when necessary, long-term care for those disabled by disease. Unless medicine is able to prevent or cure diseases that now cause chronic illnesses and impairments — thus realizing the Fries and Crapo "rectangular curve" theory — nurses will become increasingly involved in long-term care, as the population ages, and as medical technology allows life to be sustained, even under conditions of grave physical disability.

- *More nurses in ambulatory clinics, home care agencies, and extended care facilities.* Due to the increase in chronic disease and the growth of the aged population, nurses will likely become more involved in care of persons in outpatient settings, in the home, in adult day programs, and in extended care facilities. Currently 60% of all nurses (some 601,000) work in hospitals.[5] We expect that percentage to drop significantly in the next decade, as more emphasis is placed on noninstitutional services and earlier discharge of patients from acute care settings. Long-term care is currently the fastest growing segment of the health services industry. Projections indicate that the number of persons in nursing homes will double over the next 50 yr, should the same percentage of disabled and elderly use this service as do current populations.[54] Assuming the same ratio of nurses to patients, this means that twice as many nurses would be required just to keep pace with increases in the population in need.[55, 92] If the advice of some nurse leaders is taken seriously, and nurses assume a major leadership role in nursing homes, working for improved staffing and quality of care, then a significantly larger number of nurses will be involved in institutional long-term care.[3, 62]

  In addition, we anticipate an increase in nurses working in outpatient clinics and other ambulatory care settings. Efforts to control use of inpatient services are likely to result in increased reliance on treatment in noninstitutional environments. For persons in need of long-term care, home care and day health programs have become attractive alternatives, as both state and federal governments focus on efforts to divert long-term patients into services perceived to be less costly than nursing homes. We anticipate substantial increases in the number of nurses choosing to work in home care and adult day care.

- *Changes in the roles and functions of nurses.* Roles and functions of nurses are likely to be affected significantly by the prevalence of chronic illness and functional impairment. We anticipate that nurses will assume increasing responsibility for primary care, particularly for elderly persons.[59] In hospitals nurses will likely become more involved in teaching patients self-care so that acute exacerbations and disability related to chronic disease can be postponed or prevented. If nurses assume leadership roles in nursing homes, it will signficantly alter their functions and responsibilities. Greater attention might be paid to providing better medical management for patients, with nurses taking a more active role in the early detection and treatment of preventable illness and impairment. In addition, nurses might perform a central role in ensuring that institutional environments are more hospitable and less damaging to residents.[3, 62]

Probably the most significant changes in nursing roles and functions will occur for nurses working in noninstitutional long-term care.[78] At present, the overwhelming majority of nurses working in home care are oriented toward short-term intermittent care of persons recently discharged from an acute care hospital.[20] If funding restrictions are loosened to allow agencies to provide more long-term care to patients at home, nurses' roles and functions will be significantly different. Moves are currently underway to substantially alter the character of in-home services in the United States.[54] It is likely that within the next decade, home care and other noninstitutional long-term services will expand significantly.[24] In addition, the scope of benefits will likely be enlarged, with more emphasis placed on supportive services, such as housekeeping, personal care, and assistance with other essential activities of daily living.[86]

In response to the above trends, nurses' roles are likely to change in a number of important respects, among them the following: (1) Nurses will increasingly become managers rather than providers of care, as relatively more services are delivered by paraprofessionals and professionals of other disciplines, and as coordination of care becomes more complex. (2) Nurses will be less exclusively concerned with medical intervention. The range of services they perform will expand to include patient education; psychosocial counseling of patients and their families; assessment of the person's functional impairments, as well as environmental and social resources and constraints; and monitoring and supervision of care. (3) Nurses will become increasingly active in the supervision and in-service training of paraprofessionals, as these personnel supply greater amounts of direct care to the long term patient.[78, 86]

THE NEED FOR BETTER NURSE TRAINING IN GERONTOLOGY AND LONG-TERM CARE

Because of the relatively slow development of specialized training in long-term care and gerontology for nurses, and because of current and projected shortages of suitably prepared professionals, leading exponents in the field have argued for expansion of nursing education, in these specialty areas.[1, 2, 55, 59, 61] The Health Resources Administration recently developed a very comprehensive report on health personnel issues in long-term care.[55] This report makes a number of important recommendations for improving training of nurses, among them the following: (1) inclusion and strengthening of gerontologic content in initial and advanced nursing education programs; (2) development of a model curriculum in long-term care that is integrated throughout the total educational program of health practitioners; (3) interdisciplinary training in long-term care (so nurses work with other health professionals during the course of their educational experience); (4) expansion of training sites to include more clinical experience in nursing homes for nursing students; (5) strengthening of community nursing, with specific training in primary care, ambulatory care, and restorative care, so that nurses receive preparation in how to maintain clients' functional independence and family integrity; and (6) adequate in-service training programs that provide opportunities for service staff to upgrade their skills in the areas of gerontologic nursing and long-term care. Similar recommendations have been made by nurse educators, and by the Division of Nursing, United States Department of Health and Human Services.[31, 61, 76]

RESEARCH IN GERONTOLOGIC NURSING AND LONG-TERM CARE

Nursing research in the fields of long-term care and gerontology is still quite limited. Kayser-Jones, in a review of recently published gerontologic nursing research, surveyed five leading nursing journals concerned with care of the elderly.[61] Her search revealed only 44 research articles, two of which reviewed existing research in gerontologic nursing. Of the remaining 42 articles, 12 had a clinical focus, seven were concerned with attitudes of health professionals toward the aged, nine dealt with psychosocial problems of the elderly, seven addressed problems of the institutionalized elderly, three focussed on health needs of elderly persons in the community, two were on human sexuality and aging, and a final two focussed on minority aged, specifically Blacks. Kayser-Jones found this research limited in scope and in depth, and argues for better preparation of nurses in both theory and research in the field of gerontology; and expansion of nursing research on community and institutional care of the aged, more cross-cultural research on delivery of health services, and investigations that focus on such clinical problems as incontinence, confusion, immobility, and the use of sedative–hypnotic drugs in the elderly.

We agree with Kayser-Jones that nurses must become more actively involved in gerontologic nursing research. We think the same arguments hold for nurses conducting research in the broader area of long-term care. There is a great need for nursing research on a number of important topics, among them the following: (1) identification of the key factors that currently affect the delivery, organization, and quality of nursing and related long-term services, delivered in both institutional and noninstitutional settings; (2) the cost-effectiveness of different models of nursing home care and community-based long-term services; (3) clinical research on the needs and problems of elderly and disabled persons who receive long-term nursing care; and (4) the effectiveness of alternative clinical strategies designed to ameliorate problems commonly experienced by persons who require long-term care.

NURSING AS A POLITICAL FORCE FOR RESHAPING PUBLIC POLICIES

It has long been part of nurses' professional responsibility to see to it that appropriate services are provided to persons who require long-term care. To accomplish this goal, nurses must look beyond the narrow confines of nursing practice, nurse training, and nursing research. In particular, it is important that nursing play a prominent role in shaping public policies in long-term care, since such policies directly determine the amounts and kinds of services patients receive, who is eligible to receive care, and how the practice of nursing is structured in settings where long-term care is provided.

To conclude this chapter, we outline some ways in which nurses can have an impact on future policies and programs concerned with long-term care. Nurses constitute a powerful political force. Numbering over 1.4 million, nurses account for the largest number and percentage of all health professionals in the United States.[55, 81] Nurses have long made their views known on issues related to professional practice, education, health care, and nursing research. However, nurses have not used their influence as effectively to achieve needed reforms in long-term care. By working through their professional organizations and by educating legislators, nurses as individuals and in groups can bring about substantial changes in a number of critical areas, among them the following:

- *Ensuring appropriate health services for persons receiving long-term care.* In the future, it is likely there will be efforts to reduce the amount of health services provided for persons receiving long-term care. Despite the fact that long-term care—particularly nursing home care—is currently paid for out of "health monies," and relies on a "medical model" for delivery of services, there is overwhelming evidence that the amount of long-term care provided by health professionals is extremely limited. A number of authorities have argued that medical and nursing care for long-term patients is inadequate, particularly in institutional settings.[3, 55, 62, 92] A recent survey in California indicates that physicians spend less than half a minute per day with the average nursing home patient.[84] In many states, regulations governing the amount of nursing care in nursing homes are so lax that patients have only minimal contact with a registered nurse.[44, 91] Some state regulations have been modified so the requisite number of nursing hours per patient day can be met by allowing skilled nursing facilities to count hours of care provided by aides or orderlies as "nursing hours." In other states, even less stringent regulations have been adopted. For example, in California, not only does time spent by paraprofessionals count as nursing hours, but the number of hours spent by licensed nurses is *multiplied by two* in order to calculate nursing hours per patient day.[80] Attempts have been made at both the federal and state level to weaken even further — or even remove — the requirement that a specified number of hours of care by a licensed nurse be given to nursing home patients. These efforts are likely to intensify, as economic constraints force policymakers to explore different strategies for cutting the high cost of long-term care in institutions.[38, 39, 75]

Noninstitutional long-term care is currently attracting attention as a politically acceptable and less costly alternative to nursing home care. There is a danger that attempts to keep the costs of these services as low as possible may lead to an over-reliance on inexpensive homemaker and chore services, to the exclusion of health-related care, managed and, when appropriate, delivered by professionals. Nurses can play an important role in ensuring that long-term care — in both institutional and noninstitutional settings — is matched appropriately to patients' needs, by opposing legislation, policies, and regulations that narrow the range of medical and health-supportive services provided to patients. Unless nurses and other health professionals become vigorous advocates for breadth and quality of services, long-term care is likely to deteriorate as there is increasing pressure to lower health care costs.

- *Opposing further restrictions on eligibility and services for persons who need long-term care.* Eligibility and services are already extremely restricted for persons who require long-term care.[54, 78, 86] In the future, it is quite likely that state governments will attempt to contain expenditures by placing even greater limitations on who is eligible for long-term care, and the amounts and types of services that will be funded.[39] Action by nurses can be crucial in preventing such policies from taking effect. Nurses can be effective in educating legislators and policymakers about the detrimental consequences of reducing the availability and accessibility of long-term care for populations in need. Moreover, nurses can suggest alternative strategies for controlling costs, such as the revision of current reimbursement practices and delivery models, both of which encourage the use of expensive institutional services and end-stage intervention for persons with long-term disabilities.

- *Supporting efforts to establish better programs and policies for long-term care.* Current approaches to long-term care in the United States are relatively ineffective and excessively costly. Nurses could do a great deal to remedy this situation, if they were to press for changes in existing public policies and programs. Because of the widespread concern about the cost of long-term care, public officials, particularly those in state government, are attempting to explore alternative approaches to the problem. As a result, nurses and other health professionals have an unprecedented opportunity to provide guidance and direction for future policies and programs in long-term care. Larger numbers of nurses are employed in long-term care than any other type of professional. Large numbers of nurses serve as administrators or service directors in extended care facilities and home care agencies. Nurses comprise the largest numbers of professionals giving direct services to patients both in nursing homes and in noninstitutional long-term care. As a result, nurses are in a unique position to comment on the inadequacies, as well as the strengths, of current services and the organizations that deliver them.

If needed changes are to be brought about, it is important that nurses supply information to policymakers and that they actively lobby their elected officials to reform policies and programs in long-term care. Nurses, working collectively, can help move policy in important new directions, among them the following: (1) providing incentives for the development of noninstitutional long-term care, to bring in-home and other community-based services into better balance with institutional care; (2) establishing organizational structures or mechanisms to facilitate the integration of various forms of assistance, such as medical services, personal care, help with housekeeping and transportation, and financial assistance to ensure a basic minimum income, proper housing, and adequate nutrition; and (3) broadening eligibility for services, so long-term care is available to all persons with enduring and significant functional impairments.

In addition, nurses can effectively lobby for needed changes in public policies outside of health, but which vitally affect health. It is clear that the need for long-term care could be reduced significantly by providing assistance to vulnerable populations *before* illness results in a chronic condition or grave disability. Nurses and other professional groups can help support efforts to improve income levels, nutrition, housing, and health care for the disadvantaged. Such action would supplement current approaches to long-term care, by dealing with the *causes* rather than just the consequences of the problem.

The agenda outlined above is indeed an ambitious one. However, we think nurses can assume a central role in efforts to improve long-term care in the United States. At present, of all the professional groups, nurses appear to be in the best position to bring about reforms in the current system. We hope that the nursing profession will seize this valuable opportunity to provide leadership in the fields of gerontology and long-term care. If nursing fails to accept this challenge, not only will change be slow in coming, but nurses will have lost the chance to make a unique and substantial contribution to the health and well-being of all Americans, and to improve the stature of their profession in the process.

REFERENCES

1   Administration on Aging. AoA Occasional papers in gerontology, No. 1, *Human resource issues in the field of aging: the nursing home industry* (DHEW Publ. No. OHDS-80-20093). Washington, D.C.: U.S. Department of Health, Education, and Welfare, Office of Human Development Services, 1980.

2   Administration on Aging. *A preliminary report on the development and implementation of a federal manpower policy for the field of aging* (DHHS Publication OHDS-81-20048). Washington, D.C.: U.S. Department of Health and Human Services, Office of Human Development Services, AoA, Sept. 30, 1980.

3   Aiken, L. Nursing priorities for the 1980's: hospitals and nursing homes. *American Journal of Nursing*, February, 1981, 81 (2), 324–330.

4   Alford, R. *Health care politics.* Chicago, Illinois: University of Chicago Press, 1976.

5   American Nurses' Association. *Fact sheet on registered nurses.* Washington, D.C.: American Nurses' Association, Government Relations Division, Feb., 1980.

6   American Nurses' Assoication. *Legislative alert: impact of proposed budget cuts on nurse training.* Washington, D.C.: American Nurses' Association, Government Relations Division, March 16, 1981.

7   Baker, J. A. Critique of the Weissert study. *Home Health Care Services Quarterly*, Fall, 1980, *1*(3), 114–121.

8   Benton, B., Feild, T., & Millar, R. *State and area agency on aging intervention in Title XX.* Washington, D.C.: Urban Institute, 1977.

9   Berg, R. L. et al. Assessing the health care needs of the aged. *Health Services Research*, Spring 1970, 35–59.

10   Berkman, L. F., & Syme, S. L. Social networks, host resistance and mortality: a nine year follow-up study of Alameda County residents. *American Journal of Epidemiology*, February 1979, *109*(2), 186–204.

11   Breslow, L., & Enstrom, J. E. Persistence of health habits and their relationship to mortality. *Preventive Medicine*, 1980, *9*, 469–483.

12   Brody, S., Polshock, S. and Masciocchi, C. The family caring unit: a major consideration in the long-term support system. *Gerontologist.* 1978, *18*(6), 556–561.

13   Brotman, H. Projections for the aging population. In *Developments in aging: 1980*, A report of the Special Committee on Aging, U.S. Senate. Washington, D.C.: forthcoming, 1981.

14   Brower, H. A study of graduate programs in gerontological nursing. *Journal of Gerontological Nursing*, *3*(6), 40–46, 1977.

15 Bureau of Health Manpower, Manpower Analysis Branch, Health Resources Administration. *A report to the President and Congress on the status of health professions personnel in the U.S.* (HRA-78-93). Washington, D C.: U.S. Government Printing Office, 1978.

16 Bureau of Labor Statistics, U.S. Department of Labor. *Employment projections for the 1980's.* Washington, D.C.: U.S. Government Printing Office, 1979.

17 Butler, L. H., & Newacheck, P. W. Health and social factors affecting long term care policy. In H. Richmond, J. Meltzer, & F. Farrow (Eds.), *Public policies for long term care.* Chicago: University of Chicago Press, 1981.

18 Callahan, James. Delivery of services to persons with long term care needs. In H. Richmond, J. Meltzer, and F. Farrow (Eds.), *Public policies for long-term care.* Chicago: University of Chicago Press, 1981.

19 Callahan, J. et al. Responsibilities of families for their severely disabled elders. *Health Care Financing Review,* Winter, 1980, *1*(3), 29–48.

20 Callahan, Wayne. *Medicare — use of home health services: 1977,* (HCFA Pub. No. 03064). Washington, D.C.: Health Care Financing Administration, Office of Research, Demonstrations, and Statistics, January, 1981.

21 Community Council of Greater New York. *Dependency in the elderly of New York City: report of a research utilization workshop.* New York: Community Council of Greater New York, 1978.

22 Congressional Budget Office. *Long-term care for the elderly and disabled.* Washington, D.C.: U.S. Government Printing Office, 1977.

23 Congressional Budget Office. *Nursing education and training: alternative federal approaches. Budget issue paper for fiscal year 1979.* Washington, D.C.: CBO, Congress of the United States, May, 1978.

24 Curran, J. P. *People taking care of people: a report on the home health care service industry.* New York: Woody Gundy Incorporated, Sept. 29, 1980.

25 Davis, J. and Gibbon, M. An areawide examination of nursing home use, misuse, and nonuse. *American Journal of Public Health. 1971, 61*(6), 1146–1155.

26 Department of Health, Education, and Welfare, National Center for Health Services Research. *Health: United States, 1979.* Washington, D.C.: U.S. Government Printing Office, 1980.

27 Department of Health, Education, and Welfare, Office of the Assistant Secretary for Health. *Healthy People: the Surgeon General's report on health promotion and disease prevention.* Washington, D.C.: U.S. Government Printing Office, 1979.

28 Department of Health, Education, and Welfare. *Home health and other in-home services: Titles XVIII, XIX, and XX of the Social Security Act.* A report to Congress, pursuant to P.L. 95-145, November, 1979.

29 Division of Nursing. *List of geriatric nurse training projects supported under Sections 820, 821, and 822 of the Public Health Service Act, fiscal year 1980.* Hyattsville, Maryland: Div. of Nursing, unpublished data, December 17, 1980.

30 Division of Nursing. *Preliminary data from the 1979 survey of community health nursing.* Washington, D.C.: U.S. Department of Health and Human Resources, Health Resources Administration, unpublished data, 1981.

31 Division of Nursing. *Second report to the Congress, Nurse Training Act of 1975.* (DHEW Publ. No. HRA-79-45). Washington, D.C.: Health Resources Administration, Bureau of Health Manpower, March 15, 1979.

32   Division of Nursing. *Surveys of public health nursing, 1968–1972.* (DHEW Publ. No. HRA-76-8). Washington, D.C.: U.S. Government Printing Office, November, 1975.

33   Dunlop, B. *Long-term care: need versus utilization.* Washington, D.C.: Urban Institute, working paper 0975-05, May 1974 (revised, 1975).

34   Enthoven, A. C. *Health plan: the only practical solution to the soaring cost of medical care.* Menlo Park, California: Addison-Wesley, 1980.

35   Estes, C. L. *The aging enterprise.* San Francisco: Jossey-Bass, 1979.

36   Estes, C. L. New federalism and aging. In U.S. Senate Special Committee on Aging, *Developments in aging: 1974 and January–April, 1975.* Washington, D.C.: U.S. Government Printing Office, 1977.

37   Estes, C. L. Social policy for elders in the 1980's. *Generations: Journal of the Western Gerontological Society,* May 1980, *4*(1), 4–5, 50.

38   Estes, C. L. & Harrington, C. Fiscal crisis, deinstitutionalization and the aged. *American Behavioral Scientist,* forthcoming, 1981.

39   Estes, C. L., Lee, P. R., Harrington, C., Gerard, L., Kreger, M., Benjamin A. E., Newcomer, R. and Swan, J. *Public policies and long term care for the elderly.* San Francisco: Aging Health Policy Center, University of California, January 1981.

40   Estes, C. L., & Noble, M. L. *Paperwork and the Older Americans Act: problems of implementing accountability.* Staff information paper prepared for use by the U.S. Senate Special Committee on Aging, Washington, D.C.: U.S. Government Printing Office, 1978.

41   Feder, J., et al. *National health insurance: conflicting goals and policy choices.* Washington, D.C.: Urban Institute, 1980.

42   *Federal Register.* National long-term care channeling demonstration program: intent to initiate program. Federal Register, December 21, 1979, *44,* 75720–75723.

43   Fisher, C. Differences by age groups in health care spending. *Health Care Financing Review.* Spring, 1980, *1*(4), 65–90.

44   Flagle, C. D. Issues of staffing long-term care activities. In Millman, M. L. (Ed.), *Nursing Personnel and the Changing Health Care System.* Cambridge, Massachusetts: Ballinger, 1978, 227–236.

45   Foley, H. *Personal communication to C. Estes on federal legislation supporting geriatric training for health professionals.* Washington, D.C.: March, 1981.

46   Fox, P., and Clauser, S. Trends in nursing home expenditures: implications for aging policy. *Health Care Financing Review.* Fall, 1980, *2*(2), 65–70.

47   Fries, J. F., & Crapo, L. M. *The rectangular curve: aging, changing, and the barrier to immortality.* Stanford, California: Stanford University Press, 1980.

48   General Accounting Office. Report to the Congress by the Comptroller General of the United States. *Entering a nursing home — costly implications for Medicaid and the elderly* (PAD-80-12). Washington, D.C.: GAO, November 26, 1979.

49   General Accounting Office. *History of the rising costs of the Medicare and Medicaid programs and attempts to control these costs; 1966–1975* (MWO-76-93). Washington, D.C.: U.S. Government Printing Office, 1977.

50   General Accounting Office. Report to the Congress by the Comptroller General of the United States. *Home health — the need for a national policy to better provide for the elderly* (HRD-78-19). Washington, D.C.: GAO, December 30, 1977.

51   General Accounting Office. Report to the Congress by the Comptroller General of the United States. *The well-being of older people in Cleveland, Ohio* (HRD-77-70). Washington, D.C.: GAO, April 19, 1977.

52   Gibson, R. M. National health expenditures, 1979. *Health Care Financing Review*, Summer 1980, *2*(1), 1–36.

53   Health Care Financing Administration, Office of Research, Demonstration, and Statistics. *Health Care Financing program statistics: Medicare—participating health facilities, 1979*. (HCFA Publ. No. 03060). U.S. Department of Health and Human Services, HCFA, 1980.

54   Health Care Financing Administration. *Long term care: background and future directions* (HCFA 81-20047). Washington, D.C.: U.S. Department of Health and Human Services, HCFA, January, 1981.

55   Health Resources Administration. *Health personnel issues in the context of long-term care in nursing homes*. Washington, D.C.: Public Health Service, HRA, August 18, 1980.

56   Health Resources Administration, Bureau of Health Resources Development. *The supply of health manpower: 1970 profiles and projections to 1990*. Washington, D.C.: U.S. Department of Health, Education, and Welfare, December 1974.

57   *Home Health Line. Decade report—1980*. Washington, D.C.: Home Health Line, 1980.

58   Johnson, W. L. *Supply and demand for registered nurses: some observations on the current picture and prospects to 1985, Parts 1 and 2*. (Publ. No. 19-1837 and 19-1838). New York, New York: National League for Nursing, 1980.

59   Kane, R., et al. *Geriatrics in the United States: manpower projections and training considerations*. Santa Monica, California: Rand Corporation, May 1980.

60   Kayser-Jones, J. S. A comparison of care in a Scottish and a United States facility. *Geriatric Nursing*, January/February, 1981, *2*(1), 44–50.

61   Kayser-Jones, J. S. Gerontological nursing research revisited. *Journal of Gerontological Nursing*, April, 1981, *7*(4), 217–223.

62   Kayser-Jones, J. S. *Old, alone and neglected: care of the institutionalized aged in Scotland and the United States*. Berkeley: University of California Press, 1981.

63   Kovar, M. G. Elderly people: the population 65 years and over. In National Center for Health Statistics, *Health: United States, 1976–1977*. Washington, D.C.: U.S. Government Printing Office, 1977.

64   Kutza, Elizabeth. Allocating long term care services: the policy puzzle of who should be served. In H. Richmond, J. Meltzer, and F. Farrow (Eds.), *Public policies for long-term care*. Chicago: University of Chicago Press, 1981.

65   Lee, P. R. and Estes, C. L. Eighty federal programs for the elderly. In C. L. Estes, *The aging enterprise*. San Francisco: Jossey-Bass, 1979.

66   Lee, P. R., & Estes, C. L. Public policies, the aged and long term care. *Journal of Long-Term Care Administration*, Fall 1979, *7*(3), 1–15.

67   Lee, P. R., Estes, C. L., et al. *The federal government, health policy and the health care of the disadvantaged*. Paper presented before the Commission on Civil Rights, Washington, D.C., April 15, 1980.

68   Levine, E. Nursing supply and requirements: the current situation and future prospects. In Millman, M. L. (Ed.), *Nursing personnel and the changing health care system*. Cambridge, Massachusetts: Ballinger, 1978, 23–45.

69   Lowi, T. *The end of liberalism*. New York: Norton, 1979.

70   Markus, G. *Nursing homes and the Congress: a brief history of developments and issues*. Washington, D.C.: Library of Congress, 1972.

71   Meltzer, J. and Farrow, F. Federal policy directions in long term care. In H. Rich-

mond, J. Meltzer, and F. Farrow (Eds.), *Public policies for long-term care.* Chicago: University of Chicago Press, 1981.

72   Miller, S. M. *The political economy of social problems: from the 1960s to the 1970s.* Paper presented at the annual meeting of the Society for Study of Social Problems, New York, August, 1976.

73   National League for Nursing. *Community health agencies with vacancies in registered nurse positions, April 1977 and 1978.* New York, New York: National League for Nursing, Community Home Health Agencies—Community Health Services, unpublished data, 1980.

74   Newacheck, P. et al. Income and illness. *Medical care,* December, 1980, *18*(12), 1165–1176.

75   Newcomer, R. J., Harrington, C., & Gerard, L. *A five-state comparison of selected long term care expenditure and utilization patterns for persons aged 65 and older.* Working paper no. 11. San Francisco: Aging Health Policy Center, University of California, 1981.

76   Nichols, E. and Hallburg, J. Preparation of leaders in gerontological nursing: the program at UCSF. *Journal of Gerontological Nursing, 6*(3), 162–164, 1980.

77   Panneton, P. and Wesolowski, E. Current and future needs in geriatric education. *Public Health Reports.* January-February, 1979, *94*(1), 73–79.

78   Reif, L. Expansion and merger of home care agencies: optimizing existing resources through organizational redesign. *Home Health Care Services Quarterly,* Fall, 1980, *1*(3), 3–36.

79   Richmond, G. M. An analysis of non-institutional long term care planning methods for care in the home. *Home Health Care Services Quarterly,* Winter, 1981, *1*(4), 5–44.

80   Ricker-Smith, K. *A Challenge for public policy: the nursing home experience in California's Golden Empire Region.* Sacramento, California: Golden Empire Health Systems Agency, unpublished report, 1980.

81   Roth Aleda et al. *1977 national sample survey of registered nurses* (HRP-0900603). Springfield, Virginia: National Technical Information Service, 1977.

82   Schatzkin, A. How long can we live? A more optimistic view of potential gains in life expectancy. *American Journal of Public Health,* 1980, *70*(11), 1199–1200.

83   Soldo, B. J. America's elderly in the 1980's. *Population Bulletin,* November, 1980, *35*(4), 3–47.

84   State of California, *California Health Facilities Commission,* Long Term Care Effectiveness Standards Task Force. Sacramento, California: unpublished data, May 1981.

85   Syme, S. L., & Berkman, L. F. Social class, susceptibility and sickness. *American Journal of Epidemiology,* July 1976, *104*(1), 1–8.

86   Trager, B. Home health care and national health policy. *Home Health Care Services Quarterly,* Spring 1980, *1*(2), 1–103.

87   U.S. House of Representatives, Select Committee on Aging, Subcommittee on Health and Long-Term Care. *Nurse Shortage and its impact on care for the elderly* (Comm. Pub. No. 96-255). Washington, D.C.: U.S. Government Printing Office, 1981.

88   U.S. Senate, Committee on Human Resources, *Subcommittee on Aging hearings: oversight and extension of the Older Americans Act.* Washington, D.C.: U.S. Government Printing Office, 1978.

89   U.S. Senate, Special Committee on Aging, Subcommittee on Long-Term Care. *Nursing home care in the United States: failure in public policy* (report No. 93-1420). Washington, D.C.: U.S. Government Printing Office, 1974.

90   U.S. Senate, Special Committee on Aging, Subcommittee on Long-Term Care. *Role of nursing homes in caring for discharged mental patients.* (Supporting paper no. 7). Washington, D.C.: U.S. Government Printing Office, 1976.

91   Vladeck, B. C. *Unloving care: the nursing home tragedy.* New York: Basic Books, 1980.

92   White House Conference on Aging, Technical Committee on Health Services. *Health care needs of the elderly,* draft report. Los Angeles: Division of Research in Medical Education, University of Southern California, February 1, 1981.

BRUCE C. VLADECK

10

NURSING HOMES: A NATIONAL PROBLEM

No one seems to like nursing homes very much, but we probably cannot do without them. A consensus exists — indeed, has existed for at least a decade — that most of the frail elderly are better cared for in noninstitutional settings, yet the supply of nursing home beds grows faster than the availability of noninstitutional services. In these apparent paradoxes lies the nub of what might be called the nursing home problem. By exploring these paradoxes, it is possible to both identify significant aspects of the nursing home problem and derive some hypotheses, if not predictions, on its future transformations.

Somewhere between 1.25 million and 1.5 million people are housed in somewhere around 16,000 or 17,000 nursing homes, at an annual total expense approaching $20 billion. Since 1975 expenditures for nursing homes have grown more rapidly than any other of the rapidly growing components of national health expenditures, and that one fact constitutes the nursing home problem for some observers. More than half of all nursing home expenditures arise directly from public programs, and those expenditures have been increasing faster than almost any other public expenditures.[1] That, from the perspective of public policy, clearly *is* the core of the nursing home problem.

All of the statistics in the preceding paragraph are estimates, approximations, or informed guesses. As difficult as it may be for those familiar with hospitals, health manpower, or similar activities to imagine, no one really knows just how many nursing homes there are in the United States, or just how much they cost. Indeed, there is an enormous amount about nursing homes that is simply not known, at least in any systematic way, and what is

The views expressed herein are solely those of the author, and should not be attributed to the New Jersey State Department of Health or any other organization.

known by policymakers, health professionals, and the general public contains considerable misinformation and misconception.

Nursing homes most often reach the short agenda of public attention as the result of highly visible scandals — of which the one that broke in New York City in 1975 remains the gaudiest example. Opportunities for private profit at the expense of the care rendered to the helplessly frail are so intrinsic to the basic structure of nursing home care — in which private entrepreneurs are paid to take care of strangers who cannot take care of themselves — that scandals are bound to recur. To the considerable extent that they constitute the sum of public knowledge about nursing homes, however, such scandals have led to other kinds of distortions, as the public and its representatives have sought to make the worst cases impossible, and thereby may have frustrated efforts at the best.

At this writing, long-term care policy in the United States is probably in the greatest period of flux it has encountered since the enactment of Medicare and Medicaid in 1965. What appeared to be a developing professional and policy consensus about long-term care policy was embodied to a limited degree in the Medicare provisions of the Omnibus Budget Reconciliation Act of 1980, and to a far greater degree in a series of legislative proposals introduced during the same Congress. Separate initiatives were underway in the Executive Branch. But the enormous dislocation in American social policy resulting from the 1980 elections will affect nursing homes as much as other service institutions. In particular, the Omnibus Budget Reconciliation Act of 1981 will lead to significant changes in Medicaid, the lifeblood of the nursing home industry, in ways that as yet are hard to predict, while shifts in Executive Branch attitudes and personnel will also have a profound effect. The emerging consensus of 1980 has been submerged in the tides of 1981 reaction; even if those tides soon begin to recede, the consensus may have already dissolved.

THE DEMOGRAPHIC PROBLEM

In explaining the development of the modern nursing home system, the first point that must be emphasized — that can not be emphasized enough — is that it constitutes a sort of response to a phenomenon literally without precedent: the extraordinary change in the age composition of the population of modern, industrial societies. Never before in human history have there been so many old people (using the conventional criterion of 65 yr and older) nor so many of the very old (over 75).

While the "greying of America" has become something of a popular cliche, generalized perceptions of the problems posed by this demographic change tend to focus on the concerns of the majority of the elderly: income support (especially Social Security), retirement, medical care costs, and so forth. It is less widely recognized that the relatively small minority of the elderly who are seriously functionally impaired, or over 75, is growing at a much faster rate than any other segment of the population, over or under 65. And that is the population most at risk for long-term care services. In 1950 fewer than five million Americans were 75 or over; by 1990, there will be more than 15 million.

Thus, it is widely believed that the growth of nursing homes and related institutions is attributable to the breakdown of family structures, community supports, and other social mechanisms, yet all the available evidence strongly suggests that two-thirds of the frail elderly are cared for by family, neighbors, or friends.[2] The proportion could never have been very much higher. There are just so many more frail elderly persons that the absolute number of people in need of purchased long-term care services has grown faster than any other service-requiring population.

The typical nursing home resident is a white widow or spinster in her early 80s. More than 80% of all nursing home residents are over 75, and three-quarters are women. Only one in ten has a living spouse. Almost all have multiple, chronic medical conditions, and somewhere around half have serious mental or emotional difficulties. Most do not have very much money.[3] If there were no nursing homes, the needs of this population would still pose the most serious difficulties for social policy.

It should also be emphasized that it is only very recently that we have begun to recognize the frail elderly as a specific subpopulation within society with distinct needs and problems. The inadequacy of nursing homes and nursing home care can, in large part, be attributed to the failure, until the last few years, of most health care professionals and policymakers to focus on long-term care of the frail elderly as a distinct problem. We have no national long-term care policy in part because the recognition that it might be a good idea to have one dates back less than a decade. The first generation of professionals specifically trained for long-term care are mostly at the early stages of their careers. Long-term care services are still delivered by professionals trained in acute care settings (and to a far greater degree by nonprofessionals not formally trained at all), operated primarily by entrepreneurs with still less professional background, and overseen by public officials more oriented towards acute medical services, on the one hand, or welfare programs on the other, than long-term care *per se*.

The effects of ignoring social problems are not always benign. Society abhors a vacuum. The long-term care system that has grown up in the absence of coherent public policy or defined professional norms is both very unsatisfactory and very expensive, but like Mt. Everest, it is there, and there to stay.

THE NURSING HOME PROBLEM

From the standpoint of the population it primarily serves, the typical contemporary American nursing home, as an institution, makes no sense. The average resident stays for a year and a half, yet most nursing homes are profoundly unhomelike. Indeed, by law they must be substantially more fireproof, aseptic, and compartmentalized than any satisfactory home can be. The very process of admission to a nursing home generally creates (or reflects) an emotional or social dislocation likely to compound preexisting psychosocial problems; yet hardly any nursing homes provide formal mental health services (other than medications generally prescribed by internists or general practitioners), while none are required to offer psychosocial supports, although many try, and some do a good job. Nursing homes are presumably health care institutions, yet the typical nursing home resident gets less attention from physicians than the typical elderly nonresident. The primary medical diagnoses of long-stay nursing home residents tend to be directly or indirectly iatrogenic. Frail elderly people cared for outside nursing homes, even when they receive fewer services, tend to live longer.[4]

The structure and organization of nursing homes are more explicable if one conceives of them as pale carbon copies of general hospitals, and historically that is what they are. The arrangement of semiprivate rooms along a corridor dominated by a nursing station, the organization of staff and professional responsibility, the fiction that care plans flow from written physician orders, even the kinds of record keeping — all follow logically and genetically from the general hospital model. Yet general hospitals are the way they are because they have been organized to do specific things, which are not what nursing homes do.

Most obviously, people do not go to the hospital to stay. Indeed, 10% of all the people who go to hospitals do so to have babies or to be born. The indignities, inconveniences, and discomforts one can tolerate in a short acute stay — because one expects they will be compensated for by the resolution of an acute problem, because one has no choice, and because one knows it will be temporary — can become unbearable irritants in a nursing home, where a resident knows she is probably stuck for the rest of her life.

Hospital patients consume a lot of ancillary services, which are generally provided by separately organized departments whose work is coordinated, if at all, by individual attending physicians. Nursing home residents, who spend most of their time, in the words of some knowledgeable observers, "(1) in the facility and (2) doing nothing," receive mostly personal care and some nursing, yet nursing homes are required to have separately organized departments for a range of services, including physical therapy, occupational therapy, audiology, social services, and the like, which most residents never receive.[5] The results have been a senseless fragmentation of care organization and some of the worst financial abuses, such as phantom "consultants" billing for phantom services supervising departments that never treat patients.

It acute care hospitals, quality assurance, while only recently recognized as a separate formal function, has long been a by-product of the professional needs and concerns of the physicians and nurses who work in them. Physicians functioning as independent entrepreneurs have a number of incentives, ranging from professional liability to a desire to keep their customers happy, to be concerned about the quality of services provided in the hospitals where they practice. But physicians are largely absent from nursing homes, and quality assurance in long-term care has consistently been, and remains, the most intractable and fundamental problem.

If hospitals are physicians' workshops, the health professionals with the primary, continuous, and central responsibility for patient care and quality assurance in nursing homes are registered nurses. This is the wrong chapter in this volume for an extended discussion of the present and future of professional nursing in long-term care institutions, but the uniqueness of nursing's role in nursing homes deserves emphasis here. In most nursing homes, the primary *de facto* (if not in *de jure*) clinical responsibility lodges with the nursing director, and that is both a symptom of the historically low status of nursing homes within the health care sector and the source of great future promise for both nursing and nursing homes.

THE HOSPITAL PROBLEM

While nursing homes are profoundly unlike hospitals — though they are perhaps not unlike enough, considering the differences in institutional mission — it is hard to understand the current role of nursing homes in the health care system without understanding their relationship to the needs of hospitals and those who have made policy about hospitals. Just as Voltaire argued that, if God did not exist, he would need to be invented by man to serve theological purposes, so what we call a nursing home is largely an invention of people concerned about hospitals. And the thinking about nursing homes continues to be governed by the perceptions and prejudices formed in the hospital sector that apply poorly, if at all, to long-term care.

Institutions offering essentially residential services for the dependent elderly, often supplemented with some degree of health services, and even a segregated "infirmary," have existed in this country for at least a century.[6, 7] The longest traditions belong to voluntary, not-for-profit organizations, many associated with denominational or fraternal groups, but the history of for-profit nursing homes (originally supervised commercial boarding homes operated by licensed nurses) goes back at least as far as the 1930s.[8] But the modern nursing home, in terms of both its physical configuration and its financing, has been defined largely by people who were preoccupied with hospitals.

Like so much else in contemporary American health care, the physical appearance of most nursing homes can be traced historically, in a direct causal line, to the Hill-Burton program. Hill-Burton, more formally the Hospital Survey and Construction Act of 1946, was of course hospital-oriented legislation, conceived and managed by people whose primary expertise lay with hospitals. When it was amended in 1954 to provide up to $10 million annually in grants and loans for nursing home construction, that authority was extended only to nursing homes operated "in conjunction with a hospital."[9] More importantly, the mechanics of Hill-Burton required the development of physical construction standard that, thanks to the federal arrangements of Hill-Burton, served as the model for state codes as well. The hospital-like standards adopted by hospital-oriented Public Health Service officials in the 1950s remained the basis for the physical standards for today's nursing homes.

In part because it was a hospital-oriented program, Hill-Burton assistance was available only to public and nonprofit institutions. Relatively few nonprofit hospitals took the federal government up on its offer after 1954 to attract them into the long-term care business, and voluntary homes for the aged were slow to redefine themselves as health care institutions. So the predominantly for-profit character of the nursing home industry was largely unaltered by Hill-Burton. What did change was the status of nursing homes as institutions serving both health and social service needs. After 1954 they were to be defined primarily as health care institutions.

Along with this change in definition came a change in perceived function. The mid-1950s were the zenith of "progressive patient care" as an ideology in hospital services, and with growing recognition of the increase in the elderly population and the concomitant increase in chronic illness, there was perceived to be a growing need for "post-acute" inpatient services to care for those people, predominantly elderly, who no longer needed the level of care provided by a general hospital but were not yet capable of being sent home. The need for such a level of service appeared to be embodied in the growing number of patients in general hospitals who posed disposition problems. They did not seem to really belong in the hospital any longer, and the hospitals certainly did not want to have to continue taking care of them, but they were not capable of going home or had no homes to go to.

Nursing homes had long been providing care for the dependent elderly, but these developments in the hospital industry led to a redefinition of their role as a kind of receiving site for post-acute hospital patients with continuing medical needs. Nursing homes were thus drawn ineluctably into a medical service model — albeit as the tail end — as places where people were sent (from hospitals). Henceforth, the "need" for nursing home services would be determined largely by the size of the "backlog" of patients awaiting discharge from general hospitals, and the cost-benefit of nursing homes would be calculated with reference to the *per diem* costs of acute hospital care.

A moment's reflection will reveal the implications of seeing nursing homes as posthospital receiving facilities rather than service-rich residences for those admitted from the community. To best serve the acute care hospital system, nursing homes must be capable of providing relatively intensive medical and nursing services (intravenous administration; oxygen and suction; specialized nursing care); must provide for continuity of care by maintaining the relationship between patients and their attending physicians; and must have a relatively rapid patient turnover, to ensure the availability of beds whenever the hospital needs to get rid of a post-acute elderly patient. To best meet the needs of long-term residents, nursing homes should have abundant generic personal care staff, strong medical direction, and as much stability as possible in resident population. In fact, about a third of all nursing home residents are admitted directly from hospitals and roughly half directly from the community.[10] The institutions to which they are admitted, half-fish and half-fowl, are specially oriented to the specific needs of neither group.

The redefinition of nursing homes to suit the needs of general hospitals reached its apotheosis in the development of the Medicare extended care benefit and the initial implementation of that benefit. Eager to ensure a potential cost savings for their hospital insurance program, the framers of Medicare provided coverage of up to 100 days of "post-hospital extended care," provided that care was part of a single "spell of illness" involving an acute hospitalization of at least 3 days.[11] By converting the last days of an acute stay into extended-care days in an extended care facility, the theory went, Medicare would save money by paying lower *per diem* rates.

As has been demonstrated elsewhere, the basic logic underlying that belief was fallacious; more to the point here are the effects efforts to translate that logic into practice had on nursing homes in the late 1960s.[12] Because there were hardly any institutions in the United States in 1966 equipped or oriented to provide the service for which the Congress had just created an entitlement, Executive Branch officials certified as providers more than 2,000 existing nursing homes that gave primarily residential services. The demand for such services was, of course, far greater than that for the much narrower post-acute step-down, and Medicare's expenses for extended care were soon running fivefold greater than any conceivable savings from reductions in acute day cares. The extended care benefit was soon cut back by administrative fiat.[13]

In the meantime, however, Medicare's experience had had an important fallout effect on Medicaid. Nursing homes had been reimbursed, to a very limited degree, as health care services by welfare-related benefit programs since 1950. Policymakers had some conception of the difference, at least in theory, between custodial and medical institutions, so when public support of health care for the poor was expanded, first by the Kerre-Mills program in 1960, then many times over by Medicaid in 1965, nursing home benefits were limited to "skilled nursing homes." Medical services, Congress seemed to feel, should be covered by health programs with federal matching funds, but residential services should remain with state welfare agencies. Yet skilled nursing homes turned out, in practice, to be anything that met the basic Hill-Burton-derived physical standards and that employed at least a couple of registered nurses. The characteristics of the facility, rather than the needs of its occupants, determined reimbursement status, and since the facilities' characteristics had been defined to meet the needs of a largely nonexistent population, many institutions providing primarily residential services qualified for Medicaid reimbursement.

Today federal law and regulation recognize three classes of long-term care facilities: skilled nursing facilities (SNFs), intermediate care facilities (ICFs), and residential or domiciliary care facilities (DCFs). SNFs and ICFs are both reimbursable under Medicaid, but only SNFs qualify for Medicare. DCFs, ostensibly providing no medical services, are eligible for neither. While a considerable body of law and regulation attempts to distinguish SNFs from ICFs, and SNF patients from ICF patients, as a practical matter the distinction only has such force as individual states choose to give it. State governments not only administer Medicaid, they are also responsible for the licensure and certification of health care facilities under federal as well as state programs. California has essentially no ICFs; Oklahoma only six SNFs among 350 licensed nursing homes. In New Jersey, most nursing homes have a single long-term care license, although individual Medicaid patients are assessed as needing either skilled or one of the two levels of intermediate care. In those states, of which New York is perhaps the most notable example, that have attempted to enforce a serious and relatively rigid boundary between SNF and ICF level services, the cost can be a considerable hardship on patients and facilities. Multiple "levels" of care may make sense in a hospital context, where nurse staffing, in particular, needs to be responsive to shifts across a broad range of patient care need intensities. Levels of care are sub-stantially less appropriate in long-term care, where the course of a patient's needs can be anything but unidirectional, and where moving a patient from one physical setting to another in response to possibly transient changes in the patient's condition can have seriously dysfunctional effects.

As noted above, a central difference between hospitals and nursing homes lies in the characteristics of quality assurance efforts, and the mainte-nance of adequate quality care has been a never-ending problem for nursing homes. As opposed to much acute medical care, good nursing home care is highly personal, subjective, physically intimate, and low in technology. It is also all too rare. As a partial response to this chronic problem, those con-cerned with nursing homes and the well-being of their residents sought, in the late 1960s and early 1970s, to partially address the problem through reim-bursement. Again, there was a partial analogy to hospitals. And again, that analogy was probably faulty.

Since its inception, Medicaid, like its predecessor programs, has paid for the greatest bulk of nursing home care. While Medicaid only supplies 50% of the industry's revenues, it pays the bulk of expenses for at least two-thirds of nursing home residents at any given time (that apparent discrepancy is largely accounted for by the fact that Medicaid pays the *difference* between a recipient's nursing home costs and her own income; the 50% figure is thus net of the required contributions of recipients' incomes). In keeping with its welfare origins, Medicaid customarily paid flat or negotiated *per diem* rates to providers, rates that were often extremely low. This low level of reimburse-ment, it was widely believed (and widely contended by nursing home provid-ers), made it uneconomic, if not impossible, for many operators to provide decent care. Hospitals, by contrast, were reimbursed by Medicaid (as by Medicare) on the basis of their "reasonable costs," and this reimbursement philosophy, while undoubtedly expensive, was widely perceived to have con-tributed to major qualitative improvements in hospital care.

Thus, as the result of efforts by those seeking to upgrade nursing home care, Section 249 of the Social Security Act Amendments of 1972 required states to adopt reasonable cost-related methods of reimbursing nursing homes under Medicaid. Implementation of this provision was delayed at the federal level until 1978, although many states moved more expeditiously. The primary apparent effect was a substantial increase in state expenditures over and above normal inflation rates. The quality of services also improved, but it is impossible to attribute a significant independent impact to reimbursement, especially since new regulatory standards and enforcement mechanisms, also mandated by the 1972 Social Security Act Amendments, were being put into place at the same time. The language of Section 249 was substantially modi-fied by Congress in 1980.[14]

THE LONG-TERM CARE PROBLEM

Less than half of the frail elderly receiving long-term care are in institutions; most of the rest are at home, receiving informal services and assistance from family and friends.[15] Most of those in need of long-term care would prefer to remain at home; and indeed, the use of nursing homes is strongly but inversely correlated with income. Those who can afford services outside institutions presumably "vote with their feet" to remain out. Yet public programs spend billions on institutional care and only a comparative pittance on services required to help people remain in their homes, even though some studies suggest that the latter is significantly cheaper, at least for a given public program.[16] In many instances, because of what they will pay for and what they will not, Medicare and especially Medicaid actually encourage people who could remain at home with appropriate support to enter institutions.

Even if policymakers were to choose to do nothing about these apparent contradictions, the population at risk for long-term care services is growing so rapidly that something will, eventually, have to give. In fact, these apparent contradictions have been nowhere more obvious than in the circles occupied by those who make policy, but initiative has been frustrated by two basic concerns.

The first is anxiety over what might be termed excess demand. The fact is that most of those now at home receiving some form of long-term care are receiving it without direct public subsidy at all. Provision of public subsidies, in addition to those now available for nursing homes, could cost as much as $25 billion a year within 5 yr—$25 billion *new* dollars, unless reliable and tested controls were available. They are not. In-home services may, under the proper circumstances, substitute for nursing home care at lower cost, but until substitution rather than addition can be assured, policymakers will tread lightly.[17]

Second, but obviously related closely, is the fact that *any* new policy initiative requires incremental expenditures in the first few years, and incremental dollars of any kind have been unavailable in recent years, as the annual increases in the cost of the existing Medicare and Medicaid budgets have run into the billions of dollars. It may be wise, in the abstract, to invest a few hundred million today in hopes of saving many billions in the future, but public officials do not run for reelection in the abstract.

Nonetheless, the latter part of 1980 brought a number of public initiatives in long-term care. Of most immediate significance to nursing home residents, new federal regulatory standards, several years in the making, were prepared for final adoption. While inadequate and partial in many ways, the proposed new standards substantially strengthened the protection of residents' rights; clarified the role of medical direction and partially redefined the role of nursing directors to make more explicit their captainship of the care team.

The Budget Reconciliation Act of 1980 removed the limitations on home health visits under Medicare; substantially loosened requirements for qualifying for those benefits, including elimination of the requirement for prior hospitalization; authorized the use of "swing beds" for long-term care in underutilized rural hospitals; and potentially eased the pressure for new nursing home construction by authorizing Medicare and Medicaid reimbursement to hospitals at less than 80% occupancy for patients awaiting nursing home placement at rates based on locally prevailing SNF rates. There was also initiative in the Executive Branch, as the Department of Health and Human Services embarked on a $50 million program to test local "channeling" agencies — an effort, in part, to test alternate solutions to the excess demand problem — and to develop a national data base on the needs of the frail elderly population. Finally, legislation was introduced in Congress, and hearings were held, on proposals to expand public coverage of long-term care services outside of institutions, either by providing generous incentives for state Medicaid programs to offer community care services to those who would otherwise be eligible for nursing home care, or by adding a long-term care Title XXI to the Social Security Act.

The 1980 elections and fiscal 1982 budget process derailed much of this momentum. The new nursing home regulations were withdrawn, and will never reappear. The budget for the channeling demonstrations was cut by more than half. Most of the people in the Executive Branch who knew anything about long-term care left. Most importantly, reductions were imposed on the federal contribution to Medicaid.

Because federal requirements for state Medicaid programs were also modified, and perhaps most notably because — thanks to the remarkable efforts of the staff of the Health and Environment Subcommittee of the House Commerce Committee — much of the Medicaid Community Care Act proposed in 1980 was incorporated into the 1981 Reconciliation Act while hardly anyone was looking, 50 state governments are now reexamining their long-term policy.

But they have very little money with which to act, and all the signs suggest they will have still less money in the future. Meanwhile, the population needing services continues to grow at an alarming rate. Under the best of circumstances, it would take a heroic and largely unprecedented effort at building institutions and redirecting public policy to provide first-rate long-term care services for all those who will come to need them in the 1980s and 1990s. The best of circumstances are not likely to prevail.

REFERENCES

1 Gibson R: National health expenditures, 1979. Health Care Financing Review 2:1, (1980)

2 Congressional Budget Office: Long-Term Care for the Elderly and Disabled. Washington, DC, US Government Printing Office, 1977

3 Vladeck BC: Unloving Care: The Nursing Home Tragedy, pp. 13–17. New York: Basic Books, 1980

4 Ibid, pp 17–19

5 Manard BB, Woehle RE, Heilman JM: Better Homes for the Old, p 22. Lexington, MA, Lexington Books, 1977

6 McClure E: More Than A Roof: The Development of Minnesota Poor Farms and Homes for the Aged. St Paul, Minnesota Historical Society, 1968

7 Thomas WC Jr: Nursing Homes and Public Policy: Drift and Decision in New York State, pp 57–104. Ithaca, NY, Cornell University Press, 1969

8 Ibid

9 Vladeck, op cit, pp 42–43

10 Hing E, Zappolo A: A comparison of nursing home residents and discharges from the 1977 national nursing home survey. Advance Data from the National Center for Health Statistics 29:5, May 17, 1978

11 Vladeck, op cit, pp. 49–52

12 Vladeck, op cit, pp 82–83

13 Vladeck, op cit, pp 52–57

14 Weiner SL, Lehrer SS: The afterthought industry: Developing reimbursement policy for nursing homes. Milbank Memorial Fund Quarterly/Health and Society (in press)

15 Congressional Budget Office, op cit

16 Comptroller General of the United States: Report to the Congress: Entering A Nursing Home: Costly Implications for Medicaid, pp 43–53. Washington DC, US General Accounting Office, November 26, 1979

17 US Department of Health and Human Services. Health Care Financing Administration: Long Term Care: Background and Future Directions. Washington, DC, US Government Printing Office, January 1981

ELDONNA M. SHIELDS
ELLA KICK

11

NURSING CARE IN
NURSING HOMES

HISTORICAL PERSPECTIVE

The nursing home, or long-term care institutional setting, has evolved in response to the needs of the increasing numbers of aging people and to changes in life-style and increased mobility of younger people. Today's nursing home as an institution evolved from the old age homes and poorhouses of the early 1930s and 1940s. For the most part, these early institutions were board and room facilities for indigent older people or those who had no other place to live. The resident worked off most of the cost for board and room by doing various chores around the home as long as he remained physically and mentally able. As the residents living in these facilities grew older and became infirm or were thought to be too senile to care for themselves, care was provided that was directed toward keeping them clean, fed, dry, and quiet.

The services provided in these early long-term care institutions were much different from those offered today. No special training was required to work in these early institutions. The owner, usually a woman, wore many hats: she was cook, cleaning lady, laundress, gardener, and "nurse." If *profes-sional* nursing care was needed, the older person was admitted to a hospital. Geriatric nursing and long-term care institutions, therefore, had their origin with the almshouses or boarding homes where care was primarily custodial in nature. This is a stigma that has yet to be overcome.

In the United States in 1939 there were approximately 1,200 nursing homes with over 25,000 beds, an average of 21 beds per facility. Medicaid and

195

Medicare, introduced in 1965, provided a new source of support for long-term care facilities, and nursing homes increased in both size and number. By 1977 there were 18,300 nursing homes with over 1,384,000 beds, an average of 76 beds per facility.[1] Recently there has been a trend toward the closing of the smaller facilities and the opening of larger, often chain-operated facilities of 250 beds or more. This trend is primarily due to the costly building regulations dictated by the Medicare and Medicaid programs. Table 11-1 presents information on the size of nursing homes in 1979.

Before Medicare legislation on 1965, nursing homes were primarily owned and operated by women, many of whom were called "nurse." A few were actually operated by visionary registered nurses who recognized that the needs of older people required the skills of the professional nurse, and saw the nursing home as a setting for independence in nursing practice. However, after the 1965 amendments to the Social Security Act, men (including physicians) saw long-term care as a potential source of wealth, and stepped in to relieve the women of the heavy burden of enterpreneurship.

It was also at this time that the focus of geriatric care changed from the homelike environment where many older persons' life-styles were maintained by participation in ongoing activities; for example, older women helped peel potatoes or mend clothes, and older men helped with some of the gardening. Regulations accompanying Medicare and Medicaid changed long-term care facilities to medically oriented institutions where participating in such activities was considered abusive, and was only permitted if specifically ordered by the physician and written into the overall therapeutic plan of care.

Since the 1965 amendment to the Social Security Act, the contemporary nursing home has emerged as a stepchild of the health care system and as a low-class replica of a hospital. The medical model is the predominant mode of care in nursing homes. Admission is dependent upon a physician's order and a medical diagnosis is required to justify the need for skilled nursing care.

Although nursing was the first professional group to speak out in support of the Medicare program, little acknowledgement of the role of the professional nurse was ever incorporated into the rules and regulations that

TABLE 11-1 Size of Nursing Homes in 1979

Bed Size	Nursing Homes		Number of Beds	Average Number of Beds
	N	%		
Fewer than 50 beds	80,000	42.3	182,900	23
50–99 beds	5,800	30.8	417,800	72
100–199 beds	4,200	22.3	546,400	130
200 beds or more	900	4.6	255,400	284

Department of Health, Education, and Welfare: The national nursing home survey: 1977 summary for the United States. No. 43, DHEW Pub. No. (PHS) 79–1794, Hyattsville, Md. July, 1979.

structured nursing home care. The professional nurses' full potential, therefore, has not been realized. This omission has become a serious constraint on the availability and provision of professional nursing care in the nursing home.

In 1972 the Social Security Act was again amended to redefine the "extended care" of Medicare and the "skilled care" of Medicaid in the same terms. This resulted in two levels of federally supported care – skilled nursing care and intermediate care – thus eliminating what was previously referred to as "extended care."

A skilled nursing home was defined as "an institution primarily engaged in providing skilled nursing care and related services for patients who require posthospital medical or nursing care or rehabilitation services.[2]

This definition at least takes into consideration the need for nursing care as a criterion for admission to a skilled nursing home. However, the regulation stating that admission must be by order of a physician was maintained. This means that the physician identifies the need for skilled or intermediate nursing care. One could ask whether this is the malpractice of nursing!

According to Medicare and Medicaid regulations, post-hospital extended care, skilled nursing, or rehabilitation services are those services furnished pursuant to physician orders. Services that would qualify as skilled nursing services include the following:

1 Intravenous, intramuscular, or subcutaneous injections or hypodermoclysis or intravenous feeding.
2 Levine tube and gastrostomy feedings.
3 Nasopharyngeal and tracheotomy aspiration.
4 Insertion, sterile irrigation, and replacement of catheters
5 Application of dressings involving prescription medications and aseptic techniques.
6 Treatment of extensive decubitus ulcers or other widespread skin disorders.
7 Health treatments that have been specifically ordered by a phsician as part of active treatment and that require observation by nurses to adequately evaluate the patient's progress.
8 Rehabilitation nursing procedures, including related teaching and adaptive aspects of nursing, that are part of active treatment.[3]

It should be noted that this definition is devoid of nursing services such as health assessment, health promotion, disease prevention, development of nursing care plans, patient education, and the nurse's role in decision making. Although some nursing terminology is currently used by regulators, the total plan of care is determined by the physician, because the physician's signature on the plan of care is a requirement of the payment mechanism to the nursing home.

The physician-dominated acute care medical model orientation to the provision of skilled nursing services in long-term care still permeates the entire Medicare and Medicaid programs. It has evolved into a system of care that encourages increased dependence and disability on the part of the older person. The nursing home is, in fact, financially rewarded for iatrogenically induced dependence and disability, as reimbursement is based upon inserting the catheter, nasogastric tube, and for allowing the skin to break down. There is no recognition of, or reimbursement for, the tremendous skill involved in promoting, maintaining, or restoring bladder function, independence in feeding, and skin integrity. As a result, the cost of providing nursing home care has risen more than 500% from 1966 to 1975.[4] The appropriateness of such a system must be questioned. How can nursing care in nursing homes be improved when nursing care is not recognized in the payment mechanisms of Medicare and Medicaid as the essential health service provided in nursing homes?

NURSE SHORTAGE IN NURSING HOMES

Much information is currently available as to the shortage of nurses within our health care system. The widely publicized shortage of nurses in hospitals is even greater in the nursing home. The shortage must often quoted for hospitals is 100,000 registered nurses. However, according to the Western Interstate Commission for Higher Education (WICHE), the projected need for registered nurses in the nursing home by 1982 is between 118,000 and 243,000. The need for 118,000 registered nurses results in a minimum ratio of one nurse per 33 residents. The need for 243,000 registered nurses results in a more optimal ratio of 1:15. This represents an increase in the number of existing nursing home nurses of between 174% and 466% by 1982. In 1980 8.1% or 80,000 of all working registered nurses were employed in nursing homes, compared to 65% employed in hospitals.[5] Between 1972 and 1980 there was a 42% increase in nursing home employment.[6] However, during that period the number of nursing home beds increased dramatically, and despite an increase in nursing home nurses, a shortage of great magnitude persists.

Dr. Linda Aiken in her presidential address to the American Academy of Nursing stated.

> The use of the term "nursing" to describe most of the existing facilities that care for the health-impaired elderly is far from accurate. In fact, there is a shocking lack of health professionals working within them. Only 5 percent

of nursing home employees are registered nurses. On an average day in an average nursing home, there are only 1.5 licensed health care providers for every 100 patients in evidence – this is a section involving almost two million patients![7]

There are many reasons why there are so few nurses working in nursing homes. One, nurses who work in nursing homes often work in isolation. As evidenced in Aiken's findings in 1981, it would not be unusual to find only one licensed nurse in a nursing home of 100 residents for a 24-hr period. This person may be a registered nurse or a licensed practical nurse.

A second reason for the nurse shortage in the nursing home has to do with the low status of the nursing home nurse. The nursing home is considered by many nurses, other health professionals, and the general public as the dumping ground for older people and the dumping ground for incompetent nurses. As an example, a nurse formerly employed in a coronary care unit once said she was sent a sympathy card signed by the staff in the coronary care unit when she accepted employment in a nursing home.

A third reason has to do with the unrealistic staffing patterns that are supported by legislation in some states. As an example, in Ohio the most recent regulations that govern licensure for a nursing home accepting only private pay clients require a minimum staffing ratio that would provide the following levels of care delivery per resident: registered nurse – 1.7 min every 8 hr, or 4.8 min in 24 hr; licensed practical nurse – 8 min every 8 hr, or 24 min in 24 hr; nurses' aide – 26 min every 8 hr, or 80 min in 24 hr.[8]

A fourth reason for the nurse shortage in the nursing home is a lack of understanding of the role of the professional nurse in the nursing home. This lack of knowledge about the role of the nurse in this setting can be well understood when one realizes that in 1976 only 13% of all registered nurse programs offered content on aging. Of this 13%, only 22% required content on aging for graduation. Of the 87% that were not currently offering an aging component, 85% indicated that such a component was planned for implementation in the near future, a sign that perhaps future cohorts will be better educated in the care of older adults than the current pool of nurses.[9]

The literature also indicates that 83% of the directors of nursing in nursing homes are diploma educated, 7% are associate degree graduates, and the remaining 10% are baccalaureate graduates.[10] This creates many problems, as most diploma programs generally educate nurses to function almost exlusively in the acute care setting. When a nurse with this background is introduced to the long-term care setting, she functions much like the head nurse on a unit in the hospital. One must question the appropriateness of such practices. Perhaps an increase in the number of continuing education programs could become a part of the fringe benefits offered to attract nurses to nursing homes.

Salary and fringe benfits are other reasons cited as major deterrents to seeking employment in the nursing home. In 1977 registered nurses working in nursing homes were receiving an average hourly wage of $5.59 for full-time employment compared with $6.86 per hour for full-time nurses working in hospitals, a difference of 20%. Even grocery store cashiers who require no special educational preparation received $7.64 per hour — 28% higher than incomes of nurses employed in nursing homes![11] A 1977 survey of registered nurses in the eastern and western United States indicated a salary range $2,640 to $3,216 per year less for staff nurses working in nursing homes.[12] In addition to salary differentials, nurses employed in nursing homes receive fewer benefits than nurses working in hospitals. Given the noncompetitive wage structure for nurses in nursing homes, it will be very difficult to recruit the well-qualified nurses needed to provide leadership to help raise the standards of care.

Finally, but far from being the least important, is the issue of professional autonomy and the lack of control over nursing practice. The current Medicare and Medicaid regulations are built upon the medical model of care and, therefore, provide payment only for medically related problems. The physician is the health professional that certifies when the older person needs "skilled" nursing care. A non-nurse determines when a person no longer requires nursing care. The appropriateness of such a system must be questioned.

In addition to the underfinancing of care, the major impediment to improving the quality of nursing care in nursing homes today is the insufficient number of registered nurses educationally prepared to provide direct care to older people and their families, and also to direct others in the technical tasks that do not always require the skills of the professional nurse.

NEEDS OF INSTITUTIONALIZED OLDER PEOPLE

Most older people are in institutions because they can no longer take care of themselves. Their multiple needs are related to the influence of age on physical, psychological, social, and spiritual functional abilities. For most older people their medical diagnoses have long been established. Their remaining medical needs are for periodic review and evaluation of disease processes and prescribed medical regimen. The World Health Organization states that "other health workers, including physicians, would only be involved in the care of the patient as a result of referral by the nurse."[13]

The primary health care needs of the institutionalized older adult should be directed toward the promotion, maintenance, and restoration of optimal physical, mental, social, and spiritual function, and emphasis should be placed on maximum independence in the activities of everyday living or on care that is directed toward maintaining life with dignity and comfort until death. Health and nursing care needs cannot be determined by medical diagnoses and treatment alone. The medical needs of the older person must be structured into a matrix of needs that approach the person's care holistically.

This fact is well substantiated in a recent study by Leslie on the use of the nursing diagnosis in long-term care.[14] It was found that the nursing diagnoses were more relevant and predictive of the nursing care needs of the older adult than were the medical diagnoses. The data revealed, for example, that 90.4% of the 210 residents included in the study required nursing assistance with elimination (45.7% for bladder, 44.7% for bowel). The nursing diagnosis of impaired mobility was found with 80.4% of the residents, and susceptibility to hazards was found with 64.7% of the older people evaluated. Few of the nursing diagnoses requiring nursing care were directly related to or even implied from the medical diagnoses. The medical diagnoses identified chronic, irreversible conditions, while the nursing diagnoses described needs that nurses could work with in promoting, maintaining, and restoring health or preventing disease or disability.

The most striking comparisons between the relevance of the medical diagnosis and the nursing diagnosis can be seen in the percentage of residents with a nursing diagnosis of sensory disturbance (32.3%) and the medical diagnosis of loss of special senses (6.3%).[15] The number of recorded nursing diagnoses per older person ranged from 1 to 21, with an average of between 10 and 13, as compared with the average range of four to six different medical diagnoses found with most older adults.[16]

In order to meet the health care needs of institutionalized older adults more appropriately, a nursing model of care is required that is consistent with the following definition of nursing: "Nursing is the diagnosis and treatment of human responses to actual or potential health problems."[19] This model recognizes nursing as the primary health care service in the nursing home, and places the nurse in a position of responsibility, authority, and accountability for the nursing and health services provided to the residents. Success with this nursing model is measured against the older adult's actual level of function in relation to a broad spectrum of physical, psychological, social, and spiritual parameters, and is compared to the older person's potential level of function.

The nurse strives to promote, maintain, and restore maximum function and independence in the health behaviors essential to everyday living; uses anticipatory guidance in working with the maturational and situational events that confront the older person and the family as they continue to grow and develop; and works with the older person and the family in modifying their environment to support health. The role of medicine lies in the area of disease. The physician strives to diagnose, treat, cure, and rehabilitate the person who is ill and to prevent disease.

Nursing and medicine become interrelated and work together collaboratively when health and illness coexist within the same person. The nurse determines the influence of the disease and its medical treatment on the efficiency of health behaviors and the ability of the older person to maintain them independently. For example, the use of diazepam (Valium) with the older person may decrease anxiety and agitation; however, the muscle relaxant side-effects will also decrease the efficiency of mobility.

The nurse intervenes when there is an imbalance between what is needed to efficiently maintain a specific health behavior and the older person's ability to maintain it independently. The study cited earlier by Leslie would be supportive of this approach.[17]

When using this conceptual framework, the elements of the health care system on which nursing would focus in practice, education, and research are the *promotion, maintenance, restoration of health* and the *prevention of illness and disability*. The specific nursing services provided would include the following:

- Health appraisal.
- Health education.
- Health counseling.
- Health monitoring.
- Anticipatory guidance.
- Technical services.
- Treatment management.
- Consultation.

The cost of providing each of these nursing services could be identified to reveal the overall cost for nursing care for each resident and family. This may provide the data needed for a more appropriate allocation of funds to meet the nursing and health care needs of the older person.

The nursing model of care could be implemented realistically in the nursing home if the concept of primary nursing, as currently used in many hospitals, were modified. The professional nurse (primary nurse), instead of doing *all* the assessing, planning, implementing, monitoring, and evaluating of nursing care for each resident assigned to her, would delegate nursing care to a nursing assistant who is permanently assigned to the primary nurse. Both the primary nurse and the nursing assistant would have the same permanent assignment regardless of the time of day or shift that is worked.

The literature indicates that the quality of care in nursing homes is dependent upon the number of registered nurses employed. In a study focusing on patient outcome as a measure of quality of care, Linn and colleagues found that

> the one variable consistently related to patient outcome was registered nurse hours. Homes with more RN hours per patient were associated with patient survival, patient improvement, and patient discharge from the nursing home. RN hours specifically were related to outcome whereas hours per patient of other service providers or the total staff/patient ratio were not so related.[18]

These findings have been further substantiated in a more recent study by Kaeser revealing more adequate patient care planning and personal care services when there were more nurses and fewer licensed practical nurses; more adequate professional interventions when there were more registered nurses and fewer aides; and more overall adequacy when there were more registered nurses, fewer licensed practical nurses, and a not-for-profit status or an owner on site as administrator or director of nursing service.[19]

The registered nurse in the above example would function as the primary nurse responsible for assessing, planning, implementing, monitoring, and evaluating the total nursing care for the residents and their families. Each primary nurse would be scheduled to be in the nursing home for 8 hr per day, 5 days per week, and would be available on call for the residents for whom she is responsible for the remaining 16 hr. The specific hours or times the registered nurse is in the nursing home may be flexible, and still provide for 24 hr registered nurse coverage. If at any time there is a change in a resident's condition that would require a modification in the plan of care, the primary nurse would be consulted to determine the specific modifications.

In addition to being the primary nurse for a panel of residents, the registered nurse would also be responsible for seeing that the aspects of nursing care delegated to the nursing assistant are appropriately carried out. It is vital that the primary nurse specifically describe the following for each aspect of care that is delegated:

- The specific care to be provided.
- How the care is provided.
- When the care is provided.
- Where the care is provided.
- Who actually provides the care.

This is especially important when delegating certain aspects of care to the resident, family, and nursing assistant.

As primary nurse the registered nurse would therefore be responsible for the following:

- Assessing the health status of the older person to identify the actual and potential needs for nursing and other health care services.
- Planning and implementing nursing care to meet the actual and potential needs for nursing and health care.
- Monitoring the older person's response to nursing and other health care.
- Evaluating the older person's response to nursing and health care.
- Communicating the plan for nursing and health care to appropriate nursing personnel and other health care professionals.

In addition to establishing the plan for nursing and health care for residents and their families, the registered nurse would also do the following:

- Supervise the care delegated by her nurse colleagues to the residents, family, or nursing assistant.
- Coordinate other personnel and health care services as determined by the total plan of care.
- Develop and evaluate standards for nursing practice, peer review and audit mechanisms.
- Participate in peer and interdisciplinary reviews.
- Identify the need for and implement staff development programs for nursing personnel.

Because these elements of nursing care are also referred to in the present Medicare and Medicaid regulations for nursing services provided in nursing homes, it seems logical and appropriate that these services become a part of the payment mechanisms for nursing care. Nursing services are currently considered as part of the reimbursement for room and board and the related activities such as dietary, housekeeping, laundry, and maintenance.

At a reimbursement rate of $40 per day per resident, the allocation of funds with registered nurse coverage at a ratio of 1:30 and nursing assistant coverage at a ratio of 2:33 per shift would be the following:

• Registered nurse	20%	$8.00 per resident day
• Nursing assistant	47%	18.80 per resident day
• Food/dietary	15%	5.60 per resident day
• Laundry	3%	1.20 per resident day
• Housekeeping/maintenance	3%	1.20 per resident day
• Administration	7%	2.80 per resident day
• Other	6%	2.40 per resident day

The fact that nursing is the primary health care service provided in the nursing home must be reflected in the budget of the nursing service department. However, few registered nurses have the expertise to determine or compete and negotiate for a budget, and then to efficiently allocate the funds in the management of human and material resources needed to provide quality nursing and health care. The director of nursing in the nursing home must become more knowledgeable in long-term care nursing administration. It is the responsibility of the profession to provide the educational programming needed to accomplish this.

STRATEGIES FOR CHANGE

Based upon these preceding issues, I would like to propose several strategies for change that have the potential for increasing the number of nurses working in the nursing home; decreasing the isolation in which the nurse often works; improving the image of the nursing home, nursing care, and the nurse choosing to work in this setting; improving the salary and fringe benefits paid to the nurse; and providing autonomy and control over nursing practice.

The four strategies to be discussed include the following:

1 The development of networking among registered nurses practicing within the nursing home setting; and between and among registered nurses in other practice settings.

2 The development of a mentoring system for the registered nurse that is new to the nursing home setting.

3 The use of an independently organized group of registered nurses, external to the nursing home, contracting to provide the nursing services for individual nursing homes.

4 The use of the teaching nursing home as a means for furthering the growth and development of gerontologic nursing as a practice discipline.

One approach to dealing with the isolation so often experienced by the registered nurse practicing in the nursing home setting is the development of networking. Through networking, registered nurses practicing in nursing homes within a given locale would meet collectively. This would provide the opportunity for them to develop peer relationships that would give them a sense of identity and community. A network of peers would provide the occasion to share information, review work, provide feedback, explore issues and strategies, assist each other in problem solving, and become a source of encouragement and support. A networking group could also provide the collectiveness and influence needed to improve the employment conditions so often cited as reasons for nurses choosing other areas of practice.

This type of networking has been accomplished at the national level of the American Nurses' Association (ANA) by the establishment of the Council for Nursing Home Nurses within the Division of Gerontological Practice. What is being proposed here is that similar networks also be established at the state and local levels to provide support and leadership needed to deal with the everyday issues and problems encountered in nursing homes.

Networking among registered nurses practicing in nursing homes would also provide an opportunity for the registered nurse new to the nursing home setting to develop role models to imitate and to develop more mature and growth-producing mentor relationships.

In discussing the use of a mentor in nursing it is important to differentiate between role modeling and mentoring. The major difference between a role model and mentor is the interaction between the two professionals involved. A mentor is the "accomplished, more experienced professional who extends to a young, aspiring person, within the context of a one-to-one relationship, advice, teaching, sponsorship, guidance, and assistance toward her establishment in her chosen profession."[20]

The mentor is a professional who possesses and represents the qualities that the nurse, new to the nursing home setting, hopes to acquire. The mentor facilitates and influences the younger nurse's advancement within the profession by enchancing professional skills and intellectual development. The mentor also provides counsel and moral support during times of stress and encouragement during risk-taking situations.

The role model, on the other hand, is an "individual who demonstrates by skills and techniques, personal organization of values, philosophical beliefs and attitudes, and overall style, behavior that is viewed by another and contrasted with her own performance. The role model is observed and compared as a standard of excellence from which the individual can learn, imitate, identify, and somehow magically incorporate into nursing."[21]

The role model, therefore, fosters imitation, which is important early in the professional's career. However, it "assumes that the imitator will achieve only the level of performance and skill which has been demonstrated."[22] With mentoring, there is a relationship between the two professionals that fosters professional growth and self-development. It is the difference between giving a person a fish and teaching the person to fish — the difference between eating for a day and eating for a lifetime.

Networking and mentoring should also take place among nurses practicing in nursing homes and within other practice settings. It is through this type of networking that the nurse in the nursing home setting can begin to break down the negative stereotypes that exist within the profession. Nurses within other practice settings can begin to network with each other to share information, review work, provide feedback, explore issues and strategies, and assist each other in problem solving. By so doing, all nurses within a given locale can begin to develop a sense of community or belonging, which can result in nurses working with nurses to improve the quality of nursing care available in a given community, and it can provide the collectiveness that is essential in order to advance nursing in its development as a profession.

The third strategy for dealing with the issues related to the shortages of nurses and quality of care in nursing homes is the use of contracting for nursing services. Ardith Grandebouche, R.N., president of a nursing personnel pool, believes that the service problems and shortages of nurses can be remedied only by "something different from anything in the past. . . . One of the problems is that nursing is not controlled by nursing, it's controlled by hospital administrators, by physicians, by many different forces pulling this way and that. A management contract changes that situation."[23]

The increasing popularity of outside agencies providing temporary nursing staff for many nursing homes and hospitals may be the beginning of this strategy being realized. However, in order to ensure autonomy and control over nursing practice, it is vital that nurses organize themselves to provide nursing services, and not be organized and employed by some outside, non-nursing group. When nurses are employed by temporary staffing agencies they are putting themselves and the services they are credentialed to provide in a position to again be exploited and controlled by others.

External, independently organized groups of nurses providing nursing services under contract could establish an environment supportive of professional autonomy and control over nursing practice, thereby increasing the effectiveness and quality of nursing services provided in the nursing home. When contracting for nursing services with a group of independently organized registered nurses, external to the nursing home, the delivery of nursing service would be under the control of nursing, thus creating an environment in which the nursing model could easily be implemented. The *Standards of Gerontological Nursing Practice* could be used as the guide to quality nursing care.[24]

A fourth strategy, which is designed to generate new knowledge and improve the quality of nursing and health care within the nursing home is the establishment of teaching nursing homes.

The development of the teaching nursing home, as suggested by Aiken and Butler is analogous to the strategy used by medicine in the establishment of teaching hospitals. By affiliating with medical schools and larger teaching hospitals, the teaching hospital was successful in reducing professional isolation and improving the clinical capabilities and medical care provided in smaller community hospitals.[24,26]

It is believed that since nursing is the primary health service provided in nursing homes, similar affiliations with university schools of nursing, medical schools, and teaching hospitals will also result in decreased professional isolation and improved quality of nursing and health care by offering a different perspective and fresh approach to nursing practice, education, and research within the nursing home setting. "Just as 450 teaching hospitals have become models for 7,000 community hospitals, teaching nursing homes could become models for 18,000 nursing homes."[27]

In conclusion, the nursing home does have the potential for being a very exciting, professionally challenging, and rewarding area in which to practice nursing. It is a setting where the full potential of the nurse can truly be realized, as working with older people demands the best skills that are known to the nurse. It has been said that whether our nursing homes become the dumping grounds for those older people who are physically, mentally, or socially indigent, or a community of experienced people, is determined by the nursing staff.

Can there be nursing care in nursing homes? The answer to this question lies within nursing. Our answer to it is vital — as much of the future of the profession will be determined by our response.

REFERENCES

1 National Center for Health Statistics: Overview of nursing home characteristics, 1977 national nursing home survey provisional estimates, by M. Meiners. *Advance data from vital and health statistics*, No. 35, DHEW, Hyattsville, Md. September 6, 1978a.

2 Office of Research and Statistics: *Social Security Bulletin annual statistical supplement, 1975*. Social Security Administration, Washington, D.C., U.S. Government Printing Office, 1976.

3 Department of Health, Education, and Welfare, Social Security Administration, *Federal Register*, 40(107), Tuesday, June 3, 1975.

4 Western Interstate Commission for Higher Education. *Analysis of planning for improved distribution of nursing personnel and services*. Government Printing Office, Washington, D.C. March, 1979.

5 Moses, Evelyn and Roth, Alida. "Nurse Power," *American Journal of Nursing*, October 1979. Vol. 79, No. 10, p. 1750.

6 American Nurses' Association. *Facts on Nursing*. ANA.

7 Aiken, Linda H. Nursing priorities for the 1980's: Hospitals and nursing homes. *American Journal of Nursing*. Feb., 1981, p. 239.

8 Ohio Department of Health. *Nursing and rest home law and rules*. Revised to May 10, 1977, p. 8.

9 Division on Gerontological Nursing Practice: *Gerontological concepts as presented in basic nursing education programs*. Kansas City, Mo.: American Nurses' Association, 1976.

10 Buseck, S.A. and E.M. Shields. Training of registered nurses providing patient care in nursing homes. Final report submitted to DHEW, Bureau of Health Services Research, Division of Long Term Care, Washington, D.C. December 1, 1974.

11 Department of Health, Education and Welfare: *The national nursing home survey: 1977 summary for the United States.* No. 43, DHEW Pub. No. (PHS) 79–1794, Hyattsville, Md. July, 1979.

12. U.S. Dept. of Labor, Bureau of Labor Statistics. *Occupational outlook handbook.* 1977.

13 Banker, D.E. The Role of Nursing in Care of the Elderly. In, World Health Organization, Regional Office for Europe, *Nursing aspects in care of the elderly.* Copenhagen: WHO, 1977.

14 Leslie, F.M. Nursing diagnosis: use in long term care. *American Journal of Nursing* 81:1012–1014, 1981.

15 *Ibid.*

16 *Ibid.*

17 *Ibid.*

18 Linn, Margaret W., et al. Patient outcome measure of quality of nursing home care. *American Journal of Public Health.* April 1977, pp. 337–344.

19 Kaeser, L.A. The relationship between patient care expenditures and quality of care in long term care nursing homes. Doctoral Dissertation. Cornell University, 1981.

20 Hamilton, Margaret Smith. Mentorhood: A key to nursing leadership. *Nursing Leadership*, Vol. 4, no. 1, March, 1981, pp. 4–13.

21 *Ibid.*, p. 9.

22 Smoyak, S.A. Teaching is coaching. *Nursing Outlook.* Vol. 26, No. 6, June, 1978, p. 322.

23 LaViolette, Suzanne. Agencies experiment with contracts. *Modern Healthcare.* April 1981, p. 40.

24 Division on Gerontological Nursing Practice. *Standards: Gerontological Nursing Practice*, Kansas City, Missouri, American Nurses' Association, 1976.

25 Aiken, Linda, *op. cit.*

26 Butler, Robert. The Teaching Nursing Home. *JAMA*", Vol. 245, No. 14, April 10, 1981. pp. 1435–1437.

27 *Ibid.*, p. 1435.

GENROSE J. ALFANO

12

HOSPITAL-BASED EXTENDED CARE NURSING: A CASE STUDY OF THE LOEB CENTER

Health care in the United States is, for the most part, focused on the care of people with acute, episodic illness. Hospitals have increasingly become short-term, high-technology treatment centers; patients are discharged as soon as possible to recuperate in their own homes. Ambulatory health care is also delivered primarily on an episodic basis in physicians' offices and clinics, with very loosely organized — if any — continuing care provisions. However, the burden of illness in the American population is increasingly chronic in nature, and the organization of medical care is not as effective with chronic illness as it is with acute, episodic problems.

Our primary national strategy to care for the chronically ill, frail elderly has been nursing homes. However, the nursing home concept has been a failure in terms of returning patients to independent living. Most patients who are admitted to nursing homes remain there for life. Patients with chronic illnesses who are unable to carry out their usual activities, or who are at risk of suffering serious complications but who have the potential to return to independent living, do not fit well into any of the three predominant care settings: hospital, office, or nursing home.

Hospital-based extended care is not a new concept. In the late 1950s, some hospitals established special units for patients whose acute crises had been resolved but who needed short-term rehabilitation in order to return to productive lives. Extended care was originally envisioned as a setting for "extending" those professional services of the acute care hospital that would facilitate recovery but would be less costly and less technologically intensive than acute care. The original Medicare legislation provided for extended care that would be rehabilitative in nature and be accomplished in a reasonably short period of time. Very few hospitals, however, had special units that met Medicare's requirements for reimbursement as extended care facilities. Most states tried to upgrade custodial nursing homes, which was never a successful way to organize extended care. Eventually, the concept of extended care was dropped by Medicare and replaced with skilled and intermediate nursing facilities.

Renewed interest in hospital-based, long-term care has been generated by disillusionment with nursing homes, declining occupancy rates in short-term acute hospitals, and an interest on the part of teaching hospitals in expanding training in geriatrics. Whether the concept is implemented on a broad scale depends upon the overall costs of care and the effectiveness of hospital-based extended care in returning patients to optimal levels of function.

The following case study of the Loeb Center at Montefiore Hospital and Medical Center describes the achievements of a hospital-based, extended care program based on professional nursing care as the major therapy. The model represented by the Loeb Center may eventually become an alternative to nursing home placement for many patients. It also presents the potential for greater autonomy for professional nursing practice.

LOEB CENTER PROGRAM

Loeb Center initially had the following purposes:

- To provide patients with a less rigidly structured environment in which to recover from illness once the medical crisis was over, the diagnosis had been established, and treatment plan had begun.
- To provide patients with a program of nursing care that supported their healing through a process of nurturing and through a nondirective approach to learning and awareness of self.
- To provide nursing as the central, focal therapy offered throughout each 24-hr period, with other therapies and medical care provided as needed.

The program was administered, directed, and conducted by nursing professionals. A medical consultant was appointed to ensure that the care provided was consistent with the requirements of the medical center.

The Loeb Center provides patients with interim care (post-critical phase) and prepares them for discharge. Its program is based upon several

concepts related to illness, theories of learning, nursing as essentially a nurturing process, and nurturing as a major component in healing.

Loeb Center is both patient and family oriented. This orientation is most
useful at the intermediary stage of illness in bringing about a more rapid and
sustained recovery. Loeb Center care involves in-depth training for the patient and family to permit discharge into the home. As indicated in Figure 12-
1, from January 1 to July 1, 1981 84% of patients discharged from the Loeb
Center returned to their families and homes, while less than 2% were admitted to long-term facilities. A total of 14% returned to the acute care setting, but 9% of these hospital admissions were planned readmissions for
second-stage operative procedures. Fewer than 1% died.

Patients are not admitted to the Loeb Center with the goal of residency
or solely for protection and maintenance. Patients are admitted for recovery
from an acute episode, for nursing rehabilitation, and for preparation for
discharge—all as part of a continuing hospital stay. In 1977 the average
length of stay at the Loeb Center was 14.5 days. In 1980 and in the first half
of 1981, it was 12.5 days.[1]

The program has been able to function at a cost equal to one-half the
hospital *per diem*, to shorten the patient's stay on the acute general unit, and to
better prepare persons to return to their own homes.[2] The majority function
without support from sources other than family members or significant
others, but a number are referred to existing community services.

RATIONALE FOR STAFFING

The Loeb Center is organized on the premise that nurses with broad basic
preparation in general education, a strong base in the clinical, social, and behavioral sciences, and an understanding of the principles of teaching and
learning can deliver the most economical as well as the best quality nursing
care. Lydia E. Hall, founder of the Loeb Center, recognized and identified
nursing as the principal discipline in helping persons with chronic diseases
maintain function and enhance the quality of their lives. An expert clinician
with a strong background in the social sciences, Hall incorporated Selye's
theories of stress and adaptation in the understanding of chronic and acute
illness.[3] While many talked about the integration of the biologic, social, and
behavioral sciences, Hall developed a process for nursing care based upon a
theory that incorporated the teachings of Harry Stack Sullivan, Carl Rogers,
and John Dewey.[4–6] These leaders in their respective fields served as reference sources for the formulation of an illness–wellness theory and a construct
for nursing's role as a nurturer to bring about healing.

When the Loeb Center admitted its first patients, the major organizational mode for delivery of nursing care in hospitals throughout the country

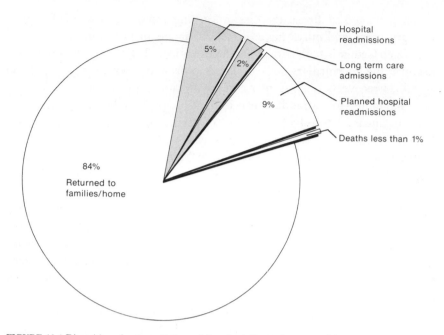

5%

2%

9%

Hospital readmissions

Long term care admissions

Planned hospital readmissions

Deaths less than 1%

84%
Returned to families/home

FIGURE 12-1 Disposition of patients discharged from Loeb Center January to July 1981.

was team or functional assignment. Division of nursing tasks or activities was considered an effective and efficient method of using persons with differing types of education and preparation—from 2 wk on the job without prior formal preparation to 5 yr of university-based professional nursing education.

Determination of patient needs rested primarily with the physician, who prescribed activity levels, diagnostic tests, treatments, medications, and procedures based upon the patient's pathology and clinical status. Nursing's function was to carry out those prescriptions wherever the patient was housed.

Nursing education curricula had long included a concept of care during hospitalization involving attention to the behavior and life-styles of people that extended beyond the solution to the immediate problems of illness. The difficulty was in implementing this concept into the actual practice of nursing in the hospital. The fractionalization of nursing care had made it almost impossible for nurses who had been exposed to the curricula to "find the time to spend with patients." Supervision of other personnel, conferences to coordinate multiple services, a shortage of nurses willing and prepared to provide clinical care, and a seeming indifference on the part of many registered nurses to deal with problems other than the most tangible and technical all fostered a stop-gap system of care that dealt with each patient problem in isolation and independent of each other.

In 1963, when Lydia Hall at the Loeb Center proposed the delivery of nursing care by registered nurses *only* and encouraged use of the case concept employed in public health nursing, it represented to some a reversal — and to others a revolution — in care concepts.[7,8] Recognizing the fact that medication should have a direct effect on the functioning of patients, it seems logical that the nurse who gave the medicine should have the opportunity to evaluate the effect. Recongizing that physical care given by the nurse would have a consequential effect on vital signs and symptomatology, it seemed more efficient to have the person who participated in these activities sufficiently skilled and able to assess the extent and implications of the effect. It was imperative to assess and evaluate the extent and types of activities and treatments that would foster rather than impede full function and that would enhance rather than threaten life. The complexities of these interrelationships meant that nursing could no longer be regarded as a list of activities ranging from the simple to the complex, but must be viewed as a process in which all activities contributed to the ultimate outcome.

A massive reeducation and reformation of nurses' attitudes was a necessity as this concept began to be but into practice. It was said that nurses would not want to give physical care or assist patients to carry out the basic activities of daily living, and that this was a waste of nurses' education, talents, and skills. It was commonly believed that physicians would not accept an organizational pattern in which nurses determined a patient's eligibility for a program of continuing hospital care. It was predicted that the Loeb Center would become nothing more than another "nursing home" and too expensive an operation for the services it would deliver.

Initial referrals to the Loeb Center did indeed include patients with problems that seemed unsolvable and would result in permanent institutionalization and patients for "rest and protective measures." However, Associated Hospital Service of New York (Blue Cross) agreed to reimburse patients for Loeb Center care on a trial basis while studying types of admissions, justifications for hospitalization, and determination as to whether the Center's program presented a savings to the plan. Initially, because of the newness of the program, and the fact that it was untried, most patients were referred after the 21st day of hospital care. At that time, the major Blue Cross contract provided total reimbursement for 21 full days and 180 half days. The Loeb Center *per diem* cost had been calculated to approximate one-half the hospital *per diem*. This meant that patients who were on half days would be saving some money if they were transferred to Loeb after the 21st day.

As use of the Loeb Center program increased, physicians, patients, and nurses began to notice a difference resulting from the Center's care. People who had been judged unrehabilitatible were improving and were able to function well enough to return to their homes. Patients who had long histories of frequent readmissions to the hospital were increasing their span of time out of hospital. Gradually a core of physician "users" built up: doctors found that their patients were happier and did better as a result of their Loeb experience. In November 1964 *Medical World News*, in an article entitled "More Care, Fewer Patients," described the Loeb Center as follows:

"Combining maximum nursing attention with minimal hospital routine, the unique program at the Loeb Center in New York speeds rehabilitation after the acute stage of illness."[9]

The Associated Hospital Service of New York, in a survey of the Greater New York area in 1965 found that the hospital readmission rate of patients discharged from the Loeb Center was one-fifth that for comparable patients discharged directly from the hospital to home care programs. Evaluations of the Loeb Center have consistently demonstrated that this facility and program provides an important and effective service for patients, plus providing an opportunity for health care providers in all disciplines to realize their skills and contributions more fully.

EVALUATION

If, as the evidence suggested, the Loeb Center program could reduce the overall cost of hospital care, improve the quality of nursing care, and satisfy patients, nurses, and medical staff, then other centers of professional nursing with similar programs should be developed. However, it was recognized that only through a well-designed research effort could hard evidence be obtained to evaluate the efficacy of the Loeb Center program and the desirability of establishing such a program elsewhere.

In 1974 the Loeb Center completed an 18-mo follow-up study of the outcomes of care funded by the Department of Health, Education and Welfare (HEW). The aims of the study were as follows:

1　To compare the outcome of hospitalization in a group of patients hospitalized at the Loeb Center for part of their stay with a comparable group of patients who received all of their nursing care in a conventional environment.

2　To study the outcome of hospitalization in a longitudinal manner in order to observe both the short-term and long-term aspects of rehabilitation after hospitalization.

3　To compare the outcome of hospitalization, using a variety of outcome criteria classified broadly as morbidity and mortality experience, employment, home and community activities, activities of daily living, verbal behavior, and level of anxiety.

4　To determine if a stay at the Loeb Center could account for a favorable

outcome being experienced (*i.e.*, did the Loeb Center make the difference?).

5   To suggest explanations for differences in the outcome that would
provide hypotheses to be tested in future studies of variations in nursing
practice and their effects on patients.

STUDY DESIGN

The study was designed to satisfy two major aims of the investigation: to
contrast two comparable groups of patients exposed to different nursing environments and programs, and to use a wide variety of outcome criteria to
assess differences between groups over a long period of time. These considerations led to a design that embodied the features of both experimental and
survey research.

The research design called for studying a group of patients exposed to
the Loeb Center program and environment and a control group without such
exposure. To provide the proper contrast, the two groups would have to be
comparable in terms of other characteristics predictive of the outcomes of
hospitalization. Then, differences in outcome could only be attributed to differences in exposure.

Admission to the Loeb Center is a function of two processes: the patient's physician must request the admission, and the patient must satisfy the
admission criteria of the Loeb Center. The unquantifiable criteria a physician
uses to choose specific patients for referral, plus the Loeb eligibility requirements, were considered sources of potential bias if one were to contrast patients admitted to the Loeb Center with those who spent their entire stay
elsewhere. Hence, the population was defined as all patients who were
referred and eligible for admission to the Loeb Center. By a random process,
a group of patients from this population would be selected to enter Loeb Center, while the remainder would act as controls. In support of this definition, it
was recognized that not all hospitalized patients would benefit from the Loeb
Center setting. Further, it would be extremely meaningful if both the Loeb
Center patients and control patients had exhibited the need for intensive professional nursing care, as well as satisfying a basic criterion for a Loeb admission—evidence of a favorable prognosis for a return to the community.
Excluded from the study population were subjects with a prior stay at the
Loeb Center.

Patients admitted to the Loeb Center represented a wide variety of
clinical diagnoses. Since many were rare in terms of their relative frequency,
and with outcomes varying widely by type of condition, inclusion of all patients was avoided. The study population definition was further refined to
include only those patients with the more frequently occurring diagnoses.

Concurrently, these were to be conditions of major community importance, reflecting different prognoses for a return to a prehospitalization level of health and activity.

Patients with coronary artery disease (CAD) represented the larger of the two groups selected. Eligibility for inclusion required that a CAD patient satisfy one of the following criteria:

1   A proven myocardial infarction based on electrocardiographic (ECG) evidence or blood chemistries (or both), with or without a secondary complication.

2   A questionable myocardial infarction or coronary insufficiency, with no straight myocardial infarction ECG evidence.

3   Demonstrable coronary insufficiency.

4   Congestive heart failure based on coronary sclerosis, with or without a history of myocardial infarction.

5   Rhythm disorders, coronary artery disease, or previous infarcts affecting the conduction system, with or without a pacemaker.

Eighty-five percent of the CAD referrals satisfied the first criterion. Excluded from the CAD group were those patients with angina due to reasons other than coronary sclerosis (*e.g.*, anemia, valvular disease, hypertension). Also excluded were those with any surgical intervention for coronary artery disease, except for pacemaker implantation.

The second major group were those patients with a fracture of the femoral head or neck where the injury was of traumatic origin. Subjects with fractures of pathologic origin were considered ineligible.

After referral to the Loeb Center and determination of the patient's eligibility, allocation to a specific group depended upon the result of an arithmetic manipulation of the terminal digits of an accession number assigned at admission. The allocation method was withheld from physicians making referrals, and from those who determined the patient's eligibility for admission to the Loeb Center.

The patient's allocation was revealed to the attending physician after eligibility for admissions to the Loeb Center and to the study was determined. If a referring physician or a patient declined participation, the allocation procedure was still followed (*i.e.*, a nonparticipating control subject would not be admitted to the Loeb Center, while a nonparticipating Loeb Center subject would).

The initial sampling scheme called for a 50:50 allocation to the Loeb Center and control groups on a random basis as patients entered the study. Subsequently, two revisions were made. Because of the demand for acute beds and bed availability at the Loeb Center, two patients were randomly allocated to the Loeb Center for every one admitted to the control group. Secondly, the original procedure did not insure a 50:50 allocation of the patients of each attending physician. Due to inequities in allocation ratios, and subsequent complaints, a separate allocation scheme was adopted for each referring physician.

FINDINGS

Evaluation findings support the premise that Loeb patients fared better and at less overall cost.[2] The following is a summary of major findings:

COST OF HOSPITAL STAY. Loeb Center patients remained in the institution on an average of 5.5 days longer than control patients. However, average costs for the control group exceeded the Loeb Center group because costs in the Loeb Center were only half the hospital *per diem*.

HOSPITAL READMISSION. There was a significantly longer interval between discharge and readmission for the Loeb Center group. Coupled with the fact that control group subjects experienced more multiple rehospitalizations, the findings tend to support the premise that the overall cost of care is less when Loeb Center is appropriately substituted for a portion of the acute care stay.

The Loeb group averaged 1.56 episodes of rehospitalization as compared to a mean of 1.84 in the control group, a statistically significant difference. The report further indicated that 63% of the Loeb subjects who were rehospitalized had a single episode, *versus* 47% of the control group — again a statistically significant difference. The study also measured the elapsed time from the discharge date of the initial hospitalization to readmission. The Loeb subjects were readmitted on the average almost 7 wk later than the controls — 28.1 wk *versus* 21.3 wk. In addition to measuring the average number of elapsed weeks to rehospitalization, the study suggested a difference in the pattern of the rate in which rehospitalization occurred over the 18-mo period. The probability of being hospital free was always greater for the Loeb Center group at any time during the first 72 wk after discharge. However, as indicated in Figure 12-2, after 72 wk post-discharge, both groups were similar. This leads to speculation that additional exposure to ongoing nursing care from the Loeb Center on an ambulatory basis might result in even fewer rehospitalizations. A second-phase evaluation, discussed later, is underway to test this.

NURSING HOME ADMISSION. Nursing home admissions were significantly fewer among Loeb Center patients. Only 1.4% of Loeb Center patients entered a home, compared to 11.9% of the control group. Almost all of the nursing

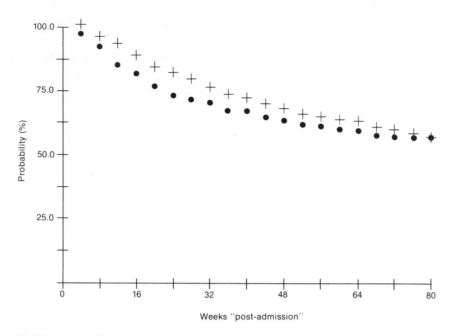

FIGURE 12-2 Probability of not having experienced a rehospitalization by a specified time after the index admission. CAD participants only. + Loeb; • control.

home admissions among the control group were made directly from the hospital, suggesting that the Loeb Center stay substituted for nursing home admission.

MORTALITY. There were no significant differences between the groups in mortality.

RETURN TO WORK. Although both groups were comparable in functional levels, the Loeb Center patients were more likely to return to work and maintain social group activities. As indicated in Figure 12-3, three-quarters of all Loeb Center patients who were workers were reemployed, compared to 63% for the control group.

NURSE RECRUITMENT AND RETENTION

How did we get nurses initially, and do they stay? Since there had never been a facility such as the Loeb Center, most nurses saw the Center as the usual nursing home. In 1963, much as now, nursing homes were not held in good repute and had trouble attracting qualified and competent nurses. Initially we also had difficulty recruiting nurses. With the aid of some very strong and loyal friends on faculties of various schools, we began to attract young graduates from accredited nursing schools in all three programs—diploma, associate's degree, and bachelor's degree. Word spread that the Loeb Center was a place where nurses could practice the kind of nursing they had been taught, and for a number of years recruitment efforts thrived. It is interesting to note that our major source for recruitment has always been from generic baccalaureate programs.[10]

Nurses had to learn to work with each other in peer, rather than hierarchical, relationships. They had to learn to confer with physicians on the goals of care, anticipated outcomes, and measures to promote and support the patient's achievement of those outcomes. Nurses also had to learn perhaps the most important truth—that patients were achievers, and that nurses were facilitators, teachers, supporters, and nurturers.

With time it became easier to identify the qualities in nurse applicants that predicted those who would do exceptionally well, those who would be willing to conform but not committed either to a philosophy of their own or that of the institution, and those who would be unhappy. Our major concern about unhappy staff members was not that they would disagree with the program, but that they would cut corners in the care of patients. That concern also held true for the noncommitted, who were more likely to measure the amount of work they did rather than the benefits of care to patients.

It is important at the Loeb Center that nurses work collegially and interdependently. There is, in the traditional sense, no one in charge, no one to

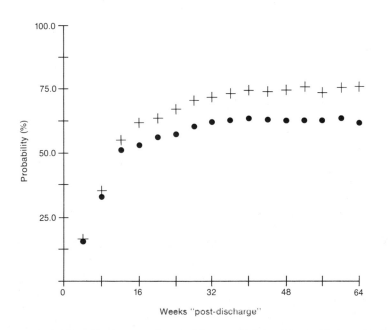

FIGURE 12-3 Probability of having returned to work by a specified time following discharge. Previously employed CAD responders. + Loeb; • control.

direct others in the care they give. There are only professional colleagues, some of whom are more knowledgeable and experienced than others, and who have additional skills, competencies, and knowledge to help their fellow professionals develop further.

With a system prevalent throughout the nation in which nonprofessional personnel were giving most of the daily care to patients, and the nurses were acting as medication givers, technicians, supervisors, and coordinators of unit activities, most nurses had little exposure or experience in working collegially with their peers. Curricula included courses in leadership of nonprofessional personnel, or in management of patient care, not in how to work collaboratively with others. It is still necessary to help all nurses who come to work with us to develop a sense of awareness of the competency and skill of their peers; to help them learn how to coordinate their efforts so that the result, while dependent upon individual contributions, is greater than any single contribution; and to help them form a mutual support system for each other, as well as for patients and their families.

It is this competence and skill in the areas of clinical and psychosocial nursing that engenders the respect and cooperation of the medical staff and most benefits patients and families. Physicians soon recognize that they can confer and consult with the nurses in solving patient care problems that are not immediately responsive to the standard medical regimens. Patients and families come to regard the nurse as a source of support and guidance as well as an advocate.

Most of our nurses leave the Loeb Center after 1 yr or 2 yr of employment. We are not as unhappy about that phenomenon as we are about the fact that over the past few years it has become increasingly difficult for us to maintain the quality of the staff we have become accustomed to and which is necessary to provide the level of nursing care we consider essential if patients are to receive the help they need and we are to reduce costs. Our major problem retaining nurses relates to the comparatively small scale of the Loeb Center. The opportunities for promotion are limited. If Loeb had a greater variety of services and was larger so that lateral and vertical mobility could be increased, the retention rate of nurses would improve significantly.

Loeb's recruitment and retention problems have been exacerbated by the concentration in many baccalaureate programs upon health and health maintenance to the neglect of pathology and its effects on normal physiology. There is an increasing tendency in baccalaureate programs to deemphasize nursing's role in the care of the sick, particularly in hospital settings. Consequently, we find that we are employing graduate nurses who have had minimal exposure to the sick, who find they do not like to take care of persons who are ill, and who see the nurturing role as nonprofessional. Greater emphasis in professional nursing education on the care and rehabilitation of hospitalized patients should be a high priority for the coming decade. No amount of change in the system or gains in power within the system can change the fact that nursing's role is nurturing, life supporting, life saving, comforting, and rehabilitative. Nursing education must focus on these aspects of practice to prepare nurses who are willing and able to practice in a professional setting such as the Loeb Center.

STAFFING PATTERNS

On average, a nurse at the Loeb Center cares for ten patients who are located in the same area of the unit. The areas are called districts; and each district has one day nurse and one evening nurse assigned to it for anywhere from 3 mo to 5 mo. During that period patients will be admitted to and discharged from the district with an average length of stay of about 12.5 days at present and a range of 1 day to 42 days.[11]

All staff members rotate onto 4 wk of nights every 4 mo to 5 mo. During the night rotation the nurse usually has two districts or 20 patients, in the same area of the unit. Over the years staff members have not been happy about the night rotation. It would be a simple thing to appoint a permanent night staff with no rotation of tours. However, our experiences with persons permanently assigned to nights have resulted in complaints from patients, day staff, and evening staff about the nonresponsiveness or seeming indifference of persons on the night staff. This is consistent with what is reported throughout the country. In fact, the majority of all complaints concerning nonresponsiveness of staff members involve the night staff. We prefer not to isolate our night nurses.

Over the years only a small number of nurses have given night rotation as their principal reason for leaving, and we believe the retention of quality care far outweighs that disadvantage. We are presently considering the compromise of 12-hr tours for some nurses of 7:00 PM to 7:30 AM, which will maintain the association of night staff with other staff members and reduce the danger of night staff isolation.

IMPLICATIONS FOR THE FUTURE

Having carried out a successful and effective program for the past 18 yr, we believe it is time to look at ways to extend the program to provide further service. There are several good reasons to do this. Since the Loeb Center introduced into the health care system the concept of an alternate level of care for post-critical hospitalized patients, it is appropriate for us to see if there is some way our program can enhance functioning outside the institutional setting.

CONTINUING CARE COMPONENT

Based upon the evaluation findings cited earlier, we are beginning a demonstration project involving outreach into the community. With partial support from the Robert Wood Johnson Foundation, we will extend nursing care to appropriate patients after discharge in order to increase their functional levels, reduce or defer hospitalizations for acute problems, and avoid or delay nursing home admissions. We intend to evaluate the effectiveness of this program in terms of its impact on patients, functioning levels, the recruitment and retention of nurses, and overall cost.

Evaluation plans call for a controlled study using patients from Montefiore and its affiliates. Matched patients will be assigned randomly to the Loeb Center and traditional inpatient care. Of those cared for by the Loeb Center, a group would be randomly assigned to the continuing care ambulatory program in addition to inpatient care at the Center. Thus, the study would show the relative benefits of Loeb care *versus* traditional hospital care, and it is hoped, would demonstrate the additive benefits of an ongoing ambulatory program.[12]

EXTENDED CARE OR SKILLED NURSING

In our present health care system, the needs of the frail are in danger of being overlooked. There is an increasing hospital admission rate for persons in acute medical crisis, severely debilitated with little or no reserves. While technology and pharmacology have made it possible to save lives and reverse clinical acuity, the excessive cost of this care has at the same time caused third party payers to guard zealously the use of the hospital bed. Consequently, once the crisis is resolved and clinical stability has been achieved, the mandate is to return these persons to the community, assuming recuperation will occur in the home. For those who either have no home or cannot carry out the tasks of day-to-day living without physical assistance, nursing homes may be considered a solution.

We therefore find ourselves today with what may be identified as a two-level system for those who require institutional care: the acute care hospital or the nursing home. There is less and less provision for a care setting that provides for the person who is still vulnerable to complications but no longer highly unstable — that is, the recuperating patient.

In 1963 the Congressional Record of the proceedings of the Subcommittee on Veterans Affairs cited the Loeb Center for Nursing and Rehabilitation as an alternative to acute hospital care.[13] In 1966, when Medicare became effective under Title XVIII, provision was made for extended care. The intent of extended care was to provide professional rehabilitative services. As regulations were promulgated, it became apparent that if the complete intent of the law was followed, few facilities—with the exception of the Loeb Center and some rehabilitation centers—would have been eligible for participation. Consequently, regulations were modified to allow a number of nursing homes to participate. American business, noting a possibility for a monetary windfall, began building extended care facilities. Even some commercial motel chains, such as Holiday Inn, decided to enter the extended care business.

There were a number of meetings around the United States and Canada addressing issues related to extended care. It soon became apparent that the average nursing home existing at that time was not able to qualify programmatically under the criteria stipulated in the *Conditions of Participation for Extended Care*.[14] As time went on, regulations were altered until they were directed more toward ensuring the adequacy of the nursing home as a residence than they were toward providing clinical care to persons during a transient phase of illness. By 1974 all pretense of establishing extended care facilities was dropped, and facilities eligible for reimbursement for providing extended care were to be called skilled nursing facilities. Hospitals that had been considering the addition of extended care units found that the regulations, controls, and ceilings made it uneconomical to support these units. It was far better to retain the acute care beds and keep the patients in them until ready for discharge. With increasing pressure for earlier and earlier discharge from acute care beds, the concept of an interim setting—a halfway house between tertiary acute care and return to home—is receiving increasing attention.

REPLICATION

Over the years we have been repeatedly asked why the Loeb Center has not been replicated. Obviously, those of us involved with Loeb have asked the question as well.

Theis and Harrington, in a study of nurses' satisfaction with practice summarized their findings as follows:

> At the Loeb Center, the baccalaureate graduate in nursing was enthusiastic about her work and apparently considerable satisfaction from the kind of care she was enabled to give. She felt that she could practice nursing in a way that was consistent with what she had been taught and was capable of giving, and that her concept of her professional role was not only supported but enhanced by her superiors. Her behavior reflected her own convictions

as well as those of the administration. She perceived her work situation as one that allowed for flexibility and freedom in implementing individual plans for nursing care. Her morale was high and she expressed feelings of loyalty and admiration toward the administration—contrasted with the baccalaureate graduate employed as a staff nurse in the typical hospital, who seemed dissatisfied because her working environment did not permit her to use her full range of professional knowledge and skills. She felt unable to put into practice much of what she had learned, and was often frustrated because her concept of the nursing role was not congruent with what she was actually expected to do on the job.[15]

Tiffany included the Loeb Center in a study of the relationship between organizational structure and goals of hospitals and the support of the professional role in nursing.[16] The study suggests that the successful implementation of the professional nursing role at the Loeb Center was associated with an institutional philosophy of nursing autonomy and with the considerable authority afforded clinical nurses in their practice. These institutional characteristics were absent in hospitals, which could not sustain nurses in professional roles.

Despite the findings of Theis and Harrington and Tiffany, our outcome experiences of more than 18 yr, the result of the HEW study, and the positive reaction of numerous visitors representing hospital and health administration, governmental agencies, nursing education, nursing administration, physician administration, physician education, and clinical specialties of all kinds, there has not been major movement to replicate the concept and organization of the Loeb Center.

We believe a number of factors have combined to militate against replication of the Loeb model. First, and perhaps foremost, is that many people do not believe it is essential that a professional nurse provide the care, nor do they define the parameters of nursing practice as we do. Therefore, those who have tried to replicate the program, but have employed nonprofessional or less-skilled persons, have not produced the same results. Second, until recently it has been economically more attractive for most hospitals to maintain the Loeb-eligible patient in an acute care bed, rather than transfer that patient to a bed for which they receive only half the reimbursement. This factor, of course, is less applicable in those hospitals that have consistently high occupancy rates. However, in such settings there is often another problem. Where the extended care beds are not protected by certification, hospitals will transfer acute patients, or patients awaiting permanent nursing home placement, to the extended care unit when they are pressed for beds. In such a situation, the unit becomes an overflow setting and the program becomes impossible to maintain, resulting in staff dissatisfaction and turnover.

Perhaps the Loeb Center was an idea ahead of its time. The evaluation of Loeb is now in, and it is positive. Patients receiving care at Loeb fare better and consume fewer resources than comparable patients cared for within our traditional medical system. The national disillusionment with nursing homes, the nation's excess hospital bed capacity, and an increasing emphasis within American health care on the return of patients to productive and independent living may all coalesce to facilitate the replication of the Loeb model in the future.

Hospital nursing is in a state of crisis. Dissatisfaction is high among professional nurses and has resulted in rapid turnover and many hospital vacancies. The Loeb model not only benefits patients and families, but also has much to offer the nursing profession in its search for greater autonomy and professionally challenging roles.

REFERENCES

1   *Loeb Center Annual Reports* — 1977 & 1981, Unpublished.

2   Alfano, G., Levine, H., Rifkin, H., Hall, L. *Longitudinal Effects of an Experimental Nursing Process Supported By Public Health Service Grant Number NU-0038 Division of Nursing, Final Report*, Unpublished, 1975

3   Selye, Hans, *The Physiology and Pathology of Exposure to Stress*, Medical Publishers, Acta, Inc., Montreal, 1950

4   Sullivan, Harry Stack, *Interpersonal Theory of Psychiatry*, Ed. Perry and Gawel, W. W. Norton & Co., Inc., New York, 1953

5   Rogers, Carl, *Client Centered Therapy*, Houghton, Mifflin Co., Boston, 1965

6   Dewey, John, *Interest and Effort in Education*, Houghton, Mifflin, & Co., Boston, 1913

7   Hall, Lydia E., "A Center for Nursing," *Nursing Outlook*, 11:805–806, November 1963

8   Hall, Lydia, E., "Quality of Nursing Care," *Public Health News*, New Jersey State Department of Health, June 1955

9   "More Care — Fewer Patients," *Medical World News*, pages 125–128, November 1964

10 Hall, Lydia E., *Annual Report*, Loeb Center for Nursing and Rehabilitation, Montefiore Hospital and Medical Center, New York, 1964

11 Alfano, Genrose, J., "The Loeb Center For Nursing and Rehabilitation: A Professional Approach to Nursing Practice," *Nursing Clinics of North America*, 4 (3): 487–493, September 1969

12 Alfano, Genrose, J., "Demonstration Project to Improve Outcomes For The Chronically Ill," Loeb Center for Nursing and Rehabilitation, Montefiore Hospital and Medical Center, New York, 1981, Unpublished

13 *Hearings: Before The Special Subcommittee On Intermediate Care Of The Committee On Veterans' Affairs House of Representatives Eighty-Eighth Congress First Session* pages 1514–1515, 1515–1562, 1963

14 "Conditions of Participation for Extended Care Facilities," *U.S. Department of Health, Education, and Welfare Social Security Administration HIM-3*, March, 1966

15   Theis, Charlotte, Harrington, Helen, "Three Factors That Affect Practice-Communications, Assignments, Attitudes," *American Journal of Nursing*, 68 (7): 1478–1482, July 1968.

16   Tiffany, Constance, *Nursing, Organization Structure, and the Real Goals of Hospitals A Correlational Study*, Doctoral Dissertation, Ann Arbor, Michigan, University Microfilms International, Indiana University 1979

BIBLIOGRAPHY

Alfano, Genrose J., "Creativity in Nursing Practice – The Challenge." *Virginia Nurse Quarterly*, 38: 7–12, Winter 1970

Bowar-Ferres, Susan, "Loeb Center and Its Philosophy of Nursing," *American Journal of Nursing*, 75 (5) 810–5, May 1975

Brown, Esther Lucile, *Nursing Reconsidered – A Study of Change*. Philadelphia, J.B. Lippincott Co., 1970, pp 156–165

Ellis, Barbara, "The All R.N. Staff: Why Not?" *Hospitals*, 52 (20): 107–8, 110–112. 16 October 1978

Hall, Lydia E. & Alfano, Genrose J., "The Patient With Myocardial Infarction: Incapacitation or Rehabilitation?" *American Journal of Nursing*, 64 (11) C20 to C25

Hall, Lydia E., *Project Report Loeb Center For Nursing & Rehabilitation At Montefiore Hospital*, Unpublished, New York, July 1964

Henderson, Cynthia, "Can Nursing Care Hasten Recovery? *American Journal of Nursing*, 64 (6): 77–80, June 1964

Leone, Lucile P., "Center For Creative Nursing: Loeb Center For Nursing & Rehabilitation, Montefiore Hospital. New York City," *Public Health Report*, 78: 347–8, April 1963

May, Rollo, *Man's Search for Himself*, New York, W.W. Norton & Co., 1953

Schorr, Thelma M., "Let's Hear It for Primary Nursing," *American Journal of Nursing*, 77 (11): 1787, November 1977

Smith, Homer William, *The Kidney: Structure and Function in Health and Disease*, Oxford University Press, New York, 1951

Wiggins, Lois Reeves, "Lydia Hall's Place in the Development of Theory in Nursing," *Image*, Sigma Theta Tau, February 1980

THE CONTRIBUTION OF NURSE PRACTITIONERS TO AMERICAN HEALTH CARE

Nurse practitioners are nurses with advanced clinical expertise and broad responsibilities for clinical assessment and treatment of commonly occurring health problems. Nurse practitioners evolved as a new type of nurse specialist within the past 15 years. And although nurse practitioners represent only 2% of nurses, there has been great excitement and controversy over their education and roles.

Nurse practitioners have been viewed by many as physician substitutes because they have assumed responsibility for some aspects of care traditionally provided by physicians. As the supply of physicians has increased in recent years, controversy has developed over the future of nurse practitioners in ambulatory care.

The papers in Part IV provide analyses of the success of nurse practitioners and forecasts of what the future holds. In Chapter 13, Ford, a founder of the nurse practitioner movement, recounts the history of nurse practitioners, evaluates their success, and speculates about their future in American health care. Lewis, a physician involved very early in demonstrating the efficacy of nurse practitioners in ambulatory care, explores in Chapter 14 the impact of the burgeoning supply of primary care physicians on the future options of nurse practitioners. Diers, in Chapter 15, synthesizes a number of studies on the effectiveness of nurse-midwives in improving access to and the quality of health services for mothers and infants. And LeRoy in Chapter 16 provides a comprehensive analysis of research on the overall cost-effectiveness of nurse practitioners.

Unlike nursing in hospitals and nursing homes where the growth potential is great, nurse practitioners face a decade of increasing opposition by other provider groups and declining growth rates in ambulatory care. One of the greatest challenges for nursing in the 1980s will be to sustain the important contributions of nurses in ambulatory care despite growing constraints. Effective and articulate communication to the public about nurses' unique contributions to health care will be imperative.

LORETTA C. FORD

13

NURSE PRACTITIONERS: HISTORY OF A NEW IDEA AND PREDICTIONS FOR THE FUTURE

INTRODUCTION OF THE NURSE PRACTITIONER

The early 1960s were turbulent times of tremendous social unrest with growing demands for rights, equity, and access to health care (and other resources) and for increased participation by consumers in decision making in matters of health and illness. The federal government and others assumed that physicians were the primary providers of all *health* care and that biomedical research was paramount to conquering disease and disability. From these erroneous assumptions national concerns for the availability and use of health manpower grew and resulted in the multiplicity of training programs for huge numbers of different types of health workers, many of whom supported the "medicalization" of health care and its biomedical fix.

The assumption about the needs for medical manpower was not the impetus for the introduction of the nurse practitioner concept. This dilemma, however, provided the opportunity to test an expanded scope of practice for professional nurses in the care of well children in ambulatory settings, traditionally a major concern and responsibility of public health nurses. But changes in nursing would have to occur if the *health* needs of people were to be met through expanded roles of nurses.

Fortunately, a mirror reflection of societal changes was occurring simultaneously in nursing. Graduate education in nursing was redirecting its focus from functional roles (teaching and administration) to clinical specialty majors. New conceptualizations about the nature of nursing and health began to appear in the literature. Increased numbers of nursing programs were initiated in institutions of higher education, and student enrollments soared. With new knowledge and sophisticated technology to assess and treat patients, the survival rate of patients was higher, though their acuity level was greater, not only during hospitalization but after discharge as well. Early discharge was required as hospital costs soared and utilization-review legislation was enacted. Government agencies, with their inevitable regulations, sought to control costs in the guise of safeguarding quality. Once again, nursing resources were called upon, this time to monitor and evaluate care through utilization-review mechanisms and inspection and accrediting agencies.

Nursing education and nursing research were also changing, albeit, not fast enough. New curriculum designs were in vogue. Special projects, such as the WCHEN Graduate Education project, were redirecting the course of the clinical majors to provide the theoretical and scientific underpinnings for advanced specialty practice.[1] Nurse faculty members began seeking doctoral preparation in a host of related fields. Nurses clamored for continuing education. The focus of nursing research was also shifted from studies of the educational processes and programs and of the nurse as a person and professional, to investigations into clinical practice problems and to inquiry in the delivery of health services to improve the nursing care of people.

It was from these trends in practice, education, and research in nursing and health care that the first nurse practitioner program was conceptualized. The dearth of physician manpower *provided the opportunity* to test new roles; it was not, however the *raison d'etre* for the initiation of the expanded role.

My personal goal was to test an advanced clinical role for the community health nurse, and, if successful, to influence collegiate nursing education programs.

The pediatric nurse practitioner program was futuristically designed within the parameters established by the nursing profession. Those parameters, which are relevant today, were the following:

- *Clinical context*. Through assessment, implementation, and evaluation, the nurse practitioner was expected to make sophisticated clinical judgments and management plans based on an historical and clinical data base, including physical and psychosocial information, on the health status of a child in the context of his family and its daily living patterns. The clinical assessment included a health and developmental history of health problems; current and past daily living patterns; and family experiences that influenced health; a physical examination including observation, inspection, palpation, auscultation and percussion; and a psychosocial appraisal.

- *Accountability*. The nurse practitioner was *primarily* accountable to the client for the quality of care provided. Further, she was expected to be accountable to herself and to her profession, to the agency that employed her, and to her team members.

- *Health focus.* The content and processes of the pediatric nurse practitioner were based on normal growth and development of children, and strategies that enabled the best use of the health system's resources; and in helping families cope with the stresses and strains of daily living, providing health teaching, counselling, and anticipatory guidance; and maintaining health and wellness to the greatest extent possible, even in those patients with serious handicaps or disabilities.

- *Investigations.* Systematic observations and inspections of patients, explorations of the clinical phenomena in the domain of nursing, and contributions to the literature of nursing were encouraged. The most common scholarly activity for nurse practitioners in the early years was, understandably, at the descriptive level of both clinical and organizational phenomena.

- *Collaboration.* While the nurse practitioner was and could be an independent practitioner, she was expected to function in a system that offered comprehensive care. This required a team relationship if total health care was to be achieved. Learning to develop true collegial relationships, including shared accountability is not easy for any of the health professionals, particularly those socialized in an era of exclusive professional autonomy. Indeed, it is a life-long developmental task that must be initiated during training.

- *Change strategies.* The nurse practitioner model required changes in nursing and medical practice and also in the regulatory systems that controlled health care delivery and professional practice. So strategies, logistics, and tactics of social change were paramount to introducing, facilitating, and evaluating our expanded role, to accommodating new roles, and to gaining an historical perspective of the progress made.

- *Self-development as a person and as a professional.* Role changes had to be internalized to engender adequate self-confidence and self-esteem to enable the nurse to withstand the stresses and strains of role change — even to benefit from them — and to ensure collegial relationships with others in the health care delivery system.

The first nurse practitioner program was initiated in 1965 to test an expanded scope of practice for professional nurses who held a baccalaureate degree in nursing and who were eligible for admission to the graduate program in nursing at the University of Colorado. In the dream of the original architects, Ford and Silver, the ideal nursing candidate was one who held a master's degree in public health nursing.[2] Though our first enrollee was a community health nurse with a master's degree, such candidates were scarce, so nurses with baccalaureate degrees in nursing who qualified for admission to graduate school were accepted. Academic standards were maintained, and the seed for the dream — the preparation of nurse practitioners in the master's programs in nursing — was planted. One of the goals within the general mission of the university was to prepare people for a life of learning and productive citizenry, and in good conscience one could not ask nurses to invest a great deal of energy and resources in dead-end careers. Both Ford and Silver were academicians in nursing and medical education who were committed to serving the needs of society and their respective professions within the context of their own institution's goals. The social time was ripe for innovation: people were demanding their rights; every institution was under pressure to be responsive; health care personnel were relatively scarce; and humanistic, rather than materialistic values, were in vogue.

Where, then, could the resistance be to preparing professional nurses to provide comprehensive care to well children, to make sophisticated clinical judgments about acutely or chronically ill children, and to perform adequately as primary practitioners in childhood emergencies? In their naivete, the architects never suspected that their own colleagues, particularly in academia, would be the real barriers to bringing about swift changes in patterns of education and health care delivery.

The pediatric nurse practitioner program at the University of Colorado started modestly as a demonstration project with an evaluation design in a continuing education format of two academic semesters; 4 mo of didactic and clinical experience at the medical center and 4 mo to 5 mo of field work in the community, followed by a year of solid practice in the role of a nurse practitioner. Funding, which originally was sought unsuccessfully from governmental sources, was granted by the Medical School Research Fund. Later private foundations, the Commonwealth Fund and the Robert Wood Johnson Foundation, contributed. Their vision and their willingness to take risks helped change the direction of nursing education and practice, altered the health care delivery system, and challenged traditional legislative, political, and professional controls. Federal funding provided continuing support after the introductory years.

The first name selected for the product was *pediatric public health nurse practitioner*. Unfortunately, the combination name seemed lengthy and cumbersome and the public health portion of the name was dropped. Therein lies a tale of resistance to change from the traditionalists in pediatric nursing, resistance that rippled from the local and regional sites to the Children's Bureau in Washington, DC. The nurse codirector of the project was a public health nurse specialist, not a pediatric nurse. This created all kinds of problems on the training site, in our efforts to seek federal funding, and in the eventual integration of the concept, content, and processes into the degree programs in nursing education at the birthplace of the nurse practitioner, the University of Colorado. Also, there were fears that pediatricians would control and devour nursing education and practice, and any interdisciplinary collaborative effort was viewed with alarm and suspicion.

All sorts of strategies were used by those resisting the inevitable change: passive resistance of the pediatric nursing faculty to full participation in the education of the nurse practitioner students; refusal of federal health agencies to fund the project as proposed; political pressure at the national level to accept a Children's Bureau–designed project as a substitute; disruptions in communication and abusive interpersonal relationships among resistant faculty and nurse practitioner students; and many incidents that consumed the energies and talents of the small but committed band of change agents. Given those barriers, it is remarkable that the idea survived, was expanded to adult and elderly care, exported world wide, and finally institutionalized in education and practice.

While there were resisters to change, there were also promoters of change. In the long run, these promotors of change were supported by a climate for innovation, provided with resources, and encouraged by some prominent national health visionaries in nursing and medicine. They developed counter-strategies to ensure the nurse practitioner's future. The first strategy was communication. This included publication in nursing and medical journals, newspapers, and magazines and exposure on television. Further presentations were made at national meetings to describe the program; the nurse practitioner's preparation, performance, and personal and professional development; her acceptance by patients, physicians, and other nurses and agencies; and the adjustments needed in health care delivery. Another strategy that fed the first was the generation of an extensive data base through collations of information and research. This was gathered from experiences, anecdotal records, evaluative studies and reports, and lately in increasingly sophisticated research on structure, process, and outcome. Another strategy was the use of the political process to gain support and funds from professional associations, employing institutions, federal, and state agencies and foundations.

Before the original project was completed, many similar programs were initiated to prepare nurse practitioners, first in pediatric care and, later, many other kinds of nurse practitioners, such as family, adult, school, obstetrics/gynecology, geriatric, and perinatal nurse practitioners. These later models included a larger component of the medical management of patients, though the essential framework of the pediatric nurse practitioner remained. However, some of the changes made in these later models lost sight of the academic standards, the initial goal of integrating the nurse practitioner concepts into the degree curricula, and the maintenance of the major conceptual and philosophical dimensions of the nursing role. This latter development created problems for nurses and nursing and delayed the institutionalization of the nurse practitioner in education and practice. The availability of funding to a host of educational and service agencies, including all types of nursing schools, medical schools, hospitals, and community agencies, also created confusion in practitioners, patients, politicians, physicians, and the public alike. The diversity and schisms found in nursing generally were now expanded to the nurse practitioner program as well, making it extremely difficult to gain a consensus for changes in standards, certification, accreditation, licensure, and the subsequent rules and regulations governing preparation and practice.

Other health care workers emerged in the 1960s, at least 240 new breeds. One of these was the physician's assistant, who quickly became confused with the nurse practitioner. True, there were similar tasks performed by each, just as there are among other articulated and traditional complementary roles. But explaining the differences in philosophy, preparation, practice, professions, licensure, legal sanctions for practice, and accountability became a full-time occupation for some of the promoters of the nurse practitioner. Further, the labeling of the nurse practitioner as a physician extender, midlevel practitioner, or new health professional all created illusions that medicine and nursing were on a hierarchical continuum of preparation and practice, with the physician and medicine at the pinnacle. Implicit in this assumption was that medicine was a generic discipline encompassing all aspects of curing and caring, comprehensive in its nature to include prevention, promotion, restoration, rehabilitation, and terminal care, and legally and professionally authoritative and all powerful.

However, the social times and technologic advancements were such as to allow, and indeed require, expanding numbers and different kinds of health workers to meet the needs and desires of an increasingly demanding public. So all types of nurse practitioner programs were inaugurated, and they proliferated. At the height of the funding, there were 200 nurse practitioner programs in the nation. Most of these used a continuing education format, though the integration of nurse practitioners concepts and skills into advanced degree curricula also began in the early 1970s. Federal funding of programs started to play a major role in advancing the concept of nurse practitioner nationwide.

Other factors, necessary to maintain the nurse practitioner, were observable. Continuing clinical practice for nurse practitioner teachers became a paramount requirement to maintain, teach, and research clinical judgment. The definitive and systematic physical assessment skills taught to nurse practitioners began to be viewed as appropriate for undergraduate baccalaureate students and practicing nurses. Primary care and health maintenance organization (HMO) patterns of health care delivery emerged. Standards of practice and education by the professional organization (American Nurses Association) were published and systems of certification of individuals and accreditation of programs were initiated. State laws controlling nursing practice began to be reviewed and revised to accommodate the expanded scope of practice.

Federal laws, designed to encourage regional planning, identified nurse practitioners as a necessary requirement for health care delivery, cost control, and
quality assurance. The excitement and sometimes fear of this new model of
nursing raised many questions and led to a proliferation of research projects
on the role of the nurse practitioner; descriptive articles of personal experiences; texts, programs, and audio-visual instructional materials; and formal
and informal evaluations of educational and practice programs.

THE IMPACT OF THE NURSE PRACTITIONER

During the decade and a half following the introduction of the nurse practitioner in 1965, the impact of the nurse practitioner is recorded in professional
and public press, on television, in legislation and in government publications,
and in practically every conceivable type of literature in health care from the
mid-1960s onward. The nurse practitioner affected health care delivery
systems, educational programs, relationships to other health care providers,
regulatory systems that control practice, program accreditation, and certification of practitioners, and professional societies of nursing and medicine.
Extensive documentation on every aspect of the nurse practitioner's preparation and performance exists. No role in nursing, or in any other field for that
matter, has as thorough an investigation and description as has the role of the
nurse practitioner.

Several comprehensive reviews of this body of literature have been published. Edmunds in 1978 presented an overview of 600 articles and studies on
the effectiveness of the nurse practitioner.[3] Her analysis was framed in developmental periods. The precursive stage (1963 to 1969) in which the efforts to
communicate the experiences of the programs, faculties, and graduates
helped win support for the continuing development of the role. The second
stage from 1970 to 1974 was one of role definition and legitimatization, in
which the competence of the nurse to assess and manage health problems was
ascertained. The third state, that of role consolidation and maturation, occurred from 1975 to the present. It emphasized and validated the quality of
care provided by nurse practitioners, their influences upon employment settings, costs, distribution, and education.

Edmunds' analysis and the annotated bibliography in the Division of
Nursing *Nurse Planning Series*, combined with extensive surveys and profiles
on the programs and performance of nurse practitioners, provide comprehensive compilations of the huge data base available.[4]

Another analysis of the many articles and studies cannot be accomplished in this historical overview. An attempt is made, however, to highlight

some studies in each period of development, commenting on the difficulties inherent in the designs and methods used, presenting general, corroborated findings, and suggesting a research agenda for the future.

During the first stage of development of the nurse practitioner, several demonstration projects and investigations were conducted simultaneously in different parts of the nation. On the east coast, at Yale University, Hathaway examined a new pattern of delivery in college health services using nurses who successfully handled health problems of students.[5] Siegel and Bryson experimented in the delivery of maternal and child services with public health nurses who function in a collaborative relationship with physicians.[6] These nurses amply showed that they could function competently as primary care takers and that patients enthusiastically accepted them as such. In 1966, an extensive study by Ford, Seacat, and Silver corroborated these findings in their maternal and child care project.[7]

In the West, when the Colorado project on the pediatric nurse practitioner was underway, Lewis and Resnick launched a scientific investigation of the care of chronically ill adult patients given by nurses with expanded responsibilities.[8] This study, often cited for its classic design using control and experimental groups, showed that those patients under the nurse practitioner guidance demonstrated increasing functionality, fewer untoward symptoms of disease, and more efficiency in the use of the health care system when compared with the control group. Connelly and colleagues, Yankauer, and Stoeckle, Farrisey, and Sweat through their studies in the East, reported similar findings on the efficacy of using nurses in expanded roles in team care and the positive responses of the patients.[9-11]

In the next phase of development, that of evaluation in role definition and legitimation stage, the nurse practitioner's clinical decision making was also extensively studied. Many investigators compared the clinical judgments made by nurse practitioners to those of physicians, and also to physician's assistants, in terms of providing care, the acceptance and compliance of patients, and the development of colleagueships with physicians and other nurses. Studies by Charney and Kitzman, Duncan and co-workers, Yankauer and associates, and a host of others added confirmation to the growing body of literature on the competence of the nurse practitioner to gather health histories and clinical data and to analyze and interpret them.[12-14] They also included analysis of the ability to make sophisticated and clinical judgments and develop a plan of care, including independent nursing management, consultation with a physician and, if necessary, referral. Patient and physician acceptance was generally excellent. Any reservations of skeptics during this period were held mainly by those who were far removed from the practice or by those who had no experience with nurse practitioners.

I can remember this period and the earlier one well because of the many memorable stresses and little support among nursing faculty colleagues. I also can remember the encouragement that Esther Lucile Brown provided when she visited the nurse practitioner program in Denver and observed the nurse practitioner in practice. Dr. Brown said, beaming, "I've just seen nursing in its finest role." Serious limitations of the evaluative studies conducted in this stage of development have been noted. Many investigators compared nurse practitioners with physicians, using concepts, standards, and criteria for *medical* practice, not broadened *nursing* and *health* care. Probably the assurance that the public and the professions needed was that nurse practitioners were not providing second class or low-quality care (assuming all physicians deliver high-quality care). Researchers were prompted to respond to questions of differences between the care medicine and nursing provided, but it is hoped that the next decade will expand conceptual designs and research methodologies to provide data on patient care outcomes.

During this period the escalation of all kinds of nurse practitioner programs was supported by federal funds, mainly in continuing education programs. Sponsorship was variable. Hospitals, clinics, neighborhood health centers, university nursing schools and medical schools all vied for funds from federal sources and foundations. Program offerings and educational patterns were variable. Every nursing and medical specialty began to educate nurse practitioners. Physician assistants also began to specialize. Most of the nurse practitioner programs used a continuing education mode, though the integration of physical assessment skills began to occur at the baccalaureate level in nursing programs. Also, master's programs in nursing began to offer full preparation for nurse practitioners, mainly in pediatrics and family care. Almost all programs, federally funded or otherwise, had an evaluation component of products, programs, and outcomes. This integration of philosophy, concept, and processes of the nurse practitioner was promoted slowly at first but with increasing rapidity by funding agencies, the federal government, and foundations. There were pressures from students, actions of professional nursing and medical organizations, demands from nurse practitioners for accreditation and certification, and changes in state practice laws. Also, there was growing recognition that despite all the monies poured into health care, the costs were escalating, episodic illness overshadowed efforts for prevention and promotion, maldistribution of manpower was still evident, and public interest in national health insurance was waning in light of inflation and energy problems.

Efforts to control costs and discourage use of expensive hospital services emerged in the guise of quality assurance legislation and regional planning authorities such as health systems agencies. The latter program identified ten parameters for planning, five of them directly or indirectly noted the deployment of nurse practitioners for patient care delivery service. Neighborhood health centers and health maintenance organizations which were introduced through federal support, moved from their limited geographic availability on the west coast to national prominence through federal support and private philanthropic organizations. These innovations in health care delivery offered an expanded arena for the enlarged scope of nursing practice. Further, the concept of primary care as a promising replacement for traditional general medical practice was gradually formulated and presented as a new option in health care that supposedly ensured access, accountability, continuity, coordination, and comprehensiveness.

By the mid-1970s, the economy began to show signs of deteriorating and national priorities began to change. Inflation and energy problems, aggravated by internal and external political situations, took precedence over earlier priorities. One of these, health care, began to fall lower on the list of national issues; only the *costs* of health care remained high on the list of public concerns.

The nurse practitioner movement was entering its third phase of role consolidation and maturation. Research into issues of legal control, costs, supply, practice, and distribution were all part of this stage of development.

Legislative changes to accommodate expanded nursing roles, sought early in the 1970s, were enacted in well over 35 states. The most recent dimension of change — prescriptive authority — was initially instituted in Oregon and Washington as independent functions of qualified nurse practitioners. It is now under consideration in many other states. Limited, or physician-dependent, prescriptive authority exists in several states, though there are few studies of the outcomes of this new overt function. Covertly, individual nurses and physicians usually work out the details of prescriptive authority in the interest of serving the patients and safeguarding their care.

Legislative control of the nurse's expanded scope of practice began benignly and has increasingly become an issue of major proportions. Nurses cannot accept legislation that places them under physicians' supervision. Nor have they generally been willing to be registered as physician's assistants in order to expand nursing's scope of practice and secure reimbursement for medical services. Efforts to word state practice laws, which allow for collaborative arrangements, colleagueships, and team relationships, are fought for. So are reimbursement plans that identify nurses as providers of care. The federal Rural Health Act passed in 1974 allowed for reimbursement for nurses only when medical acts were performed and only when they were clearly under the physician's supervision.

Studies on the costs of nurse practitioner use are in their infancy. Recently more attention has been paid to this issue, but investigations are still at their most primitive stage, with no clear data base on the economies, which I believe are possible. Some studies, like those of Schultz and McGlone, Rec-

ord and colleagues, and Miller and Byrne indicate that cost savings are possible, given certain conditions.[15–17] An interim report of the Graduate Medical Education National Advisory Committee (GMENAC) on the
nonphysician health care providers, which included nurse practitioners with
others, sums up the general findings for the decade on the nurse's expanded
role:

> The Panel reported that nonphysicians who provide primary care are
> found to do so without jeopardizing quality and are generally highly ac-
> cepted by patients. In some settings, their utilization was found to result in
> cost savings. Restrictive state laws and regulations, exclusionary reimburse-
> ment policies, and the unwillingness of physicians to delegate were iden-
> tified as constraints.[18]

The words "nonphysician" and "delegate" are keys to the major inherent
problems in the past 15 yr of extensive studies on the role of the nurse practitioner. Most of the conceptual models used to study nurse practitioner performance were based on comparisons with the medical role. Generally, delegation, productivity, and substitutability were the major interests of
investigators on comparative studies of physicians and nurse practitioners.
There has been little or no effort to identify the real health needs of people or
to conduct studies of long-range patient outcomes in terms of behavior
changes or increased functionality and their relationship to cost savings. Too
little investigation has been made into the use of health services, or to test
new organizational structures, legal mechanisms, or reimbursement plans
that would facilitate the delivery of care in a humane, effective, efficient, and
economic fashion. As Diers and Molde suggest, there is a need for methodologic rigor in sampling, in measuring the outcomes for some targeted populations, especially the chronically ill and well, in defining concisely the groups
under comparison, and in performing longitudinal studies of outcome.[19] They
further note the need for expanded sources of data, studies that use appropriate standards of care and units of analysis for cost benefits. In this third phase
of the role consolidation and maturation stage, several major, federally supported studies were undertaken for the Department of Health, Education and
Welfare. One by Sultz and associates has produced a national data base of import.[20–22] This investigation was conducted in three phases. Phase I was a nationwide, longitudinal study of the products of nurse practitioner educational
programs: number, kinds, curricula, and student characteristics. Phase II was
a follow-up study of graduates in their employment settings, their impact on
the delivery system, and the "goodness of fit" between their functions in
practice and their educational programs.

Phase III of these longitudinal studies series surveyed educational and
employment aspects of nurse practitioners and also pointed toward directions
for the future. The summary of findings of the Phase III studies places the

capstone on a decade and a half of efforts to improve health care by changing the health care delivery system and the education of nurses for expanded roles.

Phase III findings were as follows:

* 90 percent of the graduates were employed.
* Almost half of all patients served by nurse practitioners were in the lowest income category.
* The nurse practitioner movement is continuing to expand into new and different service delivery sites.
* The types of services provided, the degree of physician consultation required, and the productivity in terms of patient encounters are clearly compatible with the basic thrust of nurse practitioner preparation.
* Role autonomy continues to be a most important factor motivating nurses to obtain nurse practitioner preparation.
* Employers of nurse practitioners were almost universally satisfied; 93% considered them cost beneficial.
* The nurse practitioner was well accepted (by employers and patients).
* The nurse practitioner preparation is essentially sound and appropriate to the health care marketplace.

Finally, the investigators comment, "Those who helped to initiate the nurse practitioner movement and prevailed over considerable opposition during its earlier years can look with satisfaction on the findings of this study."[22]

But can we? In some ways we can. Consider the impact on the world at large. Probably one of the most interesting events of the past decade is the emergence of the nurse practitioner in primary care on the international scene. This visibility is evident in pronouncements by international health associations, publication in professional journals, and the influx of foreign visitors to training sites.

A skillfully prepared brochure was produced recently by the World Health Organization (WHO) and its Pan American Health Association on the role of the nurse in primary health care.[23] A 10-yr health plan adopted in 1972 by the Ministers of Health of the Americas was to extend health services to everyone in the hemisphere by the end of the decade. The preface of the publication notes, "The nurse is in a unique position to contribute to the attainment of this objective."[23] Interestingly enough, this publication addresses the need for supervision of the nurse from the perspective of the type of assistance the nurse should have in carrying out her functions. No mention is made of a requirement for medical supervision.

North of the United States, the introduction, implementation, and impact of the nurse practitioner are captured in a superb monograph by Phillis E. Jones of the Faculty of Nursing at the University of Toronto entitled *Nurses in Canadian Primary Health Care Settings*.[24] The Canadian literature is as variable as is that of the United States and other countries, ranging as Jones says "from experiential descriptions to reports of controlled experiments." Her analysis of a myriad of studies included medical care and community nursing settings and focused on activity studies of practice, workload of the nurse, practice productivity and use, patient satisfaction, professional socialization, the quality of care and patient outcomes, and the quality of life components.

The varied purposes, designs, methodologies, and data treatment of the Canadian studies preclude, as they do in the United States, comprehensive comparisons; however, the time–activities studies generally revealed that the focus of the nurse's attention was on clinical matters directly related to patient care, rather than on functional or systems management. In examining the workload studies, reviews of the Canadian attachment system are presented. The attachment plan is the assignment of a district public health nurse to work collaboratively with a physician in private practice, thus forming a team to serve a common panel of patients. Increased cooperation between nurse and physician in planning for and in providing care generally resulted in coordination, comprehensiveness, and continuous service to people. (Britain has used a similar system successfully.) The most cited group of Canadian studies usually referred to as the "Burlington Trials" corroborated many of the findings of American investigators on quality assurance, acceptance by the patients, and financial outcomes.[25-27]

From other continents, the interest and action level in the expanded role of the nurse is also high, as evident in the numerous articles published in the *International Nursing Review*, WHO publications, and the growing interest of foreign students to seek preparation as nurse practitioners, mainly for primary care.

But once again, can we be satisfied here in the United States with our progress? Yes and no. On the positive side, we've made great strides. At last count, in 1979 the following gains were evident:

- An estimated 20,000 nurse practitioners have been prepared; 90% are practicing.
- The quality of care and acceptance by patients are unquestioned.
- One hundred four master's programs and 133 continuing education programs prepared nurse practitioners.

- Increasingly the master's level clinical specialist programs are including the assessment and management components introduced by the nurse practitioner concept.
- Nurse practitioners have responded to the unmet needs in rural areas and to the care of chronically ill and elderly people.
- Nurse faculty are becoming more interested and involved in practice and in the problems of nursing service.
- Fellowships for preparing nurse faculty in primary care were established by the Robert Wood Johnson Foundation.

But we still have work to do to complete the stage of maturation and institutionalization. Despite the voluminous data, barriers still exist to the full use of nurse practitioners (and professional nurses generally) to improve health care and to deliver it at reasonable costs. Those barriers, the windmills of the mid-1960s raised by the skeptics, are becoming realities, not because they are legitimate, but because they are in the vested interests of certain groups and because of the social and economic uncertainty and conservatism of the times. There are four barriers of major import: reimbursement, legal constraints, educational support, and underuse in practice settings. Today these barriers are becoming increasingly evident due to the predicted glut of physicians in 1990; the anticipated competitive modes in health care delivery; the limitation of federal support for health services, education, and research; and the fear of the loss of power and control by some professional groups, particularly the physicians.

All of these issues are coming to public attention at a time when great imbalances between the supply and demand for professional nurses have been revealed through the public press. These imbalances are evidenced in shortages, maldistributions, and nurses' dissatisfactions with salaries and working conditions.

The nurse practitioner has been a particular target in interprofessional conflicts with medicine, especially in the delivery of primary care. The scenario is played out in many ways: the withdrawal of support of the American Medical Association from the National Joint Practice Commission; the efforts of physicians in New Jersey to prevent school nurse practitioners from practicing, and the hospital administrators' strategy to bus nurses to the State Nurses' Association to rescind the previously accepted position supporting the entry-into-practice resolution; the attempts of Arkansas physicians to control the delivery of health care to rural and deprived population by establishing restraints on the nurse practitioners working collaboratively with a physician in a rural and deprived area. Texas nurses can tell their own tales of their decade-long fight to secure adequate legislation for the practice of professional nursing. Nurse midwives in various states, New York, Tennessee and Mississippi, to name a few, have also faced serious challenges from physicians who seek to control the practice and economics of nurse midwifery.

Regretfully, all these border skirmishes create tensions and distrust among the most basic team members — nurses and physicians — so that their energies, time, and resources are diverted away from vital goals in health care delivery, from the education of future professionals, and from clinical and health services research. All the professional groups are resorting to legal and political strategies to secure their territorial boundaries, to ensure their financial futures, and to control the health care delivery systems.

Albeit, increasingly we in nursing must continue to attend to the issues at hand in reimbursement, legislative matters, and educational funding through political processes if the public is to be served well. Though we have shown what we can do when we mobilize our resources, witness the response to the threats for national training act reductions. We must develop our personal, institutional, and professional organization strategies to create an active (rather than reactive), funded, and well-oiled political machine. This will take the preparation of some special nurses for statesmanship. It will take money — contributions from nurses in the form of donations and membership dues. It will take unity in nursing so that massive support can be marshalled quickly as needed. It will take new and creative partnerships with consumer and local community groups, especially if state block grants for education and services come to fruition. And finally, it will take the establishment of a common educational base, with appropriate mechanism for accreditation, certification, and licensure.

Can we do it? Why not? Look at what we have done in the last decade and a half in introducing, implementing, and evaluating the nurse practitioner. A new and a deviant idea in nursing in 1965 has become one of the normative and recognized roles in nursing worldwide. Tomorrow all the basic skills of the nurse practitioner will probably become the traditional armentarium of all professional nurses. My own view, which is gaining support and encouraging experimentation, is that the nurse practitioner is a nurse for all settings.[28] Weston, in a recent article in *HCFA Forum* suggests that the future opportunities for nurse practitioners are in the care of the chronically ill and elderly.[29] I agree, although patients in acute care settings are demonstrating real needs as well. Aiken's superb analyses attests to this.[30, 31] So, as Sultz says at the end of his Phase II study, "The Nurse Practitioner is alive and well and flourishing throughout the United States," strong enough to have survived the onslaughts of the past, politically knowledgeable enough to overcome the present threats, and committed enough to ensure future directions to institutionalize the concept in education, practice, and research. The idea of the nurse practitioner is an idea whose time has come.

REFERENCES

1 Ford, Loretta C., Marguerite Cobb, and Margaret Taylor. *Defining Clinical Content, Graduate Nursing Programs, Community Health Nursing.* Boulder, Colorado: Western Interstate Commission for Higher Education, 1967.

2 Ford, Loretta C., and Henry K. Silver. The Expanded Role of the Nurse in Child Care. *Nursing Outlook* (September, 1967), Vol 15, 43–45.

3 Winterton, Marilyn Edmunds. Evaluation of Nurse Practitioner Effectiveness: An Overview of the Literature. *Evaluation and the Health Professions* 1:1 (Spring 1978), 69–81.

4 *Nurse Practitioners and the Expanded Role of the Nurse: A Bibliography.* Nurse Planning Information Series, No. 5, U.S. Department of Health, Education and Welfare, PHS, H.R.A., Bureau of Health Manpower, Division of Nursing, Hyattsville, Maryland. DHEW Publication No. (HRA) 79-20, HRP 0500601, November, 1978, 247.

5 Hathaway, R. The Role of the Nurse in a University Health Service. *Nursing Outlook* 10:8 (1962), 533.

6 Siegel, E., and S.C. Bryson. A Redefinition of the Role of the Public Health Nurse in Child Health Supervision. *American Journal of Public Health* 53 (1963), 1015–1024.

7 Ford, P.A., M.S. Seacat, and G.G. Silver. Broadening Roles of Public Health Nurse and Physician in Prenatal and Infant Supervision. *American Journal of Public Health* 56 (1966), 1097–1103.

8 Lewis, C.E., and B.A. Resnik. Nurse Clinics and Progressive Ambulatory Patient Care. *New England Journal of Medicine* 277 (1967), 1236–1241.

9 Connelly, J.P., J.D. Stoeckle, E.S. Lepper, and R.M. Farrisey. Physician and Nurse—Their Interprofessional Work in Office and Hospital Ambulatory Settings. *New England Journal of Medicine* 275 (1966), 765–769.

10 Yankauer, A., J.P. Connelly, and J.J. Feldman. A Survey of Allied Health Workers Utilization in Pediatric Practice in Massachusetts and in the United States. *Pediatrics* 42:5 (1968), 733–742.

11 Stoeckle, J.D., R.M. Farrisey, and A. Sweatt. Medical Nursing Clinic for the Chronically Ill. *American Journal of Nursing* 63 (1973), 87–89.

12 Charney, E., and H. Kitzman. Child-health Nurse (Pediatric Nurse Practitioner) in a Private Practice: A Controlled Trial. *New England Journal of Medicine* 285 (1971), 1353–1358.

13 Duncan, B., A.N. Smith, and H.K. Silver. Comparison of the Physical Assessment of Children by Pediatric Nurse Practitioners and Pediatricians. *American Journal of Public Health* 61 (1971), 1170–1176.

14 Yankauer, A., S. Tripp, P. Andrews, and J. Connelly. The Outcomes and Service Impact of a Pediatric Nurse Practitioner Training Program—Nurse Practitioner Training Outcomes. *American Journal of Public Health* 62 (1972), 347–353.

15 Schultz, Phyllis R., and Frank B. McGlone. Primary Health Care Provided to the Elderly by a Nurse Practitioner/Physician Team: An Analysis of Cost Effectiveness. *Journal of the American Geriatrics Society* 25:10 (October, 1977), 443–446.

16 Record, J.C., et al. *Final Report: Provider Requirements, Cost Savings and the New Health Practitioner in Primary Care: National Estimates for 1990.* Bureau of Health Manpower, Contract No. HRA. 231-77-0077. Portland, Oregon, 1979.

17 Miller and Byrne, Inc. *Final Report, Review and Analysis of State Legislation and Reimbursement Practices of Physician's Assistants and Nurse Practitioners*, Contract No. HRA 230-77-0011, National Center for Health Services Research, Office Assistant Secretary for Health, Department of Health, Education and Welfare, Washington, D.C., 1978.

18 Report of the Graduate Medical Education National Advisory Committee to the Secretary, Department of Health and Human Services. Volume VI: Nonphysician Health Care Provider Technical Panel. U.S. Department of Health and Human Services, Public Health Service, Health Resources Administration, Office of Graduate Medical Education, Washington, D.C., U.S. Government Printing Office, DHHS Publication No. (HRA) 81-656, 1980.

19 Diers, Donna and Susan Molde. Some Conceptual and Methodological Issues in Nurse Practitioner Research. *Research in Nursing and Health* 2 (1979), 73–82.

20 Sultz, Harry A., O. Marie Henry, and Judith A. Sullivan. Nurse Practitioners: U.S.A. Lexington, Massachusetts: Lexington Books, 1979.

21 Sultz, Harry A., Marie Zielenzy, Jane Matthews, and Louis Kinyon. *Longitudinal Study of Nurse Practitioners*. Phase I. DHEW publications. Hyattsville, Maryland, May 1980.

22 Sultz, Harry A., Marie Zielenzy, Jane Matthews, and Louis Kinyon. *Longitudinal Study of Nurse Practitioners*. Phase III. DPH Publications No. HRA 80-2, Hyattsville, Maryland, May 1980.

23 *The Role of the Nurse in Primary Health Care*. Pan American Health Organization, Pan American Sanitary Bureau, Regional Office of the World Health Organization. Scientific Publication No. 348, 1977.

24 Jones, Phyllis E. *Nurses in Canadian Primary Health Care Settings: A Review of Recent Literature*. Faculty of Nursing, University of Toronto, 1980.

25 Spitzer, W.O., R.S. Roberts, and T. Delmore. Nurse Practitioners in Primary Care. V. Development of the Utilization and Financial Index to Measure Effects of Their Deployment. *Canadian Medical Association Journal* 114 (1976a), 1099–1102.

26 Spitzer, W.O., W.A.M. Russell, and B.C. Hackett. Financial Consequences of Employing a Nurse Practitioner. *Ontario Medical Review* 40 (1973), 96–100.

27 Spitzer, W.O., D.L. Sockett, J.C. Sibley, R.S. Roberts, M. Gent, D.J. Kergin, B.C. Hackett, and A. Olynich. The Burlington Randomized Trial of the Nurse Practitioner. *New England Journal of Medicine* 290 (1974), 251–256.

28 Ford, Loretta C. "A Nurse for All Settings: The Nurse Practitioner." *Nursing Outlook*, 27(8):516, August 1979.

29 Weston, Jerry L. What's Ahead for Nurse Practitioners and Physician Assistants? *HCFA Forum* (December 1980), 2–6.

30 Aiken, Linda H., and Robert J. Blendon. The National Nurse Shortage. *National Journal* (May 23, 1981), Vol. 3, 948–953.

31 Aiken, Linda H. Nursing Priorities for the 1980s: Hospitals and Nursing Homes. *American Journal of Nursing* 81:2 (February 1981), 324–330.

CHARLES E. LEWIS

14

NURSE PRACTITIONERS AND THE PHYSICIAN SURPLUS

In order to avoid speculating about a prognosis before a diagnosis has been established, I shall first review the evidence supporting the contention that there is, or soon will be, a surplus of physicians in the United States. If the available data indicate that condition to be present, we can then turn our attention to the primary question, that is, Will nurse practitioners survive in such a system?

After reading the literature on the training of health manpower during the 20th century, future historians will probably conclude that planning for this sector of the economy was either nonexistent or done so poorly that it contributed little to the futile attempts to rationalize the system. At the beginning of the 20th century, Abraham Flexner reported a survey of the status of medical education in the United States.[1] He concluded that there were many schools of low or marginal quality. As a result, 70 nonacademic proprietary institutions closed their doors between 1910 and 1925, and the output of physicians declined rapidly.

The first evidence of subsequent concern with a physician shortage appeared in the form of a statement made by the National Grange to the 1928 meeting of the American Medical Association (AMA).[2] The Grange had commissioned a study of the availability of physicians in smaller communities, and concluded that there was a shortage of physicians — at least in rural areas. However, later that year, the American economy collapsed with subsequent massive unemployment. Even physicians were affected. Faced with the specter of unemployed doctors, organized medicine became concerned with a possible surplus of physicians. In his presidential address to the AMA in 1933, Lewis suggested that "there is apparently an overproduction of doctors.

. . . Careful studies indicate that there are in the United States 25,000 more physicians than are required."[3] The experiences of the Great Depression were translated into policies that guided organized medicine in its opposition to any increase in the production of physicians for the next 20 yr.

Finally, in 1953 the AMA suggested that there *was* a shortage of physicians and the number of medical schools should be expanded. By 1961 the AMA was calling for the use of federal funds for construction and support of new medical schools to alleviate this shortage.

There was even greater concern about the distribution of practitioners by type of practice. The seemingly unlimited funding for the support of research and subspecialty training in the 1950s and 1960s was associated with a continuing decline of the number of general physicians. The specialty of family practice was born after a long gestational period and from the union of persuasive and impassioned general practitioners and semifrigid establishments of medical education. (This seduction may have been one of the most significant medical manpower events of the century.) Following the report of the Ad Hoc Committee on Education for Family Practice of the AMA Council on Medical Education (the Willard Report) in 1966, and that of the Citizen's Commission on Graduate Medical Education, chaired by John S. Millis, family practice was recognized as the 20th medical specialty field by the AMA's House of Delegates in 1969.[4, 5]

The passage of limited entitlement to care by Titles 18 and 19 (Medicare and Medicaid) further exaggerated the imbalance between demand for care and the existing supply of physicians, and finally the government acted. The 1965 amendments to the Health Professions Educational Assistance Act of 1963 created the Health Professions Educational Improvement Program, which received initial funding in fiscal year 1966. After legislative authority expired in 1971, this program was renewed in the form of the Comprehensive Health Manpower Training Act (Pl 92-157). As a result of these efforts, the number of first year medical students rose from 8,760 in 1965 to 1966 to 14,044 in 1973 to 1974.[6] Incidentally, federal expenditures for the support of training for nurse practitioners increased from $420,000 in fiscal year 1971 to $7,500,000 in 1973. These programs clearly benefited from being part of the massive campaign to ensure access for all to medical care (and in particular to primary care) in the 1970s.

The first nurse practitioners were a product of the shortage of physicians and the leadership of a few nurses and physicians who perceived that nursing could assume many of the functions of patient care traditionally defined as "medical." Some of us, however, were interested in the development of this type of practitioner for reasons unrelated to the shortage of health manpower. Both groups profited from the increased funding available to develop training programs to cope with the shortage of primary care practitioners. The concept of "physician extenders" was embraced somewhat gingerly by many segments of the medical profession. While this term suggests a prosthetic device rather than a group of professionals, it fairly accurately reflects the medicocentric view of physicians.

During the latter years of the 1970s some voices were heard expressing the opinion that soon there would be a surplus of doctors. Analysis of the need for manpower in the United States was delegated within the federal government to the Graduate Medical Education National Advisory Council (GMENAC). This group was charged with reviewing data, forecasting physician manpower requirements, and recommending the mix of residency training positions needed to facilitate a requirement–supply equilibrium. Over a period of 3 yr GMENAC produced a series of staff papers (including those projecting the supply and distribution of physicians and physician extenders, and describing need-based *versus* demand-based methodologies for forecasting physician requirements). It also created, through its activities, an awareness of the increase in the number of physicians in the United States as a result of policies related to the admission of foreign medical graduates and the increase in the output of American medical schools.

In 1979 the Senate Committee on Human Resources, confronted with differing projections of future supply, requested assistance from the Office of Technology Assessment. One of the principle concerns of the Congress was the variability in the estimates of requirements. An Advisory Panel on Technologies for Estimating Physician Supply and Requirements was charged specifically with reviewing the various models used in forecasting and the implications of these predictive models. It is hard to assess the impact of the report of this advisory panel, which analyzed the different estimates but concluded most valid projections indicated a future surplus of physicians.[7] It became public at approximately the same time that the GMENAC's findings were presented.

The GMENAC report projected a surplus of physicians in all but a few categories — such as child psychiatry and preventive medicine. The report met with mixed reviews. Most specialty societies initially rejected the conclusions; some, such as the American Academy of Pediatrics, still do. Perhaps surgeons were less reactive than other groups, since the report on the Study on Surgical Services in the United States, released 3 yr earlier, had conditioned them with regard to the probable need to reduce the size of residency programs in general surgery and some of the surgical subspecialties.[8]

Regardless of the initial reaction of organized groups of physicians, most practitioners seem to have accepted the GMENAC report as confirming what they were already perceiving from their perspectives — that is, there were a lot of new physicians moving into the neighborhood. Subsequent publication of reports, such as that of Schwartz and Newhouse, which analyzed the extent to which medical subspecialists were diffusing into smaller communities, also confirmed the "street knowledge" that many young physicians, completing their residency training in metropolitan hospitals, found difficulty in establishing a practice in these areas.[9] Saturation of "ideal" practice areas has slowly occurred, and more physicians have begun looking to nearby communities of lesser size for opportunities to practice.

While there will continue to be arguments about how many doctors are too many, the available evidence suggests that saturation has already occurred in those metropolitán areas in the United States that represent the most "desirable" sites for practice – the more affluent areas of urban communities in the Sun Belt. However, a recent summary of available data suggests that there will remain pockets of the population that are "structurally underserved," that is, will not have access to care regardless of the numbers of physicians generated, because of their locations and personal characteristics.[10] In other words, the poor in those rural areas that have little appeal to physicians seeking the advantages of life in metropolitan areas will continue to be underserved during a time in which the number of encounters with physicians per year will continue to increase for other segments of the population. The evidence seems conclusive: There is or soon will be a surplus of doctors in most of the United States, in terms of patients' needs for services.

WILL NURSE PRACTITIONERS SURVIVE?

In order to develop a prognosis that is based more on objective data than subjective impressions, we shall examine a series of relevant subquestions. These include the following:

- Have nurse practitioners thrived during the interval 1965 to 1980? If so, why? What are the conditions that seem to have been most propitious for their development and multiplication? In developing this ecologic perspective, we shall also review the physiology – or pathophysiology – of the nurse practitioner movement in order to describe their vital functions. This will help us answer the following question:
- Where or how are they vulnerable? What are the major threats to their survival?
- Finally, moving from the general to the specific, how will an excess of physicians compromise their existence?

We will conclude with a prognostication of where, and which groups of nurse practitioners will survive (or be severely compromised), in terms of their functional existence, in the 1980s. The latter statement reflects a fundamental assumption, supported by some evidence, on which this discussion is based.[11] Nurse practitioners are not now, nor have they ever been, a homogeneous group of professionals with a common set of motivations, skills, or competencies. To discuss the survival of nurse practitioners as a group is no more meaningful than to describe the natural history of patients with chronic illnesses without identifying specific diagnoses.

HAVE PRACTITIONERS THRIVED OR JUST SURVIVED (1965 to 1980)?

There is obvious evidence of the viability of the nurse practitioner concept during the 1970s. Most notable is the increase in the number of training programs and practitioners during this period. A Congressional Budget Office report estimates that there were 12,700 nurse practitioners in active practice in 1979, compared to less than 1,000 in 1970.[12] This growth occurred primarily because of concern over relief of the physician shortage, which reduced the level of opposition from physicians, and the massive support of training programs for primary care practitioners of all types by the federal government.

Further evidence of growth may be found in the volume of writing produced on this subject. The nurse practitioner literature is little more than a decade old. The first articles describing the concept, its translation into reality, and the impact on patient care of nurses functioning in "new" roles were published before 1970; these were classified in the literature under a variety of headings. The subject heading "nurse practitioner" first appeared in the 1973 Index Medicus. Under that title, 41 articles were listed. The following year 50 articles appeared, and in 1975, 82 publications were listed. Since that time there has been a cyclic pattern with titles in odd years numbering from 70 to 90 and in even years from 50 to 70.

The content of the literature has changed over this decade. Among the articles listed in 1973, most of which were published in 1970 to 1971, only four represent reports of studies. The other (90%) were descriptions of programs and discussion of concepts. The terms "clinical nurse specialists" and "nurse clinicians" appeared in several titles.

Early articles were either editorial in nature or represented reports of trials of this "new practitioner." Almost all of these demonstrated (1) acceptance by patients, (2) a quality of care, as determined by process measures, that was at least equal to that provided by physicians, and (3) outcomes of care that were equal to or superior to those achieved by physicians. The 1980 listing includes 12 articles on curriculum design. Although this represents publications from 1977 to 1978, one article appeared concerned with assessing productivity. More recently, the focus has been on cost–benefit analyses. These studies have been reviewed in some detail in another chapter in this volume.

One sign of accumulation of the literature in any field is the number of reviews of the literature published, as well as studies of studies. The literature published during 1978 to 1980 contains many articles concerned with productivity, cost–benefit analyses, or reviews by investigators critiquing the works of others. The backgrounds of the authors also have changed, with increasing numbers of nonphysicians being represented in the most recent literature.

FACTORS FAVORING THE GROWTH AND DEVELOPMENT OF NURSE PRACTITIONER PROGRAMS

On the basis of personal experience (as well as an analysis of the existing literature, particularly that focusing on health policy issues), we divide the history of the nurse practitioner movement into two phases. The first dates from the earliest signs of life, in 1965, until 1970. During this period, the concept of nurse practitioners was born and nurtured by one cast of characters. A second group of actors have been involved in the second phase (1971 to 1980).

Since a movement is defined as a "series of organized activities working toward an objective," it is more accurate to speak of the second phase (1971 to 1980) as the era of the nurse practitioner movement. Factors that affected the growth and development of practitioners during these phases are shown in Table 14-1. These have been grouped into those related to (1) the personal

TABLE 14-1 Factors Affecting the Growth of Nurse Practitioner Programs in Two Eras

	1965–1970	1971–1980
Personal Motivations		
Increase in use of professional skills	++	+
Improvement of care outcomes	++	+
Independence	0	+
Professional recognition	?	+
Increase in income and status	0	+
External Factors		
Doctor shortage (substitution)	++	+
Legal status	±	−
Reimbursement policies	0	−
Productivity and cost–benefits	0	±
Professional Associations		
Medicine	±	±/−
Nursing	−	++

motivations of those involved — both physicians and nurses; (2) external or environmental factors; and (3) the orientations of the organized professions of medicine and nursing. Those who disagree with the choice of these variables are referred to reviews on the topic, including those of the Congressional Budget Office and the Institute of Medicine.[12, 13]

As indicated in Table 14-1, during the early developmental phase, the principle motivations of those professionals involved were related to the quality of patient care and increases in the ability of nurses to use fully their professional skills in the direct care of patients. The concept of independent practice, concern with status or income, and professional advancement were not characteristic of the orientations of those active in the early demonstration and training programs. These were not the thrusts or topics represented by the literature they produced during that period. A few persons have been involved throughout both phases, and the orientations of their contributions to the literature seem not to have changed over time.

Among the external factors, the principle driving force was the shortage of physicians. There was considerable debate about the legal status of the functions performed by nurse practitioners, particularly by those physicians aghast at the thought of a nurse performing publicly those activities traditionally reserved for physicians. However, the number of practitioners and demonstrations was not sufficiently large enough to represent a source of concern. Nor was there a great concern for reimbursement for services, since most of these activities were supported by research funds (governmental) within academic settings. In these, the real costs of services were hopelessly lost in the tragedies represented by the accounting systems of most ambulatory care services.

Professional orientations varied considerably. Those physicians involved with nurses in this form of collaborative practice were highly supportive, and there was little if any reference to the economic threats posed by this innovation. Most other physicians were too busy to care, or felt that the concept was fine, as long as these practitioners worked *for* doctors. One of the more interesting characteristics of this initial period was the hostility expressed by most nurses and organized nursing as a profession toward the initial practitioner — demonstration programs. Nurses, including most of the then current leaders of the profession, frequently described the role and functions of nurse practitioners as "not nursing."

Many of the most hostile physicians viewed the activities of nurse practitioners as "playing doctors." Comments recorded during our initial clinical trial of nurses in a more "dynamic role" at the University of Kansas include, "Why are you (the nurse) looking through the charts? (after explanation of the study)." "My God, what won't they think of next?" "Better watch out fellows (to medical students standing near), you may have to pick up the pieces." (December 1965.) And, a resident: "Look at this chart — this patient is going to a nurse clinic; can you imagine, they're even letting nurses write in the charts now!" (January 1966.)[14]

It is not surprising that the early pioneers and survivors of the first phase bear the scars of wounds inflicted by everyone but the patients, who were universally enthusiastic. Our own patients used to say things like, "Mrs. Resnick does everything that the doctors do, only more human." Another confided, "If I got real sick, I would see a doctor *if* Mrs. Resnick says so."

As indicated, in 1971 additional funding became available for the training of nurse practitioners. The resources necessary to create a movement, to institutionalize these programs, or to graft them into the body of nursing were put to work to this purpose. Examination of the literature during this second phase reveals increasing concern from those entering training programs in gaining not only opportunities to use their professional skills, but also to practice more independently of physicians and to ensure professional advancement, increased status, and security. These are not unexpected goals (as a matter of fact, they seem completely normal under the circumstances).

It is not implied that over time nurse practitioners as a group have become less interested in patient care, only that a broader set of motivations is now being represented. This includes those of a subgroup believing in the importance of independent practice on a fee-for-service basis as *the* criteria for judging the legitimacy of nurse practitioners as clearly defined "professionals."

External influences during the second phase also changed, as reflected in the literature. There was increasing concern with the legal status of nurse practitioners and with the reform of nursing practice acts. There was increasing debate over the issue of reimbursement of nurse practitioner services as patient care services *per se*, rather than a set of activities provided "incidental to" medical consultation. There was decreasing concern with the physician shortage, and the importance of preparing physician surrogates. Finally, this literature shows the rising concern over cost and benefits and productivity, issues that have characterized much of the health services research literature of the late 1970s.

During this period, nursing as a profession has embraced and incorporated nurse practitioner programs. All of the requisite mechanisms for ensuring professional identity, including certification of graduates and accreditation of programs, have been established under the control of nursing. Becoming a nurse practitioner is now a legitimate and important means of gaining professional status in nursing.

VITAL SIGNS—WORK AND POLITICS

One of the clear measures of viability of an educational program is the extent to which its graduates are employed and functioning in the roles for which they were trained. Between 1973 and 1976 the State University of New York at Buffalo, under contract to the Division of Nursing, conducted a national longitudinal study of nurse practitioners and their employers. Of the 1,297 nurse practitioners identified for the study universe, 1,101 responded to the initial survey. After one year, 753 of these practitioners were successfully reinterviewed. Of that group, 70.3% were employed as nurse practitioners, 9% were unemployed, and 16% were employed but not as a nurse practitioner. (Those employed as a nurse practitioner included persons who were functioning wholly or in part as nurse practitioners.) More graduates of certificate programs were employed in nurse practitioner roles *only* (55%) than graduates of master's degree programs (36%). When asked, Does the demand for practitioners exceed supply?, 71% responded in the affirmative.[15]

To our knowledge, there have been no recent national studies of the status of the employment of graduates of nurse practitioner programs. Clearly this index deserves careful monitoring by any group concerned with a possible surplus of nurse practitioners.

The two most frequently cited barriers to practice in this role by graduates and analysts are legal restrictions to practice, and reimbursement policies. There is considerable evidence that during this period nursing and nurse practitioners were politically effective in achieving changes in the laws governing the scope of practice.[16] Forty-seven states have altered their nurse practice acts. In two of the three others, nurse practitioners can function under the "delegatory" provision of the medical practice act. For those nurses who want legal authority to function independently, including the right to prescribe certain drugs, this may not represent a major victory.

Alterations in reimbursement policies have been slower to be realized. Under Medicare, only those acts performed in an ambulatory setting delegated by a physician who is on the premises may be eligible for payment. An exception is granted to those services provided in rural, designated personnel-shortage areas. In rural clinics qualifying under this rule, services may be billed for, if there is periodic review of such activities by a consulting physician.

Under Medicaid, reimbursement is permitted as determined by the state. Many states provide payment for services rendered by nurse practitioners when billed for by physicians. There is considerable variation on a state-by-state basis.

Several states have created experimental programs permitting the prescribing of certain drugs, and a few others are studying the effects of direct payment. However, one of these initiated in 1980 involving dependents of members of the armed forces (CHAMPUS) recently had to be extended because of the inadequate number of participants enrolled.[17]

THREATS TO WELL-BEING IN THE 1980s

Given the rate of growth observed in the 1970s, why should the coming decade be viewed with concern by many of us who have been involved in or observed the nurse practitioner movement since its inception and believe in the value and importance of this group of professionals? A reexamination of the table may provide some clues.

The personal motivations of participants will probably change little. Of those itemized, demand or concern for independent practice will probably diminish opportunities for survival; the desire and ability to improve patient care outcomes could serve as one of the most important defenses against those forces that would threaten their existence.

The doctor shortage obviously will no longer serve as a positive stimulus. An argument will be developed that the surplus of physicians constitutes *the* principle threat to nurse practitioners. Legal status and particularly reimbursement policies constitute barriers to effective use of nurse practitioners in 1981. Those barriers will probably increase.

In the long run, the orientations of medicine and nursing will determine the survival of nurse practitioners; that is, in the decade ahead, legislation governing the legal status and reimbursement of nurse practitioners will be passed as a result of the political forces brought to bear by those groups that have the greatest interest in the health care industry. This includes organized medicine and nursing, hospital associations, and insurance carriers. Unfortunately, consumers will have little to say about the laws and policies that affect their care.

Despite the valuable contributions to be made by nurse practitioners to the care of persons, it seems highly likely that their opportunities to make these contributions will depend on those external factors concerned with reimbursement and the orientations of physicians. Unfortunately, the former — methods of reimbursement — have been in the past a function of the latter. A 1979 Congressional Budget Office Report concludes that "practice opportunities for physicians' extenders depend heavily upon physician willingness to hire them."[12] This statement would suggest that this group sees the future of independent practice as quite limited.

If we look to the strengths of nurse practitioners, or positive forces that could be brought to bear in the political conflict, more emphasis must be placed on their impact on outcomes of care. A review of the literature for articles providing evidence of nurse clinicians' and nurse practitioners' abilities to improve the quality of patient care outcomes, or to increase the productivity of those they serve, reveals far fewer citations than those concerned with costs and barriers.

Sox, in his 1979 review of the 21 studies of the quality of care provided by nurse practitioners and physician assistants published over a 10-yr period, reports nine experiments in which patients were randomly allocated to physicians and nurse practitioners.[18] Only three of these studies examined outcomes of care as a part of their analysis of quality. However, only one measured disability and return to work as one of the outcomes of care.[19] The other two studies indicate no differences in death rates; however, no mention is made of any significant difference in the return to work of patients.

Our initial studies at the University of Kansas, begun in 1965, grew out of a desire to improve the quality of care for patients with chronic illness coming to the medical clinic. At the time, I served as director of the medical clinics and also was in charge of a home care unit that provided services through a multidisciplinary team approach. The study grew out of frustration in my inability to improve the quality of care to patients in the medical clinics, while observing the impact of interdisciplinary care rendered in the home by teams led by nurses. By providing nurses with some additional skills in physical assessment and tutorials in pharmacology, they were prepared to manage, in collaborative practice with two internists in our group, patients with chronic illnesses in relatively stable phases of the natural history of their illness.

In the Kansas study, employment among patients cared for by one nurse increased by 50%. In the other nurse clinic, the change was less significant. In these clinics, no patients who were working at the time of admission into the study became unemployed during the year. In the control groups, the rate of employment *decreased* during the same period of time.

In presenting the results from this first clinical trial of nurses in an extended role, emphasis in the publications was placed on patient acceptance and the quality of care as measured by examination of processes. Less attention was paid to the nurses' ability to achieve significant improvements in disability (as reflected in employment) and also in improving patients' ability to control certain aspects of their disease, such as blood sugar levels among diabetics and blood pressure among hypertensives. We were struck by the frequency with which patients on medication had to have their doses reduced as they became compliant or adherent to the prescribed drug program for the first time.

The results seemed to us to be clearly explainable by the collaborative nature of the practice. That is, the physicians were concerned with disease, monitoring its progression, and prescription of treatments; the nurses were concerned with the care of the person. While the physicians focused on diagnosis and disease, the nurses' primary attention was directed toward patients' problems and the development of the interpersonal relations and social support structures necessary to improve adherence and a sense of well-being. Our practices were not competitive, that is, doctor *versus* nurse, but complementary.

Runyan has described on repeated occasions the outcomes of care resulting from the practices of nurses in the extended role caring for patients who are chronically ill.[20] Measurement of intermediate outcomes such as blood sugar and blood pressure levels have demonstrated the ability of nurse practitioners to achieve goals of care that often elude physicians.

A comparison of patients receiving care from nurses in the Memphis Health Department Clinics with nonrandomized controls showed the following among nurse clinic patients: (1) a reduction in diastolic blood pressures of hypertensive patients ranging from 6 mmHg to 18 mmHg, (2) a significant reduction in the blood glucose levels of diabetic patients; and (3) a reduction in the days of hospitalization by about 50%. Those in the control groups had an increase in their hospitalization experience and no changes in the biologic parameters listed.

As suggested, the demands of some nurses for legislation permitting independent practice will probably contribute negatively to the struggle ahead. It is predicted that such demands will antagonize those physicians who are neutral or limited supporters of the nurse practitioner concept. There is, however, a possibility that the reverse could occur. The current administration has placed great emphasis on "supply-side" economics. They have expressed their intentions to remove most governmental regulations affecting the system. At the same time, there are signs of increased antitrust activities directed at physicians. Greenberg, in his Washington Report on reimbursement wars, quotes the administration:

> What ails American medicine is government meddling and the straitjacket of federal programs. The prescription for good health care is deregulation and an emphasis upon consumer rights and patient choice.[21]

Calling for the reform of Medicare "to encourage home-based care whenever feasible," the statement continues, "In addition, we encourage the development of innovative alternate health care systems and other out-patient services at the local level." Greenberg concludes:

The usual caveat is in order about the loose linkage between platform prose and presidential performance. Nonetheless, the Republican marching plan for health care is in harmony with forces that are already in motion. Non-M.D. health care providers are intensifying their demands for recognition by the dominant sources of finance for health care. And they are increasingly difficult to resist, given the thrust of court decisions, the consumer movement, and the attractions of competition in a distressed economy.

The nonphysician group that figured most prominently in the action that apparently stimulated Greenberg's report was represented by the Virginia Academy of Clinical Psychologists. Two Virginia Blue Shield plans reimbursed psychologists for services to subscribers *only* if these were billed through a physician (sound familiar?). This arrangement was challenged in Federal District Court, unsuccessfully, and appealed to the United States Court of Appeals for the Fourth Circuit. This Court, in Decision No. 79-1345, handed down on June 16, 1980, found for the psychologists.

The opinion, while being appealed, is of such relevance to the question posed in this article that it deserves partial quotation:

> The Blue Shield plans are a dominant source of health-care coverage in Virginia. Their decisions as to who will be paid for psychotherapy necessarily dictate, to some extent, which practitioners will be chosen from among those competent under the law to provide such services. . . . The issue is one of more than professional pride. State law recognizes the psychologist as an independent economic entity as it does the physician. The Blue Shield policy forces the two independent economic entities to act as one, with the necessary result of diminished competition in the health-care field. The subscriber who has a need for psychotherapy must choose a psychologist who will work as an employee of a physician; a psychologist who maintains his economic independence may well lose his patient. In either case, the psychologist ceases to be a competitor.
>
> Any assertion that a physician must actually *supervise* the psychologist to assure the quality of psychotherapy treatment administered is refuted by the policy itself. The Blue Shield policy provides for payment to psychologists for psychotherapy if billed through *any* physician — not just those who regularly treat mental and nervous disorders. It defies logic to assume that the average family practitioner can supervise a licensed psychologist in psychotherapy, and there is no basis in the record for such an assumption.[22]

Those nurse practitioners who would draw parallels to their plight should note the opinion rests upon recognition under law of *competence* to perform the services in question and the concept of unfair *anticompetitive* practices.

While the climate of competition and concern for anticompetitive actions may prevail in the 1980s, a group still must be recognized under law as competent to provide those specific services that are subject to economic discrimination by reimbursement practices.

HOW WILL TOO MANY DOCTORS THREATEN THE SURVIVAL OF NURSE PRACTITIONERS?

There is increasing anecdotal evidence that physicians are already concerned with the economic threat provided by an increasing number of their own colleagues. To date, no surveys have been conducted of physicians' attitudes and beliefs about a variety of important issues that will confront the health care system in the 1980s. Such data would be of considerable interest.

At the request of the Chair of the Department of Medicine at the University of California at Los Angeles, we conducted a survey of a sample of 30 chairs of departments of medicine in medical schools throughout the United States.[23] The results indicate a growing concern over lower bed occupancy and an awareness of increasing competition for patients with the types of "unusual" diseases or procedures usually referred to academic centers. In fact, the concern in many institutions is for a continued flow of patients with *any* problems, who can provide an increase in practice income to offset those reductions occurring in federal support of research and education. A variety of strategies are being developed by academic institutions, clinics, and other organized care facilities in order to compete for patients in a marketplace saturated with physicians.

In 1978 the Robert Wood Johnson Foundation initiated a national program to improve the care of patients with chronic illness. Certain community hospitals throughout the United States were invited to submit proposals for the support of physician-directed, nurse-managed programs of care for persons with one of several chronic diseases. The rationale was clear: Nurses have been demonstrated to provide high quality of care for patients with chronic illness. However, most of the demonstrations reported have occurred in teaching hospitals, in public health departments, or health maintenance organizations (HMOs). In order to make the advantages of this form of physician–nurse practice available to the general public, a series of projects were to be supported in community hospitals where care would be provided to the patients of private practitioners by nurses functioning in collaborative practices with the local physicians involved.

It was early 1981 before these projects became operational. By that time, the impact of GMENAC and the concern of physicians for a "surplus of doctors" was evident. While all of these eight projects are now functioning and developing satisfactorily, their directors were faced with significant obstacles in the form of resistance by members of the medical staff that was far greater than anticipated.

Being responsible for the evaluation of the program provided an opportunity to visit each of these settings and talk with members of the medical staff. Their comments, in some settings, were identical to those expressed in 1965, with one exception — no one then was concerned with the nurses "taking the bread out of (their) mouths."

As noted, there is considerable anecdotal evidence, although no documented epidemiologic surveys, of the growing resistance of physicians to the concept of the provision of direct patient care by nurse practitioners. Certainly there is considerable manifestation of the opposition of physicians individually and collectively to the independent practice of nurse practitioners. There is also concern by physicians and others about the nature of drug prescribing by nurse practitioners in those states where experimental programs have been developed that permit nurses to prescribe certain drugs.

For example, in early 1981 the California Pharmaceutical Association and the California Medical Association were troubled by the cessation of the practice of the Department of Health Services to issue citations to hospitals and clinics where nurses dispensed certain medications. They sought an opinion on legality of this practice from the Attorney General of the State of California. The legislature created amendments to the Nurse Practice Act in 1976, expanding the role of the nurse. They also authorized several pilot programs that will not be concluded until 1982 permitting nurses to prescribe and dispense drugs. The attorney general ruled that the changes in the Nurse Practice Act of 1976 do not provide the legal authority the nursing board and hospital association say was intended. The reason given was that the pilot programs would not have been authorized unless there was intention to test the concept before implementation.[24]

WHO WILL SURVIVE?

Nursing has been far more sensitive than medicine in attending to the needs of certain subgroups of patients, notably the chronically ill, the well, mothers and children, the poor, and the aged. However, as the number of physicians increases, more and more of them are becoming concerned with chronic disease care, the promotion of health maintenance activities, including the operation of wellness centers. Even geriatrics and occupational medicine, areas relatively untouched in the past by medical practitioners, seem likely to attract their share of specialists in the future.

In the era of too many physicians, it seems probable that only those nurse practitioners who can do some of the things physicians *cannot* do or will not do will continue to be in demand. For example, those organizations who believe in their cost-effectiveness will employ nurse practitioners. (This is another way of saying that they will be valued if they are able to see many patients quickly and work for less than a physician.) Other nurse practitioners will be in demand if through their services, the outcomes of patient care are improved to the point that demand is reduced for care. This will be important *only* in those settings where physicians have an incentive for reducing the total costs of care—independent practice associations or HMOs. All of these projections presume that there will not be any major changes in the laws defining areas of competence and court actions finding that medicine is engaging in anticompetitive practices with regard to nurse practitioners.

Also, those groups of nurse practitioners will survive who (1) provide services to the structurally underserved (*i.e.*, those persons physicians are unwilling or unable to serve) and (2) develop truly complementary practices in collaboration with those physicians who are primarily concerned with their patients' care, rather than the economics of their practices. It is unfortunate that none of these conditions promoting survival lends itself to implementation through policy.

It seems likely that for the time being we will continue to generate excessive numbers of physicians and nurse practitioners, even if the latter are not fully used. With some luck, appropriate combinations will occur. Those with similar values and orientations from the two professions *may* find each other and practice as colleagues ever after.

During the next several years, physicians will probably point to the lack of efficiency, excessive costs, and lack of evidence on quality of care as reasons to reduce the roles of nurse practitioners. These will provide much safer (and more ethical) grounds for debate than calling attention to their perceived economic threat—or the loss of bread syndrome. Nurse practitioners might well counter with the lack of evidence of the efficacy and quality of physicians' practices. They also may find happiness in a coalition of nonphysician practitioner groups, waging a crusade against restraint of trade or anticompetitive practices.

Nurse practitioners and organized nursing must agree on a set of strategies designed to preserve this potentially endangered species. There is little evidence, however, that those who must lead such a campaign perceive the level of threat to survival to be as great as presented here. The contributions of nurse practitioners to society is even greater than their value to nursing. Unless leadership comes from within nursing, perhaps consumers will rise to their own defense.

In the development of strategies, it will be unfortunate if those who have made the least contribution to care, or who have the least to lose (since they are not in practice), insist on meeting their ideological needs at the expense of nurse practitioners.

Unless effective strategies are employed, the future roles of nurse practitioners will be decided not by those issues related to patient care, but primarily those of economic concern to an excessive number of physicians exerting a disproportionate amount of political influence on "health" policy.

REFERENCES

1 Flexner, A. *Medical Education in the United States and Canada: A Report to the Carnegie Foundation for the Advancement of Teaching.* New York: The Carnegie Foundation, 1910.

2 McVey, W. Shortage of Doctors in Rural Communities. Journal Kansas Med. Soc., 29:312–314, 1928.

3 Lewis, D. The Place of the Clinic in Medical Practice. Journal American Medical Association 100:1905–1910, 1933.

4 Willard, J. Chairman, Meeting the Challenge of Family Practice. Report of the Ad Hoc Committee on Education for Family Practice of the Council on Medical Education American Medical Association. Chicago, American Medical Association, 1966.

5 Millis, J.S., Chairman, The Graduate Education of Physicians. Report of the Citizen's Commission on Graduate Medical Education. Chicago, American Medical Association, 1966.

6 Lewis, C.E., Mechanic, D., and Fern, R. *A Right to Health*, pp. 96–97, New York John Wiley & Sons, 1976.

7 Technologies for Forecasting Physician Supply and Requirements. Health Program, Office of Technology Assessment, U.S. Congress, March 1980.

8 *Surgery in the United States: A Summary Report of the Study on Surgical Services for the United States.* The American College of Surgeons and the American Surgical Association, Chicago 1976.

9 Schwartz, W.B., Newhouse, J.P., Bennett, B.W., and Williams, A.P. The Changing Geographic Distribution of Board-Certified Physicians. New Eng. J. Med. 303:1032–1038, Oct. 30, 1980.

10 Rogers, D.E., Blendon, R.J., and Hearn, R.P. Some Observations on Pediatrics: Its Past, Present, and Future. Pediatrics 67:775–784, May, 1981.

11 Lewis, C.E. and Cheyovich, T. Who is a Nurse Practitioner? Processes of Care and Patients' and Physicians' Perceptions. Medical Care 14:365–371, (April) 1975.

12 Physician Extenders: Their Current and Future Role in Medical Care Delivery. The Congressional Budget Office, Congress of the United States, April, 1979.

13 Scheffler, R.M., Yoder, S.G., Weisfeld, N. and Ruby, G. Physicians and New Health Practitioners: Issues for the 1980s. Institute of Medicine, National Academy of Sciences, Washington, D.C., May 1979.

14 Lewis, C.E. Final Report, U.S. Public Health Services Grant NU 00145. The Dynamics of Nursing in Ambulatory Care. National Center for Health Services Research, Hyattsville, 1968.

15 Sultz, H.A., Zielezny, M., and Gentry, J.M. A Longitudinal Study of Nurse Practitioners. Phase II. DHEW Publication 78-92. U.S. Government Printing Office (Stock Number 017-041-00128-9), Washington, D.C.

16 Robyn, D. and Hadley, J. National Health Insurance and the New Health Occupation's Nurse Practitioners and Physicians' Assistants. J. Health Politics, Policy and Law, 5:447–468, (Number 3), Fall 1980.

17 CHAMPUS News Release, February, 1981.

18 Sox, H.C., Jr. Quality of Patient Care by Nurse Practitioners and Physicians' Assistants: A Ten-Year Perspective. Ann. Int. Med. 91:459–468, September 1979.

19 Lewis, C.E., Resnick, R., Waxman, D., and Schmidt, G. Activities, Events and Outcomes in Ambulatory Care. New Eng. J. Med. 280:645–649 (March 20), 1969.

20 Runyan, J.W. The Memphis Chronic Disease Program. Comparisons in Outcomes and the Nurse's Extended Role. J American Med. Assoc. 231:27–30. Jan 20, 1975.

21 Greenberg, D.S. Washington Report, Reimbursement Wars. New Eng. J. Med. 303:538–540, August 28, 1980.

22 Ibid.

23 Lewis, C.E. Symptoms of Stress and Patterns of Coping in Academic Departments of Medicine. Presented at Chesapeake Educational/Research Trust Medical Care Symposium, New York City, April 1980.

24 Nelson, H. State Challenges Nurses' Authority to Prescribe and Administer Drugs. Los Angeles Times, April 25, 1981.

DONNA DIERS

15

FUTURE OF NURSE–MIDWIVES IN AMERICAN HEALTH CARE

Nurse midwifery is the oldest of the specialized practice roles for nurses. While midwifery's history is as old as the history of man, nurse midwifery as a professional practice field is generally said to have begun in the United States in 1925, with the introduction of English-trained nurse midwives to the hills of Kentucky by Mary Breckinridge in what became the Frontier Nursing Service.[1-3] Nurse midwifery makes an unusually good example of the issues nursing faces in addressing public policy considerations of manpower, economics, costs of care, quality and access to care, and interprofessional politics. In this chapter, then, nurse midwifery will be taken as an early instance of predictable concerns modern nursing is confronting: establishing rights to practice and payment for service; meeting the needs of people for humane, high-quality service; and participating in health care system reform.

DEFINITIONS

A certified nurse-midwife is

> an individual educated in the two disciplines of nursing and midwifery, who possesses evidence of certification according to the requirements of the American College of Nurse–Midwives [ACNM].[4]

The author wishes to express her thanks to Kate Schwob, BA, RN, for assistance in the preparation of this chapter. Helen Varney Burst, RN, MSN, CNM, provided both inspiration and critical commentary from her unique perspective as immediate past-President of the American College of Nurse–Midwives. Susan Molde, RN, MSN, and Ann T. Slavinsky, RN, MSN, gave valuable editorial assistance.

Nurse-midwifery practice is

the independent management of care of essentially normal newborns and women, antepartally, intrapartally, postpartally and/or gynecologically. This occurs within a health care system which provides for medical consultation, collaborative management and referral and is in accord with the Functions, Standards and Qualifications for Nurse-Midwifery Practice as defined by the ACNM.[5]

Nurse midwives define themselves as having been educated *both* in nursing and in midwifery. Note, however, that there is no mention of education in the practice of obstetrics or medicine. This is more than a semantic pirouette and is crucial for the development of nurse midwifery in concert with medical obstetrics. It also has the potential for clarifying roles for nurse practitioners. Nurse midwives define their territory as midwifery not obstetrics, so the scope of practice can at least be talked about as different from the practice of medical obstetrics. Therefore, nurse midwives have maneuvered themselves out of the potential control of physicians who do not, it is assumed, practice midwifery and, therefore, cannot be in the position of "supervising" midwives. (As we shall see later, such semantic niceties do not completely protect against interprofessional battles.) The collaborative and referral roles of the obstetrician are clarified by this wording as well: obstetricians practice medical obstetrics, meaning the diagnosis and treatment of disease.

Midwifery is the oldest health profession in history and an internationally recognized profession in its own right. *Midwifery* does not require nursing either as a prerequisite or as a recognized component of the profession. Midwifery is neither a nursing specialty nor a medical specialty, but rather a separate profession.[6] The nurse part of the phrase "*nurse* midwife," on the other hand, recognizes

the prerequisite foundation in nursing, differentiates the nurse-midwife from the lay midwife . . . and assures a continuing emphasis on patient education, support, and counseling. . . . The "midwife" part of the name recognizes the additional specialized preparation and functioning of the nurse-midwife, tempers the medical focus in normal obstetrics, and identifies the nurse-midwife with professional midwife counterparts the world over.[7]

In contrast to medical obstetrics, which, being the practice of medicine is aimed at cure of disease, nurse midwifery treats pregnancy, labor, childbirth, and women's health as normal, natural physiological processes, deeply imbedded in a society's value of the family. Nurse midwifery practice is based on a minimum of interference in the normal process, and a very high priority is placed on continuity of care — the same nurse midwives caring for the same patients throughout the childbearing cycle and the constant attendance of the nurse midwife during labor and delivery. Nurse midwifery practice provides primary care and aims to increase confidence and independence, dispel fear and provide an atmosphere of love and joy not possible when there are life-threatening complications requiring necessary machines or medical or surgical intervention.[8] Thus, nurse midwifery's historical concentration on the *essentially normal* allows an orientation toward patient and family participation in decision making, a focus on health maintenance and prevention, and an implicit feminist setting, of women caring for women.

Including the word "independent" in the definition of professional midwifery further separates midwives from delegated medical functions and from traditional definitions of nursing as well. Independent *management* explicitly occurs in the context of a team relationship with a physician, operationally defined by signed agreements and practice protocols. But unlike some specialized practice roles in nursing (primary care nurse practitioners), who are thought to be practicing both nursing and an "expanded" role in delegated medical functions, nurse midwives claim management of the normal patient for their own and refer management of the complicated patient to physicians.

A second important point in the definitions given is the ACNM's role in establishing standards of practice and of educational preparation. While nurse practitioner groups are, moving toward such quality control, nurse midwifery through its professional association has established rigorous criteria for review of educational programs, and enforces standards of practice so that it is possible for a nurse midwife to have certification revoked or suspended for failing to adhere to ACNM standards, including having a formal written alliance with a physician.[9]

Finally, the ACNM Statement of Qualifications, Standards, and Functions makes clear another crucial part of nurse midwifery's philosophy. In a section on standards for the practice of nurse midwifery, nurse midwives are explicitly committed, among other things, to uphold the right to self-determination of consumers within the boundaries of safe care, and to stimulate community awareness and responsiveness to the needs for delivery of quality family-centered care.[10] This dedication to consumer participation further places nurse midwifery on the cutting edge of health system reform and provides an enviable consumer–provider alliance that already has had demonstrated impact.

BACKGROUND

Whether the history of nurse midwifery in the United States is considered to forecast the political movements of nursing specialty groups, certain aspects of the past are at least symbolic of current concerns in nursing.

The first formal educational program for nurse midwives was established in New York City in 1932. Called the Clinic and School of the Association for the Promotion and Standardization of Midwifery (the Lobenstine Midwifery School), it was created to address the publicly acknowledged poor obstetric conditions in the United States as contrasted with other countries. By 1931 there was conclusive evidence of the potential of nurse midwifery from the Frontier Nursing Service. The Lobenstine Clinic and School was merged with the Maternity Center Association (MCA) in 1935. Varney notes that all of nurse midwifery education today can trace its beginnings to the MCA School, because all schools, with the exception of the program at Frontier Nursing Service, were started either by graduates or students of graduates of the MCA program.[11]

Nurse midwifery education developed slowly, however. Until 1955 there were but seven programs, three of which closed in the 1940s. Catholic University affiliated with the Catholic Maternity Institute in 1947 and is acknowledged as the first degree-granting program. (The Catholic University nurse midwifery program closed in 1969.) In 1955 Columbia University opened its graduate nurse midwifery program, followed in 1956 by Johns Hopkins and Yale. By 1965 there were nine nurse midwifery educational programs and the count had reached 21 programs by 1980 (with three others on the drawing boards).[12] Of the 21 programs listed in October 1980, 13 grant the master's degree; all others provide a certificate in nurse midwifery. (Refresher and internship programs are not included here.) However, the ACNM has standardized the nurse-midwifery component of education so that core *midwifery* competencies are the same in certificate and master's programs, a situation that does not yet prevail in certificate and master's degree nurse practitioner programs.

The ACNM was incorporated in 1955 in Santa Fe, New Mexico (because New Mexico was one of the few states with actively practicing nurse midwives, and the red tape for incorporation was minimal). Neither the American Nurses Association (ANA) nor the National League for Nursing (NLN) had been responsive to nurse midwives' need and wish to have a special focus and voice in professional organizations. While nurse midwives had had a special section in the National Organization of Public Health Nurses (NOPHN), when it merged with NLN, the section disappeared. Within the ANA, nurse midwives had no defined place, and a formal organizational response to nurse midwives' concern simply invited them to become part of a study on improvement of care to mothers and children. Thus, nurse midwives themselves created a committee on organization, surveyed their population, and eventually called a meeting in 1955 at which those present voted to create a separate organization to be called the American College of Nurse Midwifery (later changed to Nurse midwives).

Hattie Hemschemeyer, Director of the MCA School, was elected the first president of the new organization. Her first presidential message, reported in the fledgling *Bulletin* of the ACNM, could have been written in 1981:

> We nurse-midwives are a specialized group and our education, experience, and service have led us to the considered conclusion that in our present society it is neither desirable nor necessary to eliminate specialization. . . .[13]

By 1980 all states or territories except Kansas and Wisconsin were interpreted to have either specific nurse midwifery legislative statutes or regulations, or permissive laws with no specific recognition of nurse midwifery. Thirty-five jurisdictions have licensure specific to nurse midwifery.[14] In 1981 Kansas and Wisconsin both passed into the friendly column with the enacting of a new law in Wisconsin and new regulations in Kansas to support the practice of nurse midwifery.

The ACNM has carried out four surveys of United States nurse midwives since 1963.* Data in 1963 showed 11% of nurse midwives in active clinical practice. By 1967 this figure was 23%. The 1976–1977 survey (N = 1,299) shows slightly over 50% of responding nurse midwives in actual nurse midwifery practice. Data are being collected in 1981 for the next survey. More strikingly, the data show that over half of the nurse midwives included in the 1976–1977 survey had been trained since 1969, hardly surprising given the very large increase in the number of educational programs in the late 1960s and 1970s.[15, 16] The number of nurse midwifery services has grown from six in three states in the early 1960s to multiple services in 35 states, with many more in the planning stages.[17]

The 1976–1977 survey of nurse midwives concludes with the observation that "the number of American nurse-midwives has approximately doubled during each decade since the 1950s," a point that will become important later.[18]

While the 1976–1977 survey showed slightly over 50% of the respondents in *nurse midwifery* practice, the data also show another 33% of respondents in the *nurse midwifery labor force*, defined to include any nurse midwife employed in a position in which she used her nurse midwifery education and experience, plus those temporarily unemployed while in school or during a brief transition period (12 mo). Of those in the labor force but not in active

---

* The ACNM statistics are the only reliable statistics on nurse midwives in this country (85% of nurse midwives are members). Since one condition for approval of nurse midwifery educational programs is having an existing nurse midwifery service, faculty of all nurse midwifery educational programs are, by definition, practicing nurse midwives but are often counted in Health Systems Agency (HSA) and health department statistics as "faculty" assumed not to be practicing. Because ACNM provides the professional certification, it can also collect data on all certified Nurse-Midwives, whether they are members of the association or not. Indeed, ACNM published the first *Registry* of Certified Nurse-Midwives in Spring 1981.

nurse midwifery practice, the major reason for noninvolvement in clinical nurse midwifery was "no nurse midwifery positions available in my community" (26.7%), followed by "prefer current job because of the nature of the work, salary, hours" (17.5%). Of those not in the nurse midwifery labor force at all, 89 were retired or disabled, 102 were working in positions not relevant to maternal and child health, 32 would have liked to work but were not certified or needed a refresher course, with four not responding to the employment question (of a total sample of 1,299). In this group of nurses, then, nearly 99% were actively employed.

An interesting historical wrinkle in nurse midwifery is that nurse midwives long have held significant positions in state and local health departments, schools of nursing, hospitals, and other facilities, and in professional organizations, but were not recognized as nurse midwives.[19] Yet their background in the profession must have counted heavily toward their ability to help their organizations attack the problems of maternal and infant health and health service delivery.

Nurse midwifery is, then, a highly developed specialty area with a documented history of effective service and manpower production. Nurse midwifery has organized its political base outside organized nursing, and has worked to achieve separate status within state law and regulation. The field has developed strong quality control mechanisms for the approval of educational programs and entry-level certification of graduates. The number of nurse midwives has probably quadrupled between 1950 and 1980, and nearly the entire nurse midwifery population is active in the labor force. All of these themes, and certain others, provide a base for discussion of public policy issues.

NURSE-MIDWIFERY AND HEALTH POLICY

The economist Uwe Reinhardt notes that there is no such thing as one coherent national health policy. If there were, he says, it would include a health insurance policy, a health care access policy, a health manpower policy, a health care quality policy, and a health care cost policy, at least.[20] These potentially different aspects of national health policy provide a useful framework within which to discuss nurse midwifery.

NURSE–MIDWIFERY AND HEALTH MANPOWER POLICY

Predictions of nursing manpower needs tend to be based on unfilled or open positions, or numbers of hospital beds, or some other relatively data-based figure. It is not possible to use these methods to predict nurse midwifery manpower needs. The recent history of nurse midwifery in this country shows that nurse midwives have created new services.[21-29] Since there were not "open positions" to begin with, it is not possible to use the fact that there are now filled positions as an index of manpower need. In settings in which nurse midwifery has existed for some time, it is possible to calculate turnover and estimate unfilled positions, but such estimates will touch only an insignificant fraction of traditionally defined "need."

The phenomenal growth of nurse midwifery in the 1960s was in large part in response to the "baby boom," an insufficient number of obstetricians, and the need for hands.[30] Therefore, another approach to calculating manpower needs in nurse midwifery is to look at the relationship between the number of babies being born and obstetric manpower, realizing that nurse midwives are pushing their way into service delivery territory previously reserved to medical obstetrics. That is essentially the approach taken by the Graduate Medical Education National Advisory Committee (GMENAC) to the Secretary of the Department of Health and Human Services in its controversial report issued in September 1980.[31]

Since GMENAC was commissioned to study the supply of physicians, and only incidentally paid attention to nonphysician manpower supply, it is not surprising that the report assumes that physicians, including obstetricians, "own" the medical health service delivery systems and, therefore, all other categories of health service personnel needs must be calculated by reference to the physician group. Thus, the report recommends holding constant the levels of graduates of nurse midwifery training programs to the 1980 level given an "unavoidable excess" of obstetricians.[32]

The GMENAC Committee was composed of 13 physicians, three federal officials, one hospital administrator, a health economist, two lawyers, and two nurses (neither a nurse midwife). A Delphi survey was the major method chosen to determine consensus on what medical obstetric functions reasonably could be delegated safely. Medical service was defined as those activities that, if provided by a nonphysician, must be done under the supervision of a physician.[33]

The GMENAC report uses a formula that determines that a nonphysician is half as productive (measured in visits or deliveries) as a physician. Such a productivity formula fails to recognize certain realities of nurse midwifery practice. Nurse midwives provide care that is not traditional medical care, and they resist the 3-min visit mentality. One study that carefully controlled the risk status of patients who were then randomly assigned to physician or nurse midwife services, found that patients paid more visits (per patient) to nurse midwives than to the comparable physician group.[34] The authors speculate that this "overcompliance" may represent either clinician anxiety or patient need for counseling, particularly nutrition teaching. Productivity formulas based on number of visits without attention to what goes on in the visit will always count nurse midwives or nurse practitioners as less productive.[35]

Whether nurse midwives are as productive as physicians in numbers of deliveries depends a great deal on the setting in which the two operate and the extent to which nurse midwives may control physician intervention. Where interprofessional relationships, hospital policies, or other external considerations are at issue, nurse midwives "lose" deliveries to physicians in training, or to medical intervention that may not be indicated by patient status or available manpower.

The survey and model constructed on it determined that the projected supply of nurse midwives should handle 5% of all deliveries in 1990, provide all the prenatal and postpartum care for the patients they deliver (2.8 million visits), and assume a proportion of all the ambulatory maternity care required by low-risk patients (2.8 million visits), yet, presumably, not deliver this latter group. Such projections are based on the assumption that an excess of obstetricians is projected by 1990 and that production of additional nurse midwives will be held to current levels, though the proportion in active clinical practice will increase to 70%.[36]

The definition of nurse midwifery practice is quite clear in stating that nurse midwives practice *independently* in the management of essentially normal pregnancy, labor, delivery, and gynecologic care, within a health care system that provides for consultation with physicians when patient condition exceeds this limit. The team relationship propounded by nurse midwives with physicians dictates that there should be, eventually, mutual consultation and referral on cases that fall within one discipline's defined scope — the essentially normal should be referred to midwives, the abnormal should be referred to physicians.

To their credit, the authors of the GMENAC report suggest that further study is necessary to determine what nurse midwives do that is different from obstetricians. The nurse midwifery literature is, indeed, thin in linking process with outcome, although the definitions of nurse midwifery practice are widely available. Thus, the GMENAC report is a spur to nurse midwives and nurse researchers to provide data that might shed light on the empirical (as opposed to theoretical, philosophical, or political) differences between nurse midwifery and obstetrics.

Finally, the Delphi methodology assumes that a large sample of opinion-makers are participants in determining consensus on whatever issue is submitted to them.[37, 38] In the case of the GMENAC report, the Delphi panel consisted of seven persons: four obstetricians, one family practice physician, one nurse midwife, and one consumer.[39] Determining consensus on delegability of functions from such a small group, no matter how widely represen-

tative, is methodologically weak at best, when it is known that there is probably a wide range of opinion (among obstetricians and nurse midwives, if no
others) on the topic at hand. The Delphi technique produces, for each item (a
potentially delegable function in this case) a mean "score" (how delegable the
function is on a scale of, usually, 1 to 7) with ranges and standard deviations.
In several rounds of questionnaires, respondents see the scores of their fellow
Delphi panelists and may or may not moderate or change their own judgments. It should be clear that a panel of seven members would produce very
unreliable means or ranges, on sample size alone. Thus, that part of the
GMENAC report, which relies on the Delphi methodology for prediction,
must be read with suspicion.

From the point of view of nurse midwives, the estimate of delegable services is a serious underestimate of what services might be delivered by nurse
midwives in 1990, since the functions submitted to a panel of experts include
only medical functions, not the traditional nurse midwifery concerns with
health maintenance, patient teaching, self-care, or patient participation.[40]

If one were to take a simpleminded approached to manpower in midwifery, however, one might simply take GMENAC's own statistic that there
are to be 197,600 uncomplicated deliveries in 1990 (85% of all cases) and that,
at least in theory, *all* of them could be delegated to nurse midwives. Even if
there were enough nurse midwives to assume this clinical load by 1990, such
production would so revolutionize traditional obstetric care that it is possible
a society tilted toward a view of physicians as "in charge" could not support
the explosion. Obstetricians simply could not survive either economically or
technically if their practices were confined only to the abnormal, or high-risk,
cases. To suggest such a move, therefore, amounts to conversion of obstetricians into referral technicians closer to surgeons than to other medical
specialties, and suggests vast decrements of obstetrician manpower and the
possibility of physician unemployment. Yet, a recommendation like this is at
least theoretically possible, and should be considered as seriously as holding
midwifery training programs to current levels before it is discarded out of
today's political, economic, and interprofessional realities.

NURSE–MIDWIFERY AND HEALTH CARE ACCESS POLICY

The GMENAC report recognizes that nurse midwives help alleviate the
problem of geographic maldistribution of services. Using ACNM data from
the 1976–1977 survey, the report indicates that 10% of nurse midwives are
located in communities with populations under 10,000, while only 1% of *all*
physicians are in these locales.[41] It is likely that these figures are underes-
timates of the number of nurse midwives now serving in these kinds of sites
since these data do not include any nurse midwives serving in the National

Health Service Corps (NHSC), which was not functioning in 1976 and 1977). Nor do the data account for sites with inner-city underserved populations where it is also known nurse midwives are in active practice.

Langwell and others used 1979 data to conduct a national study of the practice sites of nurse midwives, using the county as the geographic unit of analysis.[42] Data were restricted to those states with enabling nurse midwifery legislation. In one analysis, the data show that counties with low ratios of nurse midwives-to-female population are all located in Standard Metropolitan Statistical Areas (which is also where medical schools and teaching hospitals are). The counties with low ratios of nurse midwives-to-female population have the highest ratio of obstetrician-to-female population. The authors conclude that "obstetricians serve in areas not served by nurse midwives, and vice versa."[43] When only counties with populations under 50,000 are considered, the data show that counties with the highest nurse midwife-to-female population ratios have the lowest population, lowest per capita income, lowest average daily hospital census, and lowest number of hospitals beds. However, these counties have the highest birth rates. The authors recommend, among other things, that nurse midwives be included in the health manpower categories used to calculate shortage areas.

Large-scale studies other than the two mentioned here have not been done with national data. Data from the Mississippi, Georgia, and South Carolina nurse midwifery public sector projects indirectly demonstrate that where nurse midwives are in place, they will be used.[44-47] Nurse midwifery services developed for a low-income neighborhood health center in New Haven, Connecticut, attracted new patients from the beginning and helped the health center become organizationally viable.[48]

In the private sector, Olsen reported on 34 mo of nurse midwifery service in a private practice in Wisconsin with primarily middle-class patients. Thirteen percent of the patients in this practice chose to be cared for completely by nurse midwives. (Others who chose the nurse midwife but were not clinically eligible for her care were excluded from data analysis.) The nurse midwifery patients tended to be slightly older than the average, had above-average education, and professional or white collar positions (including an interesting number of nursing positions).[49] Norton's study of the faculty nurse midwifery private practice at Yale concludes, among other things, that the practice created a new "market" of women and families who would not otherwise have been served in the geographic area. Of her sample (92 clients over 2 years) over 50% came from more than 10-mile distance from the practice base — this in a geographic area in which small distances are often seen as defining service areas.[50]

Despite the lack of large-scale national studies, it appears that nurse midwives do increase access to care. In the first place, nurse midwives are more likely to practice in places in which they can provide the full scope of services they are prepared to deliver. This tends to mean settings in which there are few obstetricians competing for the same patients, and this in itself expands the service delivery base.

It is both parenthetically and politically interesting that nurse midwifery services have developed so rapidly and with such relative lack of resistance in the very areas in which the childbearing population might be thought to be at the most risk — risk which would ordinarily make them ineligible for nurse midwifery care. Superficial sociologic analysis would lead one to conclude that enlightened public health interests, or a lack of obstetrical manpower, may override the resistance of other groups to expansion or introduction of nurse-midwifery services. In this context, nurse midwifery is no different from nursing specialities, for it has been well documented that the patients first turned over to nurses in expanded roles are the most sick, the poorest, the most complicated, the most socially undesireable, the most socially at risk, and this phenomenon has appeared in psychiatric nursing, primary care, and midwifery.[51-57]

In January 1980 the General Accounting Office (GAO) submitted its report to Congress, "Better Management and More Resources Needed to Strengthen Federal Efforts to Improve Pregnancy Outcome." Among its recommendations was that the Department of Health and Human Services (HHS) "encourage greater use of nurse midwife/obstetrician teams," and help eliminate barriers to nurse midwifery practice in hospitals and rural clinics.[58] The data on which the report was based includes testimony from all over the country to the effect that nurse midwives, especially in inner cities and rural areas, increase access to care for a population that otherwise would not be scrved at all, or who would come to hospitals only for the delivery of the baby.

It is not difficult to understand how nurse midwives have so increased access to care among the underserved or unserved populations, whether people are underserved by geographic limitations, socioeconomic status, or general undesirability in an academic medical care system where the essentially normal patients may be seen as uninteresting at best. In general, the poor and underserved have not had the choice of midwifery as an alternative to another form of care; it was midwifery or nothing.

A more recent social phenomenon is the rise of consumer interest in choices and alternatives to traditional forms of care. Since nurse midwifery deals literally with motherhood, it is perhaps not surprising that nurse midwifery has attracted such powerful consumer attention.[59, 60] Studies of private nurse midwifery practices in which patients chose to be cared for by nurse midwives consistently show that nurse midwifery patients tend to be older, better educated, and more often professional women than comparison groups in traditional obstetric practices.[61-64] Nurse midwifery profits from two other social movements: feminism and the interest of women in caring for themselves; and the desire for a natural, noninterventionist approach to childbearing. Nurse midwifery practices attract patients who might not be served at all by traditional obstetrics, choosing no care over what is viewed as paternal patronization.

Knowledgeable consumers also seek alternatives to hospitalization for childbirth — birthing centers or home birth services. Such services may provide not only professional nurse midwifery care, but homelike surroundings respecting the family's need to participate in the birth of the baby. Consumer groups supportive of nurse midwifery have sprung up throughout the country. Perhaps the best known of the consumer–provider alliances is National Association of Parents and Professionals for Safe Alternatives in Childbearing (NAPSAC), a group of parents and professionals of all kinds dedicated to providing a forum for communication, encouraging family-centered maternity care in hospitals and maternity and childbearing centers, establishing safe home birth programs, and providing educational opportunities to parents and expectant parents.*

Throughout its history, nurse midwifery has responded to the needs and interests of patients and potential patients. Its reputation for responsiveness has produced a new phenomenon of providers and consumers working together to achieve mutual goals. In this sense, nurse midwifery was far ahead of the thinking that produced health planning efforts localized in Health Systems Agencies.

Thus, nurse midwifery increases access to care through service in underserved areas and through a more general responsiveness to consumer need or demand. Nurse midwives in practice change the demand and create new markets for their services, even in the face of competing medical manpower. It is possible to see in nurse midwifery the beginnings of a larger movement in which nurse practitioners, psychiatric nurses, and other specialist practitioners may find themselves more, rather than less, desirable if their services are thought to be important alternatives to patients, in spite of an acknowledged oversupply of physicians.

NURSE–MIDWIFERY AND HEALTH CARE QUALITY POLICY

There is a small but growing body of literature on the quality of services delivered by nurse midwives, usually compared to traditional obstetric services or to public health statistics before and after introduction of nurse midwives

---

* NAPSAC publishes quarterly newsletters and puts on various programs and other activities. One of its most important contributions has been the publication or reproduction of a number of volumes that contain hard-to-find, crucial information on such topics as quality of care, standards of practice, and history of nurse midwifery. NAPSAC, Box 267, Marble Hill, MO 63764.

to a state or county. Levy, Wilkinson, and Marine's study in Madera County, California, showed a decrease in prematurity from 11% to 6.6% after nurse midwives were introduced to care for poor women there. More prenatal care was given more frequently to a larger proportion of expectant mothers; neonatal mortality was halved (from 23.9 per 1,000 to 10.3 per 1,000).[65] Meglen and Burst report nurse midwifery effectiveness in Holmes County, Mississippi, where in less than 3 yr the infant mortality rate was reduced from 39.1 per 1,000 live births to 21.3 per 1,000.[66] In Kentucky, the Frontier Nursing Service has kept the perinatal mortality rate to a figure less than half of what it averages for the rest of the country (6 per 1,000 compared to 14.5 to 16 per 1,000). Since 1951 the Frontier Nursing Service has not lost a single mother to birth-related causes.[67] Nurse midwifery services in southern Texas reduced prematurity rates by half, and 30 yr of nurse midwifery service to the people of Santa Fe County, New Mexico, produced a dramatic change in the perinatal death rate from 87.6 per 1,000 to 15.1 per 1,000, lower than the national average.[67-70]

In rural Georgia nurse midwives were introduced into four counties, with seven contiguous counties used for comparison. In the four years of the project, the infant mortality rate in the four experimental counties was reduced to 16 to 17 per 1,000, while it remained at approximately 23.5 per 1,000 live births in the comparison counties. The percent of low-birth weight babies — 24% before the project — was reduced to 13.8% afterwards. The number of babies symptom free at birth was 76.8% before and 92% after the introduction of nurse midwives. Before the project, only 1.6% of the patients made nine or more prenatal visits to their caregivers (11 visits are recommended). After the project 25.2% of the patients made nine or more visits. Most startling, the data from this project show that estimated perinatal care expenditures per patient decreased during the program, to a collective annual savings for the counties involved of $1.1 *million*.[71]

At North Central Bronx Hospital, whose clients come from one of New York City's most distressed areas, every patient receives nurse midwifery management. One year's data (1979) showed 88% of patients had normal spontaneous vaginal deliveries. Fewer than 30% of all mothers needed analgesia or anesthesia in labor and the neonatal death rate among infants 1,000 g or over was 4.2 per 1,000.[72]

Quality of care has been studied in settings in which nurse midwifery could be compared to routine obstetric practice. Runnerstrom's early study at Johns Hopkins Hospital compared nurse midwifery patients with patients cared for by resident house staff and found no statistically significant difference in labor and delivery profile or postpartum or newborn outcomes between the groups. Nurse midwifery patients had a higher number of clinic visits and tended to gain the optimum amount of weight prenatally.[73] At the University of Mississippi Medical Center, Slome and others documented equivalent outcomes in a group of patients cared for by obstetric residents and another attended by nurse midwives, except that there was a higher rate of forceps delivery in the resident group and a higher rate of compliance with appointments among nurse midwifery patients.[74] Corbett and Burst found that adolescents cared for by nurse midwives were less often anemic at delivery, had more normal spontaneous vaginal deliveries, and had larger babies than a comparable group of patients served by obstetric residents in a South Carolina project.[75] At Roosevelt Hospital in New York City, an autonomous midwifery service was formed. A study comparing 454 patients cared for by midwives to 500 patients cared for by attending physicians found "strikingly similar" results except that operative deliveries were more frequent in the physician group.[76] Studies comparing patients served by nurse midwives in a neighborhood health center in New Haven, Connecticut, with patients served by private physicians and by hospital clinics showed that in a population at considerable social and obstetric risk, outcomes among the nurse midwifery patients were essentially equivalent to the private patient group. The mean birth weight was highest among babies of the nurse midwifery patients.[77]

Commenting upon the nurse midwifery evaluation studies in testimony before the Subcommittee on Oversight and Investigation of the Interstate and Foreign Commerce Committee, epidemiologist C. Arden Miller of the University of North Carolina noted that "all of the studies . . . confirm that the health benefits of care as rendered by nurse-midwives stand up to scientific scrutiny exceedingly well."[78] In the same hearing, Judith Rooks, Expert Consultant with the Office of Population Affairs, HHS, said that "there is absolutely no instance of nurse-midwifery service in the United States that has compiled a bad record and if there was, one bad example would be very destructively used."[79]

In nurse midwifery the policy issues concerning use of scarce resources, technology *versus* clinical judgment, and control of patient care are becoming focused. Data are accumulating that routine use of some kinds of medical intervention (fetal monitoring, for example) appear to cause rather than prevent iatrogenic complications in otherwise normal patients.[80-84] The routine use of labor-stimulating drugs, pain medications, episiotomy, amniotomy, enemas, forceps, intravenous drips, and ultrasound as well as restrictions on patient position and mobility in labor have all been implicated in infant and maternal morbidity and mortality statistics.[85-94] Studies have pointed out the increased caesarean section rate (up to 30% in some teaching hospitals).[95-103] Guillemin has summarized the data and raised certain ethical and professional questions about the etiology of the increased resort to caesarean section.[104]

Nurse midwifery care is by definition low-intervention care, with serious attention paid to patient preferences such as position during labor, freedom to walk around while laboring, medication, delivery in side-lying position without stirrups, intact perineum, and so forth. Such ideologies are in abrupt conflict with the increasing medical dependence on technology and procedures taken to control patient experience rather than permit safe choices. Patients increasingly request and, if necessary, demand to have their rights, needs, and choices respected. There is a constant tension in situations in which nurse midwives and physicians practice side by side and where there is competition for "teaching material" for medical students and residents between the nurse-midwives' commitment to patient preference and a natural, normal process and medicine's conviction that there is no such thing as a "no risk patient."[105] Decisions to intervene or not (or in the policy sense, to support invasive intervention or not) are often translated into power conflicts — who's in charge?

It has been suggested that part of the conflict between obstetricians and nurse midwives on the variable of risk in intensive care situations is the simple fact that the physician's style of practice is episodic — he is not always there. The nurse midwife is always there, during labor and delivery and, thus, in a position to have more information about patient status than any number of brief examinations can provide. Continuity of care improves the ability to pick up subtle changes in a patient and keep on top of fetal heart-beat, labor progress, maternal comfort, and patient experience. Yet, as health care professionals, or as a naive society, we are not accustomed to valuing continuity, clinical judgment, or acute observation. Instead, technology is thought to be of highest value, and there is a basic distrust of natural processes.

(On the parenthetical theme that what's past is prologue, it should be noted that it was the invention of the obstetric forceps in 1720, which, being tools, were restricted to use by men, that effectively confined the practice of midwifery to women and midwives, the practice of obstetrics to men and doctors. Before the forceps, midwives had trained "barber surgeons" as they were called. After forceps, possession of the tool — the technology — raised the status of the men physicians and undermined the status of the women midwives.)[106]

A health policy based on quality of care, then, would have to consider the accumulated data on nurse midwifery practice and obstetrics, as well as the increasing tendency to declare *all* childbearing women at risk as new equipment and procedures can be used to define physiological processes more precisely. There are some obstetricians who believe so strongly that pregnancy is a dangerous time and labor and delivery the most dangerous of all, that they have seriously advocated requiring fetal monitoring of all laboring women, delivery in a Level III hospital of all women, and obstetrician attendance at delivery as minimal standards of care. Fortunately, such extravagances are too expensive for a cost-conscious society to afford as well as ineffective without clinical judgment, and questionably necessary with continuity of care and serious attention to patients' rights to decide. Yet, a belief in modern medicine, including misplaced or misused technology is so strong that midwifery care may be thought automatically to be "second class care," so devoid of mystery is it.

Sugarman has pointed out the dangers in the health-planning concept of "regionalization" of maternity services.[107] Regionalization is intended to provide easily accessible intensive and specialized care to the 10% to 15% of maternity and pediatric patients who might require it. Yet health-planning efforts have often thought "centralization" to be the solution, concentrating all maternity and pediatric patients in tertiary care institutions so that the technology can be immediately available, and the bed occupany rate high enough to pay for it. Such a concentration of services inevitably affects the quality of care for patients who are not in need of high-risk monitoring or treatment, because if the technology is there, it will be used.

It can be documented that nurse midwifery care is of high quality (at least as high as conventional obstetric care using traditional obstetric outcome measures.) If it can also be documented that modern obstetric care, including technologic dependence, is contraindicated for the 85% of women having essentially normal childbearing experiences, then is there not a need for more, rather than fewer, nurse midwives, and fewer, rather than more, obstetricians? What is the proper balance of professionals? Of intervention *versus* none? Granting the place of technology and science in improving pregnancy outcome for those women at serious risk, is it possible to formulate a health policy that will not curtail needed scientific and diagnostic development, but will at the same time reward documented quality of noninvasive care?

NURSE–MIDWIFERY AND A HEALTH INSURANCE POLICY

A national health policy that might be based on national health insurance now appears some years off. In time of pressure for cost containment and an antiregulatory national mood, health insurance policy has increasingly been pinned to voluntary competition with the "free market" operating to shape the health care system and control costs.

Until third party reimbursement is available directly for nurse-midwifery services, it will be impossible to determine how or if midwifery may contribute to cost savings. Indeed, lack of direct reimbursement limits consumer choice of service where nurse midwives practice outside the limits of a health care organization.[108] Direct reimbursement is now available to nurse midwives through CHAMPUS, the insurance system for military dependents, and in December 1980, amendments to the Social Security Act were passed to provide for direct reimbursement for care to Medicaid patients. Regulations have not yet been written to implement the latter change in the law. The lack of third party reimbursement for nursing and nurse midwifery has been recognized as a problem by numerous reports, including the GAO report on improving pregnancy outcome, and the GMENAC report referred to earlier.[109, 110]

The courts have taken an interest generally in the ways in which medical service delivery violates antitrust law and restrains trade by requirements that insurance reimbursement be limited to physician-directed systems. One case in Virginia has already been adjudicated with the judgment against Blue Shield of Virginia for restraining the trade of psychologists who provide independent psychotherapy services upheld by the court of appeals.[111] The Federal Trade Commission (FTC) has recently turned to nurse midwifery and the possibility that on occasion, obstetricians act in concert to restrain the practice of midwives. It is possible that a suit alleging restraint of trade by obstetricians against midwives will grow out of a well-publicized Tennessee situation discussed later.[112] A review of actions of the FTC in the medical field to date by one of the commissioners chastised organized medicine and concluded that "it is in the enlightened self-interest of health care professions to accept the basic policies of the anti-trust laws which are deeply rooted in our free-enterprise system."[113] If it is to mean anything, Costilo argues, "Free enterprise means freedom from unreasonable private restraint as well as from governmental restraint."[114]

Congress has been gearing up to consider proposals for health care cost containment for several years. For the purpose of this chapter, it is not necessary to detail all of the various strategies except to make one point: all the proposed strategies to increase competition (and thus decrease cost) are based on insurance plans, whether Health Maintenance Organizations (HMOs), independent practice associations, or health plans of other types. The concern in these plans, and the problem with them, is with the health care dollar that somebody is giving out, whether it is the federal government or private insurers, not with what the dollar is buying, except in the most general terms. Some proposals include the possibility of lower costs for insurance to actuarily defined groups (low-risk pregnant women, for instance).

HMOs have been thought to represent a good hope for decreasing costs and increasing competition with the fee-for-service private practice system. Even when HMOs employ nurse midwives, costs of care may not be curtailed unless visionary management realizes that nurse midwives are marketable. HMOs have had difficult marketing problems and have often chosen to highlight the availability of physicians for care to attract prepaid enrollment.

Some have worried that if they staffed with nurse midwives or nurse practitioners, possible enrollees would not enroll in the insurance plan, feeling that nurses are second class care. Recent experience suggests this is not the case and that, in fact, the availability of nurse midwifery care may increase enrollment.

The largest part of any HMOs costs are not in its own internal personnel, but in the hospitalization coverage that must be supplied with the plan. Nurse midwives, then, may help decrease costs in four ways: (1) by absolute dollar paid to nurse midwives as employees, which is likely to be less than demanded physician salaries; (2) by the noninterventionist practice of nurse midwives, which means fewer high-technology tests ordered for which the plan pays; (3) by the generally decreased hospital stay of nurse midwifery patients; and (4) by the attention paid by nurse midwives to prevention of complications of pregnancy, thus decreasing expenses for tests, treatment, and hospitalization.

The notion that nurse midwives or other nurses in primary care roles might be coins in a tough economic competition is just beginning to penetrate public consciousness. It is an ambivalent experience at best for nurses to think of themselves as "cheaper," yet that is precisely the value of nurse midwives in HMO-type organizations. To the extent that competition in the health care system will become the political rule, nurses are potentially a powerful force, simply by costing less and, thus, decreasing (or not inflating) premiums for prepaid practice plans.

Yet the style of nurse midwifery practice may run counter to certain economic priorities. For example, patients of nurse midwives are likely to have shorter hospital stays, which decreases bed occupancy (a particular problem to smaller hospitals) and increases costs. Nurse midwives may insist on longer visits, which may foster prevention of complications, but increase per visit costs. Nurse midwives use ultrasound and other technologies much less than obstetricians, making the cost of each test higher if there is an excess of equipment in a given area. The attention paid to prevention of complications of pregnancy also means that hospital services may not be required in such numbers if nurse midwives in competitive private practices build up a high volume. Thus, while an insurer might save money, which is in its interest, a hospital might lose money, which is clearly not in its interest. How the community balances these savings and costs with quality of care and consumer choice is an aspect of national health policy as yet not fully developed.

Incentives could be built into any new national health insurance policy to reward institutions that employ or allow the practice of nurse midwives. Such incentives could open the way for nursing specialty groups to receive proper attention for quality of service delivered as well as costs of care. Such massive changes in thinking about how the health insurance dollar should be allocated or accounted will take years, and will be resisted on all sides. Yet, there are indications for optimism even now. To remove nurse midwifery from the economic domination of medicine would go a long way to focus the interprofessional battles that now characterize nurse midwifery's challenge to entrenched authority, and bring the field into direct, rather than indirect economic competition.

BARRIERS TO NURSE-MIDWIFERY PRACTICE

Any discussion of health policy with respect to nurse midwives is incomplete without some attention paid to the barriers that stand in the way of full use of all the available nurse-midwifery manpower. The statistics cited earlier about numbers of nurse midwives and numbers involved in practice should be convincing evidence that despite barriers to practice, nurse midwives have developed in both the size of the group, and the scope of the services over the past decades.

The barriers to nurse midwifery practice come principally from organized medicine. Despite national positions taken by the American College of Obstetrics and Gynecologists (ACOG) in conjunction with ACNM, individual groups of physicians, local medical societies, and others affiliated with these groups have mounted sometimes disastrous campaigns to undercut the practice of nurse midwifery.[115] Congressman Gore and Congresswoman Mikulski held hearings of the Subcommittee on Oversight and Investigations of the Committee on Interstate and Foreign Commerce of the House of Representatives on December 18, 1980. A full day of testimony produced the following reports:

- In Tennessee, the active opposition of a local medical society effectively terminated a private practice of two nurse midwives and one physician. The physician's malpractice insurance was questioned, and no hospital would grant the nurse midwives privileges, even though they were simultaneously faculty of the Vanderbilt School of Nursing in which capacity they worked with and delivered low income pregnant women from the University Hospital Clinic.
- In New Jersey, new regulations were written to govern nurse midwifery that effectively curtail the full scope of nurse-midwifery practice. These regulations, which were fought vociferously by a well organized group of nurse midwives and consumers, were put through by the Board of Medical Examiners and supported by the local branch of ACOG. They specify, among other things, that nurse midwives may cut and repair

episiotomies without physician supervision, but may not repair second degree lacerations (which are clinically the same thing); that nurse midwives may not care for patients under the age of 16 or over 35. In a burst of hostility, the regulations originally specify that women delivering babies out of hospital may not use any drugs for pain relief. Finally, the regulations stipulate the Certified Nurse Midwives may only practice family planning in a physician's office or in a licensed facility, and only if a physician is present in the building, truly an unnecessary practice and one which only raises costs, and duplicates services.

- Also in New Jersey, the state medical society actively opposed the creation of an out-of-hospital birth center run by nurse midwives. The local chapter of ACOG sent letters to all of the obstetricians and gynecologists in the state urging them to "protect the women of today from the risks forgotten by their grandmothers — since the certified nurse-midwives are showing a growing desire to deliver babies out-of-hospitals, and worse yet, they are practicing family planning without a physician present."

- In Bethesda, Maryland, a private practice group of nurse midwives and obstetricians were denied continuation of their hospital privileges despite a 1-yr successful pilot program with no maternal nor infant mortality. The putative reason given was the practice's offering of a choice of home or hospital birth to clients. While the Department of Obstetrics voted to discontinue privileges, the vote was never officially communicated. Nurse midwives were given only 5 minutes to present their program and were not allowed to be present during the discussion or voting.

- Maternity Center Association (MCA) of New York City opened an out-out-hospital birthing center in 1975. MCA has been resisted throughout its short new life by six of the seven university obstetric departments in the City, State Medical Society of New York, and numerous hospitals. The nurse midwives who attend births at MCA still cannot obtain hospital privileges at the hospital used for back-up of the practice.

- Massachusetts resisted a change in state law to permit the practice of nurse midwifery until 1977 when it was finally overturned. Still, obstetricians connected with teaching hospitals in Boston and medical schools have opposed the practice of nurse midwifery in free standing birth centers located near hospitals.*[116]

Many hospitals still require the presence of a physician in the delivery room when nurse midwives are delivering the babies, whether the medical condition of the patient merits the physician's presence or not. One community hospital ambivalently requires physician attendance during the hours of 7:00 AM to 7:00 PM, but after 7:00 PM, physicians are not required to be

* In June 1981, legislation was passed to allow certified nurse midwives to practice in out-of-hospital childbirth centers licensed by the State Department of Health.

present, even though the nurse midwives and their practice are the same throughout the 24-hr day.

Resistance to nurse midwifery takes many forms. In some states, there have been successful efforts to construct practice acts or other laws to constrain nurse midwifery practice. Professional practice privileges are an eternal issue to nurse midwives as hospitals bow to the wishes of obstetricians who have sometimes feared economic competition. Physicians who have affiliated themselves with nurse midwives have been threatened with withdrawal of their practice privileges or increases in their malpractice insurance rates.

There are already indications that the kind of resistance nurse midwives have faced from organized medicine is becoming generalized to nurse practitioners and clinical nurse specialists as well. In June 1981, the AMA House of Delegates adopted several resolutions against "midlevel health practitioners," noted during debate to include nurse practitioners and nurse midwives. One resolution calls for the AMA to "work to eliminate federal funding for training of further numbers of midlevel practitioners." A second resolution calls for the AMA to "recommend to all hospital staffs that admission history and physicals be performed only by physicians" and floor debate indicated that the delegates intend the resolution to be directed against nurses, among others. Finally, a third resolution calls for "elevating the prestige and status of registered nurses who are devoted to direct patient care, particularly bedside care," taken as a direct attack on nurses in expanded roles of all kinds.[117]

Resistance comes from other sources as well. In some instances, nurse midwives have been fought by nurses themselves, either when the involved nurses were acting on behalf of physicians or when they act out of misunderstanding of some issues. Where nurse midwives have sought separate licensure as *midwives*, the state nurses associations have resisted this move, arguing that the practice of midwifery is "covered" under an expanded nurse practice act. Legal arguments aside, it is clear to those who have participated in such arguments that the issue here is but a piece of a larger national nursing issue that pits generalist nurses against specialists and *vice versa*.

Hospital malpractice risk managers are the newest sources of resistance to nurse midwives (or nurses in expanded roles). Some have alleged that nurse midwifery practice (or nurse practitioner practice) will increase the hospital's liability for malpractice risk, a statement that cannot be justified on the basis of data. In the 56 yr of nurse midwifery practice in the United States, there has never been a case of settled malpractice against a nurse midwife. In fact, malpractice insurance companies do not even have a way to calculate experience-based premiums for nurse midwives or institutions that employ them.

The kind of resistance that comes from unknowledgeable consumers seems to be wearing away rapidly. Stories about nurse midwifery are now common in local press, Sunday supplements, women's magazines, and other media. Nurse midwifery has been featured on "Good Morning America," on the Public Broadcasting System, on "30 Minutes" (ABC TV), in *Women's Day* Magazine, and the *Ladies Home Journal*. Word-of-mouth has stimulated public attention to nurse midwifery services, and word-of-mouth quickly works to produce potential patients for services. Consumers of health services of all kinds are increasingly sophisticated and willing to seek out and fight for the kinds of service they desire. Nurse midwifery has developed rather closer alliances with organized consumer groups than nursing specialties and the power of the provider–consumer alliance is notable.

CONCLUSIONS

To arrive at a reasonable understanding of health manpower need, or to define demand for nurse midwives, is beyond the powers of predictive science. What is clear is that traditional notions of manpower prediction will not work in this field. Even clearer is that the automatic assumption that the supply of obstetricians sets the limit on the need for or use of nurse midwives is unfounded. Rather, it might be thought that the supply of nurse midwives might be used as the standard against which manpower needs and quality of care in medical obstetrics might be determined.

On the other hand, nurse midwifery makes a nice test case for thinking about specialist practitioner groups in nursing, for the issues are very much the same. Nurse midwifery has just hit them earlier. For example, it is now accepted that between 70% and 90% of the problems presented to primary care providers in internal medicine, family practice, and pediatrics can be successfully managed by nurse practitioners. This compares favorably with the 85% of pregnancies that are essentially normal. Thus, nurse practitioners are in the same political and professional relationship to their colleague physician groups as are nurse midwives to obstetricians. Yet, nurse midwifery has made rather stronger progress toward professional autonomy, responsibility, accountability, and authority through institutional approval of educational programs, nationally credible certification, and separate licensure.

Similarly, the data on effectiveness of nurse practitioners shows as uniformly as does the outcome data on nurse midwifery that care is as good as, if not better than, comparable physician care. Nurse midwifery is a rather smaller conceptual and methodologic field, however, so the research data are more of a piece.[118] Yet nurse practitioners might take a page from nurse midwifery's book to make more prominent the existing data, and propose additional studies that might serve as a partial base for a national health policy.

Health policy predicting or even theorizing will be incomplete until the possibility is entertained that the American health care system may need to stand on its head and recognize nurses as primary providers. Primary nursing is revolutionizing hospital practice to return the authority for patient care in hospitals to the nurse–patient team.[119, 120] Nurse practitioner primary care and nurse midwifery may do the same in ambulatory settings.

REFERENCES

1 Breckinridge, Mary. *Wide Neighborhoods: A Story of the Frontier Nursing Service.* New York: Harper, 1952.

2 Browne, Helen E. Frontier Nursing Service and its Implications for Other Rural Areas. In *The Midwife in the United States: Report of a Macy Conference.* New York: Josiah Macy, Jr. Foundation, 1968, 75–77.

3 Varney, Helen. *Nurse Midwifery.* Boston: Blackwell Scientific Publications, 1980, 17.

4 American College of Nurse Midwives (ACNM). "What is a Nurse-Midwife?" (Pamphlet). Washington, D.C.: American College of Nurse Midwives, 1980.

5 ACNM, *loc. cit.*

6 Burst, Helen V. The American College of Nurse Midwives: A Professional Organization. *Journal of Nurse-Midwifery* 25:1 (January-February, 1980), 4–6.

7 Varney, *ibid.*, 21.

8 Varney, *ibid.*, 22.

9 Varney, *ibid.*, 28–29.

10 ACNM Statement of Qualifications, Standards and Functions. In Varney, *ibid.*, 28–30.

11 Varney, *ibid.*, 19.

12 ACNM-Approved Basic Education in Nurse-Midwifery. *Journal of Nurse-Midwifery* 25:5 (September-October, 1980), 20.

13 Hemschemeyer, Hattie. Sends Message to Members. *Bulletin American College of Nurse Midwifery* 1:2 (1965), 5.

14 Patterns of Legislation and Actual Practice of Nurse-Midwifery in the United States. *Journal of Nurse-Midwifery* 25:4 (July-August, 1980), 19–20.

15 American College of Nurse Midwives. *Nurse-Midwifery in the United States: 1976–1977.* Washington, D.C.: American College of Nurse Midwives, 1978.

16 Rooks, Judith B. and Susan H. Fischman. American Nurse-Midwifery Practice in 1976–1977: Reflections of 50 Years of Growth and Development. *American Journal of Public Health* 70:9 (September, 1980), 990–996.

17 Varney, *ibid.*, 24.

18 ACNM, 1980, *ibid.*, 1.

19 Varney, *ibid.*, 7.

20 Reinhardt, Uwe. Nursing Personnel in the Context of Health Manpower Policy. In Millman, Michael (Ed.) *Nursing Personnel and the Changing Health Care System.* Cambridge: Ballinger, 1978, 15.

21   Meglen, Marie. A Prototype of Health Services for Quality of Life in a Rural County. *Bulletin of Nurse-Midwifery* 17:4 (November 1972), 103–113.

22   Murdaugh, Sr. Angela. Experiences of a New Migrant Health Clinic. *Women and Health* 1:6 (November-December, 1976), 25–28.

23   Levy, Barry S., Frederick S. Wilkinson and William M. Marine. Reducing Neonatal Mortality Rates with Nurse-Midwives. *American Journal of Obstetrics and Gynecology* 109:1 (January 1, 1971), 51–58.

24   Reid, Michael L. and Jeffrey B. Morris. Perinatal Care and Cost Effectiveness: Changes in Health Expenditures and Birth Outcomes Following the Establishment of a Nurse-Midwife Program. *Medical Care* 17:5 (May, 1979), 491–500.

25   Lubic, Ruth Watson. The Maternity Center Association's Childbearing Center. *Journal of Reproductive Medicine* 19 (1977), 294.

26   Meglen, Marie and Helen V. Burst. Nurse-Midwives Make a Difference. *Nursing Outlook* 22:6 (June, 1974), 386–389.

27   Thiede, Henry A. A Presumptious Experiment in Rural Maternal and Child Health Care. *American Journal of Obstetrics and Gynecology* 111:5 (November 1, 1971), 736–742.

28   Dillon, Thomas F., Barbara Brennan, John F. Dwyer, Abraham Risk, Alan Sear, Lynne Dawson and Raymond Vande Wiele. Midwifery, 1977. *American Journal of Obstetrics and Gynecology* 103:8 (April 15, 1978), 917–926.

29   Diers, Donna. Nurse-Midwifery as a System of Care: Provider Process and Patient Outcome. In Aiken, Linda (Ed.) *Health Policy and Nursing Practice.* New York: McGraw-Hill, 1981, 73–89.

30   Hellman, L.M. Nurse-midwifery in the United States. *Obstetrics and Gynecology* 30:6 (June, 1967), 883.

31   Graduate Medical Education National Advisory Committee. *Report to the Secretary, Department of Health and Human Services. Vol. VI: Nonphysician Health Care Provider Technical Panel.* Washington, D.C.: U.S. Department of Health and Human Services (Pub. No. HRA 81-656), September 30, 1980.

32   GMENAC, *ibid.,* 28.

33   GMENAC, *ibid.,* 6.

34   Slome, Charles, H. Wetherbee, M. Daly, K. Christensen, M. Meglen and H. Thiede. Effectiveness of Certified Nurse-Midwives. *American Journal of Obstetrics and Gynecology* 124:2 (January 15, 1976), 177–182.

35   Diers, Donna and Susan Molde. Some Conceptual and Methodological Issues in Nurse Practitioner Research *Research in Nursing and Health* 2:2 (June, 1979), 73–84.

36   GMENAC, *ibid.,* 27.

37   Helmer, O. *The Systematic Use of Expert Judgment in Operations Research.* Santa Monica: The RAND Corporation, 1963.

38   Helmer, O. and E.S. Quade. *An Approach to the Study of a Developing Economy by Operational Gaming.* Santa Monica: The RAND Corporation, 1963.

39   Kraus, Nancy. What Happens to CNM's if There Are Too Many Obstetricians in 1990? (editorial). *Journal of Nurse-Midwifery* 26:2 (March-April, 1981), 1–4.

40   Kraus, *ibid.,* 2.

41   GMENAC, *ibid.,* 25.

42   Langwell, Kathryn, Stephen Wilson, Robert Deane, Robert Black and Kwaifong Chui. Geographic Distribution of Certified Nurse-Midwives. *Journal of Nurse-Midwifery* 25:6 (November-December, 1980), 3–11.

43   Langwell, *et al.*, *ibid.*, 9.

44   Reid and Morris, *ibid.*

45   Meglen and Burst, *ibid.*

46   Slome, *et al.*, *ibid.*

47   Corbett, Margaret Ann and Helen V. Burst. Nurse-Midwives and Adolescents: the South Carolina Experience. *Journal of Nurse-Midwifery* 21:4 (Winter, 1976), 13–17.

48   Diers, *ibid.*

49   Olsen, Lois. Portrait of Nurse-Midwifery Patients in a Private Practice. *Journal of Nurse-Midwifery* 24:4 (July-August, 1979), 10–17.

50   Norton, Sheila. Nurse-Midwifery Private Practice as a System of Care. Unpublished Master's Thesis. New Haven, Connecticut: Yale University School of Nursing, May, 1981.

51   Chen, S.P., V.H. Barkauskas, V.M. Ohlson and E.H. Chen. Documented Clinical Experiences of Primary Care R.N. Students: A Preliminary Report. *Nursing Research* 26:3 (September-October, 1977), 342–348.

52   Schulman, John and Carol Wood. Experiences of a Nurse Practitioner in a General Medical Clinic. *Journal of the American Medical Association* 219:11 (March 13, 1972), 1453–1461.

53   Meglen, *ibid.*

54   Meglen and Burst, *ibid.*

55   Corbett and Burst, *ibid.*

56   Chappell, J. and P.A. Drogos. Evaluation of Infant Health Care by a Nurse Practitioner. *Pediatrics* 49:6 (June, 1972), 871–877.

57   Slavinsky, Ann and Judith B. Krauss. Mutual Withdrawal . . . or Gwen Tudor Will Revisited. *Perspectives in Psychiatric Care* 18:5 (September-October, 1980), 194–203.

58   General Accounting Office Report to the Congress. *Better Management and More Resources Needed to Strengthen Federal Efforts to Improve Pregnancy Outcome.* January 21, 1980.

59   Arms, Suzanne. *Immaculate Deception – A New Look at Women and Childbirth in America.* Boston: Houghton Mifflin, 1975.

60   Corea, Gena. *The Hidden Malpractice: How American Medicine Mistreats Women.* New York: Jore Publications (Harcourt, Brace, Jovanovich), 1977.

61   Norton, *ibid.*

62   Dillon, *et al.*, *ibid.*

63   Brennan, Barbara and Joan R. Heilman. *The Complete Book of Midwifery.* New York: Dutton, 1977, 40–46.

64   Rising, Sharon. The Consumer-Professional Balance. *Journal of Nurse-Midwifery* 21:3 (Fall, 1976), 25–27.

65   Levy, Wilkinson and Marine, *ibid.*

66   Meglen and Burst, *ibid.*

67   Ernst, Eunice M. and Karen A. Gordon. 53 Years of Home Birth Experience at the Frontier Nursing Service, Kentucky: 1925–1978. In Stewart, David and Lee Stewart (Eds.) *Compulsory Hospitalization: Freedom of Choice in Childbirth*, Vol. II. Marble Hill, Missouri: NAPSAC Reproductions, 1979, 505–516, 512.

68   Murdaugh, *ibid.*

69   Lang, Dorothea. What is the Future for Certified Nurse-Midwives? In Hospi-

tals? Childbearing Centers? Homebirths? In Stewart, Lee and David Stewart (Eds.) *21st Century Obstetrics Now* (2nd Ed.), Vol. I. Marble Hill, Missouri: NAPSAC Reproductions, 1978, 89–104, 91.

70 Stewart, David. Skillful Midwifery: The Highest and Safest Standard. In Stewart, David (Ed.) *The Five Standards for Safe Childbearing*. Marble Hill, Missouri: NAPSAC Reproductions, 1981, 111–154, 119.

71 Reid and Morris, *ibid.*

72 Haire, Doris. Improving the Outcome of Pregnancy Through Increased Utilization of Midwives. *Journal of Nurse-Midwifery* 26:1 (January-February, 1981), 5–8.

73 Runnerstrom, Lillian. The Effectiveness of Nurse-Midwifery in a Supervised Hospital Environment. *Bulletin of the American College of Nurse Midwives* 14 (1969), 40–52.

74 Slome, *et al., ibid.*

75 Corbett and Burst, *ibid.*

76 Dillon, *et al., ibid.*

77 Diers, *ibid.*

78 Miller, C. Arden. Testimony to the Subcommittee on Oversight and Investigation of the Interstate and Foreign Commerce Committee, U.S. House of Representatives. Washington, D.C., December 18, 1980, 139.

79 Rooks, Judith, RN, MPH, CNM. Testimony to the Subcommittee on Oversight and Investigation of the Interstate and Foreign Commerce Committee, U.S. House of Reperesentatives. Washington, D.C., December 18, 1980, 153.

80 Shenker, Lewis. Clinical Experiences with Fetal Heart Rate Monitoring of One Thousand Patients in Labor. *American Journal of Obstetrics and Gynecology* 115:8 (April 15, 1973), 1111–1116.

81 Goodlin, Robert C. and Hanns C. Haesslein. When is it Fetal Distress? *American Journal of Obstetrics and Gynecology* 128:4 (June 15, 1977), 440–447.

82 Chan, Wan H., Richard H. Paul and Judy Toews. Intrapartum Fetal Monitoring: Maternal and Fetal Morbidity and Perinatal Mortality. *Obstetrics and Gynecology* 41:1 (January, 1973), 7–13.

83 Starkman, Monica, N. Fetal Monitoring – Psychologic Consequences and Management Recommendations. *Obstetrics and Gynecology* 50:4 (October, 1977), 500–504.

84 Haverkamp, A., Thompson, H., McFee, J. and Cetrulo, C. The Evaluation of Continuous Fetal Heart Rate Monitoring in High Risk Pregnancy. *American Journal of Obstetrics and Gynecology* 125:3 (June 1, 1976), 310–320.

85 Varney, *ibid.*, 195.

86 American Academy of Pediatrics Committee on Drugs. Effect of Medication During Labor and Delivery on Infant Outcome. *Pediatrics* 62:3 (September, 1978), 402–403.

87 Whitley, Nancy and Esther Mack. Are Enemas Justified for Women in Labor? *American Journal of Nursing* 80:7 (July, 1980), 1339.

88 Carr, Katherine C. Obstetric Practices which Protect Against Neonatal Morbidity: Focus on Maternal Position in Labor and Birth. *Birth and the Family Journal*, 7:4 (Winter, 1980), 249–254.

89 Stratmeyer, M.E. Research in Ultrasound Bioeffects: A Public Health View. *Birth and the Family Journal* 7:2 (Summer, 1980), 92–100.

90 Caldeyro-Barcia, Roberto. The Influence of Maternal Position on Time of

Spontaneous Rupture of the Membranes, Progress of Labor, and Fetal Head Compression. *Birth and the Family Journal* 6:1 (Spring, 1979), 7–15.

91   Shearer, Madeleine. FDA Action on the Brackbill-Broman Report on Long-Term Effects of Obstetric Medication: Implications for Informed Consent. *Birth and the Family Journal* 6:2 (Summer, 1979), 119–124.

92   Anderson, Sandra F. Childbirth as a Pathological Process: An American Perspective. *MCN – The American Journal of Maternal Child Nursing* 2:4 (July-August, 1977), 240–244.

93   Cogan, Rosemary and Evelyn Edmunds. The Unkindest Cut? *Journal of Nurse-Midwifery* 23:2 (Spring-Summer, 1978), 17–21.

94   Fischer, Shirley R. Factors Associated with the Occurrence of Perineal Lacerations. *Journal of Nurse-Midwifery* 24:1 (January-February 1979), 18–26.

95   Placek, Paul, and Selma Taffel. Trends in Ceasarean Section Rates in the United States, 1970–1978. *Public Health Reports*, 95:6 (November-December, 1980), 540–548.

96   *Evaluating Benefits and Risks of Obstetric Practices – More Coordinated Federal and Private Efforts Needed.* Washington, D.C.: General Accounting Office, 1979.

97   Marieskind, Helen I. *An Evaluation of Ceasarean Section in the United States.* Washington, D.C.: US DHEW, Planning and Evaluation/Health, 1979.

98   Rosen, M. *Consensus Development Conference on Caesarean Childbirth, Draft Report of the Task Force on Caesarean Childbirth.* Washington, D.C.: US DHHS, 1980.

99   Flaksman, Richard, John Vollman and D. Gary Benfield. Iatrogenic Prematurity Due to Elective Termination of the Uncomplicated Pregnancy: A Major Perinatal Health Care Problem. *American Journal of Obstetrics and Gynecology* 132:8 (December 15, 1978), 885–888.

100 Mann, Leon and Janice Gallant. Modern Indications for Cesarean Section. *American Journa of Obstetrics and Gynecology* 135:4 (October 15, 1979), 437–441.

101 Donowitz, Leigh and Richard P. Wenzel. Endometritis Following Cesarean Section. *American Journal of Obstetrics and Gynecology* 137:4 (June 15, 1980), 467–469.

102 Ledger, William J. Aftermath of a Cesarean. *Hospital Practice* (September, 1978), 41–43.

103 Bottoms, Sidney, Mortimer Rosen, and Robert Sokol. The Increase in Caesarean Birth Rate. *New England Journal of Medicine* 302:10 (March 6, 1980), 559–563.

104 Guillemin, Jeanne. Babies by Caesarean: Who Chooses, Who Controls? *Hastings Center Report* 11:3 (June, 1981), 15–18.

105 Dillon, *et al., ibid.*

106 Ehrenreich, Barbara and Deirdre English. *Witches, Midwives and Nurses – A History of Women Healers.* Old Westbury, New York: The Feminist Press, 1973.

107 Sugarman, Muriel. Toward *Really* Improving the Outcome of Pregnancy. *Birth and the Family Journal* 6:2 (Summer, 1979), 109–118.

108 Hackley, Barbara K. Independent Reimbursement from Third-Party Payors to Nurse-Midwives. *Journal of Nurse-Midwifery* 26:3 (May-June, 1981), 15–23.

109 General Accounting Office Report, *ibid.*

110 GMENAC Report, *ibid.*, 45–47.

111 Virginia Academy of Clinical Psychologists vs. Blue Shield of Virginia (6/16/80). Cited in *U.S. Law Week* 49:1 (July 1, 1980), 2001.

112   McCarty, Patricia. Nurse Midwives Forced Out of Practice. *American Nurse* 13:2 (February, 1981), 1.

113   Costilo, L. Barry. Competition Policy and the Medical Profession. *New England Journal of Medicine* 304:18 (April 30, 1981), 1099–1102.

114   Costilo, *ibid.*, 1102.

115   Joint Statement of the American College of Nurse Midwives and the American College of Obstetricians and Gynecologists, and Supplementary Statement. See Varney, *ibid.*, 27–28.

116   Subcommittee on Oversight and Investigations, *ibid.*

117   AMA: Cut Federal Funds for Advanced Nurse Ttraining. *Health Planning Report* (Newsletter of the American Health Planning Association) (June 17, 1981), 8–9.

118   Diers and Molde, *ibid.*

119   Manthey, Marie. *Primary Nursing.* St. Louis: Mosby, 1980.

120   Marram, Gwen, M.W. Barrett and Em O. Bevis. *Primary Nursing* (2nd ed.). St. Louis: Mosby, 1979.

LAUREN LeROY

16

THE COST-EFFECTIVENESS OF NURSE PRACTITIONERS

During the mid-1960s, amid widespread concern over a perceived physician shortage, the concept emerged of using nonphysician health professionals to provide medical services traditionally provided only by physicians. The use of these new groups of providers was seen as a way to increase the availability of health care services, particularly primary care. Nurse practitioners constitute the largest single category of these nonphysician health professionals. Accounting for the variation in training, legal requirements, and actual practice experiences of nurse practitioners, the Graduate Medical Education National Advisory Committee (GMENAC) broadly defined the nurse practitioner role as follows:

> Nurse practitioners (NPs) are registered nurses who have formal training which prepares them to have an expanded role and level of responsibility in the provision of primary health care. Their functions may include health status assessment, physical examinations, formulation of a care plan, counseling, management, referral, and coordination. Training is typically provided in a specialty area such as family practice, pediatrics, adult, or obstetrics-gynecology.
> The nursing profession has traditionally been regarded as having an independent sphere of practice, owing to its unique body of nursing knowledge. Some nurses are currently engaged in independent practice, where they may provide nursing services such as teaching and counseling, home nursing, injection of medications prescribed by a physician, and blood pressure readings.[1]

By the end of 1979, roughly 16,000 nurse practitioners had graduated from formal training programs.[2] Although there is no single data source on specialty distribution, GMENAC developed the following estimates:

Table 16-1. Nurse Practitioner Specialties

Specialty	Percent of All NPs
Family	30
Pediatrics	25
Adult	20
Maternity	10
Midwifery	10
Psychiatry and Other	5

Almost all nurse practitioners, therefore, are primary care providers.

Demand for nurse practitioner training is high, as reflected by the current high proportion of applicants to available training positions.[3, 4] At the same time, budgetary constraints and concern about the physician surplus may diminish future training opportunities. Assuming continuation of existing trends, however, GMENAC estimates the supply of nurse practitioners to be about 39,000 by 1990.[5] By comparison, the number of physicians is expected to rise from 374,800 in 1978 to 535,750 by 1990.[6] This increase is more than four times the total number of nurse practitioners projected for 1990.

COST EFFECTIVENESS ANALYSIS

Encouragement of nurse practitioners as an innovation in the delivery of primary care services is based on their potential to improve access and to lower costs without compromising quality. This promise derives from several basic assumptions, such as the following:

- Nurse practitioners can perform basic and routine medical care tasks traditionally performed by physicians.
- Physicians working in concert with nurse practitioners will thus be free to focus on more serious and more complex medical care problems.
- Training costs for nurse practitioners are cheaper than for physicians.
- Lower costs associated with nurse practitioner services will result in lower prices for the services provided.
- Improved access resulting from the addition of nurse practitioners to the health care team will increase the frequency of early detection of disease and thus reduce medical care expenditures.[7]

A number of issues, however, concerning appropriate training, task delegation, performance quality, physician and consumer acceptance, costs, productivity, and barriers to practice have constrained realization of this potential. The importance of these issues is illustrated by their dominance in published research. Only in the last few years have questions of cost-effectiveness become the focus for analysis.[8-10]

To conduct a cost-effectiveness analysis, one must be able to identify and compare alternative ways of doing the same thing. Because nurse practitioners and physicians are not interchangeable, assessing the cost-effectiveness of nurse practitioners must focus only on those medical tasks that both they and physicians can provide, excluding the additional, complementary services they provide as part of their role as nursing professionals. Given both the inadequacies of available data and the importance of complementary functions for understanding the full potential role they could play in the health care system, the scope of this paper is broader than a strict cost–effectiveness analysis.

Assessment of the cost-effectiveness of nurse practitioners must account for, at a minimum, the specific services they are qualified to provide, performance quality, productivity, task delegation experience, changes in physician practice behavior after the introduction of nurse practitioners, employment costs, impact on average expenses per patient visit, training costs, price effects, and revenue generation ability. The discussion that follows examines each of these factors. Both the analysis and conclusions drawn from it reflect the limitations of available data. While there exists a rather extensive body of literature on nurse practitioner practice, Schweitzer notes some general problems that appear consistently in the studies: narrowness of site coverage, lack of comprehensiveness of variables considered, and weakness of research design.[11] Studies often focus on a single site or small nonrandom groups of sites. A number of studies focus on nurse practitioners shortly after entering practice, thus ignoring issues related to retention and maturity. The impact of factors unique to particular types of practice settings and the sensitivity of the analysis to modest changes in key variables often do not receive adequate attention. Finally, from the perspective of cost-effectiveness analysis, perhaps the most serious problem is the dearth of information specifically defining what medical care tasks nurse practitioners are qualified to perform. Without this data, comparative analysis between them and physicians is limited.

On the basis on available data, it appears that nurse practitioners do alter the production of medical services in a manner that can improve access and reduce production costs. At the same time, a reduction in the price of medical care services or in overall medical expenditures from the introduction of nurse practitioners appears to be a less likely result. Without a reduction in price that reflects lower costs, the financial benefits derived from the cost-effective attributes of nurse practitioners accrue primarily to the physician or to the employing institution. This is similar to the experience with many new advances in medicine that are cost saving. Under these circumstances, benefits to the consumer come primarily when the introduction of nurse practitioners results in improved access.

SERVICES PROVIDED BY NURSE PRACTITIONERS

In order to determine the cost-effectiveness of nurse practitioners, it is necessary to know what they are qualified to provide and whether those services are substitutive or complementary to those provided by physicians. This key question is one on which available data are clearly inadequate. Most studies refer to services provided by or delegated to nurse practitioners in terms of office visits rather than definitive tasks. They describe services they are performing rather than those they are qualified to perform.[12] Instead of specific tasks, studies are more likely to categorize services generally into those physician services that nurse practitioners either can or cannot provide safely.

There are some studies that attempt to define areas of medical practice or diagnoses managed by nurse practitioners. While the study samples are often very small, their findings, accompanied by more general conclusions drawn from the bulk of available research, suggest several patterns as follows:

- Physicians and nurse practitioners have both a complementary and substitutive relationship.[13]
- Nurse practitioners are capable of safely providing a high percentage of primary medical care services.[14]
- Studies that document current performance reveal that the practice setting is the major determinant of services provided by nurse practitioners.[15, 16]

According to Coulehan and Sheedy, the medical practice of a nurse practitioner trained in diagnosis and treatment of general medical conditions includes wellness care, stable chronic disease (hypertension, diabetes, obesity, arteriosclerotic heart disease, arthritis, chronic depression, psychophysiological reactions), and acute self-limited conditions (colds, sore throats, acute viral syndrome, minor trauma, rashes, skin infection). Of the 15 most common diagnoses for the study sample, nurse practitioners handled 50% or more of the following conditions: upper respiratory infections, otitis media, soft tissue trauma, and gonorrhea. They managed one-third to one-half of patients with muscle or back strain, dermatitis or eczema, hypertension, diabetes, obesity, and urinary tract infection.[17] Again, it must be noted that these reflect services the nurse practitioners provided within the constraints of the practice setting, not necessarily the range of services they were qualified to provide.

In terms of specific tasks, the limited available data indicate that nurse practitioners can perform medical functions basic to primary care, such as taking medical histories, performing routine physical examinations, carrying out simple diagnostic procedures, ordering routine laboratory tests, and interpreting their results. Nurse practitioners can administer injections, apply dressings, casts, and splints, and can perform life-saving measures in emergency situations. Restrictions on drug prescribing is an issue being reviewed by a number of states. Current constraints on drug prescription represent one of the most sensitive unresolved issues regarding tasks allowed to be performed by nurse practitioners, both because of the integral role of prescribing in medical care and the implications of such constraints for professional independence.[18]

PERFORMANCE QUALITY

The quality of services provided by nurse practitioners is crucial to their acceptance by both physicians and patients. Indeed, this issue has been studied more than any other. Evaluations of nurse practitioner services repeatedly confirm their high quality.[19-23] The quality of medical care services provided by nurse practitioners is at least comparable to the quality of services provided by physicians. Furthermore, in some cases, nurse practitioners following protocols have shown performance superior to physicians in symptom relief, diagnostic accuracy, and patient satisfaction.[24]

In its study of the federal Physician Extender Reimbursement Experiment, System Sciences, Inc., used nationally recognized disease treatment protocols to evaluate the quality of care provided to patients by physician–physician extender teams and by physicians only. The results favored the teams and also revealed higher quality ratings for physican–nurse practitioner teams than for any other group.[25]

PRODUCTIVITY

It is difficult to measure productivity in strictly economic terms when applied to health manpower. Because inputs and outputs of the medical care production process are difficult to define and measure, it is common to develop proxy measures for what actually occurs when patient and health professional come together. The output most commonly associated with health professional services is defined in terms of patient visits. Productivity of physicians and nurse practitioners usually is measured by the number of patient visits per unit of time. Holmes and associates noted the inability of this measure to reflect either the complexity or the volume of services provided during a patient visit, or the relative contributions made to patient care when more than one professional is involved.[26]

While there is little doubt that the efficient use of nurse practitioners can improve the productivity of the delivery of medical services, it is essential to distinguish between potential impact and actual experience. As Reinhardt points out, determination of physician productivity must account for both technical feasibility in the production process and the probable economic behavior of the physician. One needs to know not only what is technically feasible but also what combination of inputs physicians are likely to choose and to what extent physicians will attempt to maximize the output that is technically attainable with that combination of inputs.[27] The physician, perhaps in collaboration with the administrator in an organized setting, generally determines how the nurse practitioner will be used as an input in the production of medical services. While the debate continues regarding the independence of nurse practitioners, current reality shows them to be functionally dependent on the physician. Berki defines this relationship as one of "constrained substitutability," with the physician determining most of the constraints.[28]

The extent to which tasks are delegated from physician to nurse practitioner, the amount of time it takes a physician or nurse practitioner to perform the same task, and the impact of the introduction of nurse practitioners on physician behavior are key productivity-related variables in the cost-effectiveness calculation. In a review of 15 studies that used physician office visits as a measure of delegability, Record concluded that between 75% and 80% of adult primary care services and up to 90% of pediatric primary care services could be delegated to new health professionals including nurse practitioners. The purpose of the Record study was to estimate different combinations of physicians and nonphysician professionals that could produce given levels of primary care services. Cost estimates associated with the various configurations revealed potential cost savings in cases with higher assistant participation from one-half to over 1 billion dollars, which amounted to 19% to 49% of total primary care provider costs.[29]

In the Northern California Kaiser–Permanente Medical Care Program, a health maintenance organization (HMO), nurse practitioners conducted a Health Evaluation Service (HES) consisting of automated multiphasic health testing followed by a physical examination and health appraisal. Of the patients who entered the Kaiser system through HES, 74% were managed without physician referral. Of those referred to a physician, two-thirds went to a specialty clinic, thus having the nurse practitioner visit substitute for an initial primary care physician visit. Moreover, pelvic exams conducted through the HES replaced 5,207 visits to the gynecology clinic during the study period.[30]

It is obvious from these and other studies that nurse practitioners can assume a high proportion of primary medical care tasks.[31-34] The studies also

reveal substantial variation among practices, making the translation of specific expectations for task delegation to widespread experience more difficult.
Record outlines a number of factors accounting for that variation, including
type of practice setting, structure and age of practice, provider role strain,
legal and reimbursement constraints, and level of demand.[35]

While nurse practitioners can substitute for physicians in providing
many primary care services, the time they spend in managing a patient visit is
significantly higher than that spent by physicians. Recent research has shown
that nurse practitioners spend up to 65% more time per patient visit and see
60% as many patients per day because of their longer time per visit, a shorter
workday, and more time devoted to patient telephone consultation and administrative activities.

Estimates of increases in the productivity of physician practices that
include nurse practitioners range from 20% to 90%.[38-40] In some cases, these
estimates reflect actual experiences; others are the result of computer simula-
tion models that determine productivity increases based on optimal staffing
patterns for performing medical care tasks. Given that they measure potential
rather than actual experience, the latter generally yield higher estimates. The
greatest productivity increases come when the nurse practitioner has primary
responsibility for a subset of patients and when triage is performed with the
nurse practitioner referring complicated cases "up" to the physician rather
than the physician delegating routine medical problems "down."[41]

In developing its projections of physician requirements, GMENAC estimated the amount of medical care services that could be delegated to
nonphysician health professionals. It adjusted initial estimates downward to
what it considered a feasible level based on assumptions about the future supply and productivity of these professionals. The GMENAC recommendations call for considerable increases in the proportion of medical care
services to be provided by nonphysician health professionals. These
professionals currently provide about 7% of all child medical care.
GMENAC recommends an increase to 15% of the total ambulatory workload in 1990. with nurse practitioners providing 75% of that care. For all
adult medical care, the amount would increase from the current 4% to 12% in
1990, with nurse practitioners providing half of the care.[42]

EMPLOYMENT COSTS

To determine the cost-effectiveness of nurse practitioners, both the amount
of time spent by them to perform a given service and the cost per unit of time
must be compared with that of physicians. Available cost data are limited,

and what data exist often come from studies of small samples that are not comparable. An additional difficulty in comparing costs arises because most physicians are self-employed and compensated for their services on a fee-for-service basis, while virtually all nurse practitioners are salaried.

The basic costs of employing nurse practitioners include salary, fringe benefits, and physician supervision. Available salary figures often combine data for nurse practitioners and physicians' assistants. The average salary of nurse practitioners was estimated in 1978 to be about $13,800.[43] Using 1975 data, the Congressional Budget Office (CBO) determined that median hourly earnings of nurse practitioners and physicians' assistants was about $6.00 as compared with $24.00 for physicians.[44]

The amount of time reported for physician supervision and consultation varies considerably among practices. Within a given practice, variation in consulting time is a function of the reason for the consultation, whether the physician sees the patient or only confers with the nurse practitioner, and the practice experience of the latter. The actual time per consultation ranges from less than 1 min to approximately 8 min.

In its review of available studies, the CBO determined that supervision and consultation of nurse practitioners and physicians' assistants require between 10% and 20% of physician time. With CBO estimates of hourly earnings, this adds between $3.00 and $5.00 to the nurse practitioners' and physicians' assistants hourly salary cost.[45]

It should be recognized that the salary level of nurse practitioners is in part a function of the demand for their services. As Berki points out, with some caveats, demand for physician primary care services can be considered a direct demand expressed by the patient. The physician, however, must "initiate," "express," and "legitimate" the demand for nurse practitioners, therefore making this a derived demand.[46] Goldfarb finds that the factors that depress wages of physician extenders are stronger than those that raise them, resulting in a prevailing wage level that bears little relationship to productivity and, on average, leaves them underpaid.[47]

The costs associated with nurse practitioner practice go beyond direct compensation and supervision. The need for additional staff support, space, and equipment may accompany the decision to hire a nurse practitioner. Moreover, their style of practice has cost implications. A number of studies have found that nurse practitioners perform more diagnostic tests than do physicians and have different patterns of medication use.[48, 49] Available evidence also suggests that the use of protocols can diminish the tendency toward excess use of diagnostic tests. [50, 51]

In addition to spending more time per patient, nurse practitioners may log more visits per patient in a given time period. Since the salary and supervision costs are significantly lower than for physicians, the increased return visits are not necessarily a problem from the practice's perspective, although they do consume the patient's time. However, as Spector and associates discovered, a disproportionate increase in visits can raise the overall cost per patient beyond the point where the use of nurse practitioners is cost-effective for the practice.[52] Others stress that, in terms of overall medical expenditures, such practice patterns may be cost-effective if they reduce hospitalizations.[53]

When all of these cost factors have been considered, nurse practitioners have been found to perform comparable medical care tasks at a lower total cost than physicians. Lewis and Resnik found this to be true for inpatient and ambulatory services for all patients.[54] In the Kaiser–Permanente Medical Care Program that instituted HES, which is operated by nurse practitioners, entry costs (health appraisal, follow up, and referral) for the HES group were $43.09 as compared to $61.41 for patients using physicians as the point of entry. Costs of overall medical resources used over 12 mo by cohorts of patients with comparable health status were $98.63 for the HES group and $131.18 for the physician group.[55] Studies on private physician practices, while not specifically addressing the cost issue, indicate similar experiences. [56, 57]

AVERAGE EXPENSES PER PATIENT VISIT

Even allowing for supervision costs, nurse practitioners can provide selected services at a lower cost than physicians. This, however, does not necessarily translate into lower average expenses per patient visit, which are a function of total practice expenses and patient volume.[58] A number of studies have documented increases in patient visits in practices using nurse practitioners.[59-61] In discussing this point, the CBO refers to the System Sciences study that showed practice expenses for solo physicians with nurse practitioners or physicians' assistants to be 74% higher than for solo physicians alone. At the same time, patient volume in these practices was 146% higher, resulting in an average expense per patient visit 29% lower than that for solo physicians alone.[62]

While experience has shown that nurse practitioners lower average expenses per patient visit by as much as one-third, the manner in which the physician or institution uses them and the way in which physicians use any time freed through task delegation will determine whether a potential saving is realized. If nurse practitioners are used to provide services complementary to those of the physician rather than substituting for the physician, the potential reduction in average per-visit expenses may be diminished or lost. In such cases, however, the complementary services can imply quality enhancement, a different (and implicitly better) visit for the same cost.

In order to achieve the saving that comes from any efficiencies introduced by the use of nurse practitioners, a practice employing one must either expand its volume of patient visits or maintain its volume and reduce its physician input. The latter option is obviously more feasible in an institutional setting where physicians are hired as salaried employees than in physician office practices where physicians are self-employed and simply would not hire a nurse practitioner in such cases.

If physicians continue to see the same number of patients, nurse practitioners may reduce average per-visit expenses by increasing patient volume sufficiently to more than cover costs accompanying their introduction into the practice. Reduction in physician effort (in terms of patient visits per hours worked), however, may occur for several reasons. Physicians may be seeing patients with more complex problems that demand more time per visit. They may devote more time to hospitalized patients. Some physician time is required for supervision and consultation with the nurse practitioner. And the presence of nurse practitioners may allow physicians to take more leisure time. For whatever reason, if physicians reduce their patient load, the average expense per patient visit increases. At the same time, however, it should be recognized that if the number of patients seen by the physician per day decreases because of more time spent per patient or the delivery of more complex services, the "patient visit" produced becomes a different product that may justify a higher cost.

TRAINING COSTS

Training costs indirectly affect employment costs and the costs to society of nurse practitioners. These costs are important because much of them are publicly subsidized and they may have some influence on salary expectations. Nurse practitioners obviously benefit from public subsidies for their training, just as do other health professionals. They enter the job market with a lower personal investment in training than would have existed without subsidization. This, in turn, means they are seeking a return on an investment that does not reflect the full costs of their training, thus benefiting their employers through lower salary costs.[63]

Training expenditures for nurse practitioners are substantially lower than those for physicians, as shown in Table 16-2. The figures do not include the costs of initial nursing education. At the same time, they also do not reflect costs associated with physician training beyond medical school. Until detailed cost data on training for the specific sets of services both groups can provide are available, only these gross comparisons of training costs are possible.

TABLE 16-2. Net Training Expenditures for Physicians and Nurse Practitioners (NP) Academic Year 1978–1979 (in Dollars Per Student)

	Annual Cost*	Total Cost
Physician		
Mean	14,200	60,700
Range	7,600–20,800	30,200–83,100
Nurse Practitioner		
Mean	12,900	10,300
Range	5,300–31,000	3,000–32,000

* For comparative purposes only. Many NP programs are less than 1-yr long.

Congressional Budget Office: Physician Extenders: Their Current and Future Role in Medical Care Delivery, pp. 27–28. Washington DC: US Government Printing Office, April 1979.

Nurse practitioner programs also are less dependent on federal subsidies than other health professions education programs. This makes the programs potentially less vulnerable to changes in federal training suppport, although it can be assumed that many programs do receive public subsidies at the state level, which also might diminish if federal policy no longer encouraged the training and use of new health professionals.

MEDICAL CARE PRICES

Lower costs associated with nurse practitioners do not necessarily translate into lower prices for their services. Moreover, productivity gains for physicians who employ nurse practitioners may not lead to a reduction in physician fees. Therefore, consumers cannot necessarily expect to benefit from a reduction in average charges in practices with nurse practitioners. Because the market for medical care services does not conform to the competitive model, a reduction in expenses need not be followed by a decline in prices.[64–66]

Few physicians surveyed by the General Accounting Office (GAO) reported any reduction in fees for nurse practitioner services.[67] Moreover, the CBO cautions that use of nurse practitioners to provide complementary services rather than to increase volume could lead to even higher average per-visit charges. Existing data lead to the conclusion that where prices for patient services do decline after introduction of a nurse practitioner, the change is insufficient to lead to more than a modest reduction in average charges per patient visit. The tendency for nurse practitioners to order more diagnostic tests can further increase practice revenues if the tests are performed in the physician's office. In addition, if they assume some of the non-reimbursable physician services (such as telephone consultation, prescription refills), it frees physician time to provide reimbursable services. Therefore, in the majority of cases (no price change or modest price change), the nurse practitioner's income generation potential is enhanced by the fact that additional reimbursable services are being provided and that prices may be excessive in relation to the costs of physician–nurse practitioner practices. Whether their introduction might cause fees to increase less rapidly, thus leading to a relative decline in prices, has not been examined.

There is little reason to expect physicians to charge a lower price for nurse practitioner services or to reduce their fees if the use of nurse practitioners leads to a reduction in physician time required per patient visit. There is no incentive for physicians to do so. Bicknell and colleagues write, "On grounds that they bear ultimate responsibility, most U.S. physicians employing assistants expect to continue receiving their customary fees from all patients, including those examined and treated by the assistant. The result betrays the promise of primary care assistants. Instead of bringing a reasonable dimension to primary care costs, inadvertently the assistants may maximize the worst in the fee-for-service system."[68]

With current physician pricing behavior, nurse practitioners are not only a cost-effective addition to physician practices, but often a profitable investment for the physician. Nurse practitioners' income generation potential gives the physicians more flexibility in maximizing their combined income and leisure objectives. Alternatively, physicians could choose to increase their incomes by maintaining their previous level of effort and generating even more revenue from an increased volume of patients. This alternative appears to be much more prevalent.[69] Most studies of revenue generation and profitability found higher expenses for practices incorporating nurse practitioners than for physician-only practices, but also found physician–nurse practitioner revenues to be sufficiently higher to show greater profit.[70–74]

The amount of profit realized through the employment of nurse practitioners varies considerably among practices. In a separate study of 26 nurse practitioners in pediatric practices reported by Yankauer and associates, in 1972, average annual gross revenues they generated exceeded their expenses by an average of $2,500.[75] In a study of pediatric nurse practitioners in 1969, Schiff and co-workers found that the nurse practitioner generated net revenues of about $6,000 after 1 yr of practice.[76] Schwartz examined the revenue-generating experiences of three different types of practices in California employing nurse practitioners. He found that the average annual net revenue of a nurse practitioner in rural solo private practice in 1974 was $18,653, resulting in an increase by more than one-third in the employing physician's income.[77] Use of nurse practitioners also can relieve the physician to spend time on more highly remunerative activities such as specialized procedures and inpatient care, thus contributing to higher profits. Even with limited third party reimbursement for assistant services, only one major study cited this as a financial problem for physicians employing nurse practitioners.[78]

From the physician's perspective, nurse practitioners are a cost-effective addition to the practice. That the financial benefits gained from their use are not passed on to consumers is well documented. As noted earlier, the potential increase in income afforded the physician is a major incentive for nurse practitioner employment. Given that income increases are usually the result of expansion in the volume of patient visits, consumers may benefit from improved access to services. While this has been the experience of practices in areas with few available health resources, it is unwise to assume that increased volume, regardless of its character, generally leads to improved access.

Finally, the price effects of nurse practitioner employment in prepaid organized systems should be treated separately. The productivity gains are likely to result in cost savings in such systems. Given that such organizations provide specified services in return for monthly capitation payments, they may choose to expand their scope of benefits or increase physician salaries or leisure rather than to pass the savings to the consumer in the form of reduced premiums. Which action they choose depends on how they assess their competitive advantage over similar practices in the area and standard insurance carriers.[79]

MEDICAL CARE EXPENDITURES

Practices employing nurse practitioners generally see more patients than those without them, increasing volume by as much as 50% to 60%.[80] Prices charged for services in these practices do not differ significantly from physician-only practices even though average per-visit practice expenses tend to be lower. Given current employment and pricing patterns, nurse practitioners do increase medical expenditures beyond what would have occurred without them. Because of their small numbers, their current impact on total expenditures is marginal. If they were slated to play a substantially larger role, with no other changes in the current health services delivery system, their impact on overall medical expenditures would grow.

The increase in medical care expenditures associated with nurse practitioners may be outweighed by the benefits their presence brings through increased access. In a recently reported survey, 57% of physicians who employ nurse practitioners cited the extension of services to more people as the nurse practitioner's major contribution to medical services delivery.[81] Improved access occurs not only from the general increase in volume of patient visits in such practices, but also because nurse practitioners tend to serve more low-income and non-metropolitan patients, who traditionally have had diminished access to physicians.[82] Nurse practitioners in underserved areas can free overextended physicians to focus on complex medical problems and consultant services. At the same time, improved access to primary care services may reduce expenditures for costly specialized services and hospitalization. To the extent that nurse practitioners contribute to the expansion of primary care services, the increase in expenditures accompanying their use could be offset by such savings.

COST-EFFECTIVENESS: ACTUAL OR POTENTIAL?

That individual nurse practitioners can be cost-effective is documented in numerous studies. Generalizing that experience to the total nurse practitioner population and basing future projections on individual experiences are more difficult. Their number is expected to increase by roughly 150% in the next decade, and yet physicians will still outnumber them by 14 to 1.

Given the nature of the United States health care system and realistic expectations for future structural change, it is uncertain how many nurse practitioners will find employment commensurate with their training and whether society will benefit from their cost-effectiveness potential. In their longitudinal study, Sultz and colleagues found that only 50% of those employed functioned purely as nurse practitioners. Others were either performing mixed functions or providing only traditional nursing services. Given their small numbers and current employment experience, the total impact of nurse practitioners, even if beneficial, will be modest.

The structure of the health care system is often cited as the major factor inhibiting nurse practitioners from achieving their full-potential. According to Bicknell and associates, the "hospital-based, specialist-intensive, resource-rich" system is incompatible with primary care practice and resistant to innovations that augment primary care capacity.[83] Patterns of financing that cover the costs of an inefficient delivery process, medical education that discourages delegation of responsibility, and the prominent role of physicians in defining the boundaries of practice for other health professionals inhibit the growth and efficient use of a professional that may encroach on territory traditionally reserved for physicians.

Within the existing structure, incentives to employ nurse practitioners vary according to practice arrangement, physician payment mechanisms, and budget constraints. In general, the financial incentive for physicians in private practice to hire one is diminished because physicians earn high incomes and have not been constrained by competitive market forces to produce services in the most cost-effective manner. On the other hand, employment of nurse practitioners can offer attractive benefits to physicians. They allow physicians to expand their practices both to improve patient access and increase income. They provide the physician an opportunity for more leisure time or a more leisurely work pace. Finally, many physicians who employ nurse practitioners stress their contribution to upgrading the quality and comprehensiveness of care.

The rapid expansion in medical school enrollments and projected increases in physician supply add a new dimension that may overshadow other factors influencing nurse practitioner employment opportunities. Physician supply is growing, and there are thousands more in the educational pipeline who must be absorbed into the system rather than be replaced by new, more cost-effective types of health professionals. Among the effects of this increase in physicians could be a restriction in employment opportunities for nurse practitioners. Some argue that they will fare better than other nonphysician health professionals because of their nursing background and scope of practice.[84] Regardless, there already are signs of physicians, particularly specialists, redefining the scope of their practices in response to diminished numbers of patients requiring their specialized skills. Aiken and co-workers recently concluded, "Despite the current shortage of generalist-physician services, continuing specialist participation in primary care will lead to sufficient generalist medical services by the mid-1980s."[85] Physicians may be recapturing primary care responsibilities that not so long ago they considered delegating. Moreover, it has been suggested that practicing physicians who perceive an oversupply of physicians may hire young physicians to perform the tasks that nurse practitioners perform.[86]

Organized settings, particularly those that operate on fixed budgets (prepaid group practices and some clinics), have a much greater incentive to employ nurse practitioners. It is to their financial advantage to produce services with the most efficient combination of inputs, substituting lower-priced personnel for higher-priced physicians whenever possible. The value such organizations place on nurse practitioners is reflected in the fact that 80% of all nurse practitioners are employed in organized settings.[87] Organized settings have the advantage of greater flexibility in modifying personnel arrangements to gain the benefits from substitution. Beyond fulfilling their objectives for leisure time, physicians in private practice are unlikely to reduce their time inputs to achieve a more efficient operation. Where physicians are salaried employees, however, the efficiency objectives of the employing organization may lead to a reduction in their time, numbers, or income. Future changes in practice arrangements and the preferences of or pressures on new physicians to enter organized practice settings will have an impact on future opportunities for nurse practitioners.

The use of nurse practitioners results in productivity gains and cost reductions. Yet their future participation in medical care delivery is uncertain. Available evidence indicates that their incorporation into organized settings, particularly HMOs, has contributed to more cost-effective service delivery. The experience in private physician practices is less promising. Demand for nurse practitioners in that setting has been limited; while the public benefits from increased availability of services, the cost-effectiveness of nurse practitioners in such settings has not reduced prices. Moreover, since most nurse practitioners are employed in organized settings, employment opportunities are limited by the fact that the majority of physicians practice in the private practice, fee-for-service sector.

Government subsidy of nurse practitioner training has not been accompanied by policies to ensure the promise of these health professionals once in practice. Moreover, policies that may inhibit their use, such as those supporting expansion in physician supply, have been enacted simultaneously with policies encouraging their development. There are changes, short of a national health insurance scheme with incentives to restructure health services delivery, that would facilitate the efficient use of nurse practitioners. Modifications in current reimbursement policies to compensate for their services in a manner that reflects their lower costs would affect prices. It also, however, might reduce opportunities for placement in physician private practices. Opportunities for nurse practitioners to practice more independently (through removal of legal and reimbursement constraints and granting of limited powers to prescribe and dispense drugs) could provide consumers with a lower cost alternative for receiving the primary care services that both they and physicians can provide. The expansion of prepaid group practice and other medical care organizations that operate on fixed budgets would provide more employment opportunities for nurse practitioners in settings that use them more efficiently.

In evaluating the role of nurse practitioners, it is insufficient to assess their cost-effectiveness without also looking at who gains from the savings. Are the financial benefits of lower training and employment costs to be shared with the public or reaped only by employers? Under the current fee-for-service system, are the modest salaries of nurse practitioners exploitative given their income generation capacity? The organization and financing of health services in the United States encourage inefficiency in the delivery of medical care. Reforms that would optimize the efficient use of nurse practitioners have implications for the cost-effectiveness of other components of the system as well. Nurse practitioners can be integrated into the existing system, as they have for the past decade, with perpetuation of existing inefficiencies.

From a public policy perspective, it must be asked whether improved access, resulting from employment of nurse practitioners but unaccompanied by lower prices, is worth the further inflation in medical care expenditures. This is the choice as the system currently functions. Given the overriding concern for containing health care costs, assessment of nurse practitioners should consider not only their performance within the constraints of the current system, but also their potential role in an integrated strategy of reform to meet public policy objectives.

REFERENCES

1 Graduate Medical Education National Advisory Committee. *Report of the Graduate Medical Education National Advisory Committee*, Volume VI: *Nonphysician Health Care Provider Technical Panel*. DHHS Publication No. (HRA) 81–656. Washington, D.C.: U.S. Department of Health and Human Services, 1981.

2 *Ibid.*

3 System Sciences, Inc. *Nurse Practitioner and Physician Assistant Training and Deployment Study: Final Report.* Contract No. HRA–230–75–0198. Bethesda, MD.: System Sciences, Inc., September 1976.

4 Bliss AA and Cohen ED (eds.). *The New Health Professionals.* Germantown, Md.: Aspen Systems Corporation, 1977.

5 Graduate Medical Education National Advisory Committee. *Op. cit.*

6 Graduate Medical Education National Advisory Committee. *Report of the Graduate Medical Education National Advisory Committee*, Volume II: *Modeling, Research, and Data Technical Panel*. DHHS Publication No. (HRA) 81–652. Washington, D.C.: U.S. Department of Health and Human Services, 1981.

7 Congress of the United States, Congressional Budget Office. *Physician Extenders: Their Current and Future Role in Medical Care Delivery.* Washington, D.C.: U.S. Government Printing Office, April 1979.

8 *Ibid.*

9 Record JC (ed.). *Provider Requirements, Cost Savings, and the New Health Practitioner in Primary Care: National Estimates for 1990.* Contract No. 231–77–0077. Washington, D.C.: U.S. Department of Health, Education, and Welfare, 1979.

10 LeRoy L. The Costs and Effectiveness of Nurse Practitioners. In: *The Implications of Cost-Effectiveness Analysis of Medical Technology.* Washington, D.C.: Office of Technology Assessment, July, 1981.

11 Schweitzer SO. The Relative Costs of Physicians and New Health Practitioners. In: *Provider Requirements, Cost Savings, and the New Health Practitioners in Primary Care: National Estimates for 1990.* JC Record (ed.). Washington, D.C.: U.S. Department of Health, Education, and Welfare, 1979.

12 Record JC. *Op. cit.*

13 *Ibid.*

14 *Ibid.*

15 Glen, JK and Goldman J. Strategies for Productivity with Physician Extenders. *Western Journal of Medicine* 124 (1976), 249–257.

16 Lewis CE and Cheyonich TK. Who is a Nurse Practitioner? *Medical Care* 14 (1976), 365.

17 Coulehan JL, and Sheedy S. The Role, Training, and One-Year's Experience of a Medical Nurse Practitioner. *Health Services Reports* 88 (November 1973), 827–833.

18 Congress of the United States. *Op. cit.*

19 Sackett DL, Spitzer WO, Gent M and Roberts RS. The Burlington Randomized Trial of the Nurse Practitioner: Health Outcomes of Patients, *Annals of Internal Medicine* 80 (February 1974), 137–140.

20 Lewis CE, and Resnik BA. Nurse Clinics and Progressive Ambulatory Patient Care, *New England Journal of Medicine* 227 (December 7, 1967), 1236–1241.

21 Komaroff AL, Sawayer K, Flatley M and Browne CM. Nurse Practitioner Management of Common Respiratory and Genitourinary Infections, Using Protocols, *Nursing Research* 25 (March–April 1976), 84–89.

22 Burnip R, Erickson R, Barr GD, Shinefield H and Schoen EJ. Well Child Care by Pediatric Nurse Practitioners in a Large Group Practice, *American Journal of Diseases of Children* 130 (January 1976), 51–55.

23 Lawrence D. Physician Assistants and Nurse Practitioners: Their Impact on Health Care Access, Costs, and Quality. *Health and Medical Care Services Review* 1 (March/April 1978), 1–12.

24 Greenfield S, Komaroff AL, Pass TM, Anderson H, Nessim S. Efficiency and Cost of Primary Care by Nurses and Physician Assistants. *New England Journal of Medicine* 298 (February 9, 1978), 308.

25 System Sciences, Inc. *Survey and Evaluation of the Physician Extender Reimbursement Experiment, Final Report.* Bethesda, Md.: System Sciences, Inc., March 1978.

26 Holmes GC, Livingston G, Bassett R and Mills E. Nurse Clinician Productivity Using a Relative Value Scale, Vol. XII, *Health Services Research* (Fall 1977), 269–283.

27 Reinhardt UE. *Physician Productivity and the Demand for Health Manpower.* Cambridge: Ballinger Publishing Company, 1975.

28 Berki S. The Economics of New Types of Health Personnel. In: *Intermediate-Level Health Practitioners.* V Leppard and E Purcell (eds.). New York: The Josiah Macy, Jr. Foundation, 1973, 110–111.

29 Record JC (ed.). *Op. cit.*

30 Feldman R. Taller SL, Garfield ST, Collen MF, Richart RH, Cella R, and Sender AJ. Nurse Practitioner Multiphasic Health Checkups, *Preventive Medicine* 6 (1977), 301–304.

31 Silver HK, et al. The Pediatric Nurse Practitioner Program: Expanding the Role of the Nurse to Provide Increased Health Care for Children, *Journal of the American Medical Association* 204 (April 22, 1968), 298.

32 Spitzer WO, Sackett DL, Sibley JC, Roberts RS, Gent M, Kergin DJ, Hackett BC and Olynich A. The Burlington Randomized Trial of the Nurse Practitioner *New England Journal of Medicine* 290 (January 31, 1974), 251–256.

33 Coulehan JL and Sheedy S. *Op cit.*

34 Schulman J and Wood C. Experience of a Nurse Practitioner in a General Medical Clinic, *Journal of the American Medical Association* 219 (March 13, 1972), 1453–1461.

35 Record JC (ed.). *Op. Cit.*

36 Division of Research in Medical Education, University of Southern California. *Collection and Processing of Baseline Data for the Physician Extender Reimbursement Study.* Final Report, August 31, 1978.

37   Congress of the United States. *Op. cit.*

38   Golladay F, Miller M and Smith K. Allied Health Manpower Strategies: Estimates of the Potential Gains from Efficient Task Delegation, *Medical Care* 11 (November-December 1973), 457–469, 1973.

39   Holmes GC et al. *Op. cit.*

40   Holmes GC, Livingston G and Mills E. Contribution of a Nurse Clinician to Office Practice Productivity: Comparison of Two Solo Primary Care Practices, *Health Services Research*, (Spring 1976), 21–33.

41   Smith KR. Health Practitioners: Efficient Utilization and the Cost of Health Care. In: *Intermediate Level Health Practitioners.* V Leppard and E Purcell (eds.). New York: The Josiah Macy, Jr. Foundation, 1973, 135–151.

42   Graduate Medical Education National Advisory Committee. Volume VI. *Op. cit.*

43   Wallen J. Delegability. Background paper prepared for the Non-Physician Health Care Provider Work Group of the Graduate Medical Education National Advisory Committee. May 9, 1978.

44   Congress of the United States. *Op. cit.*

45   *Ibid.*

46   Berki S. *Op. cit.*

47   Goldfarb MG. *Economic Aspects of the Use of New Health Practitioners.* New Haven: Yale University School of Medicine, 1974.

48   Congress of the United States. *Op. cit.*

49   Flynn BC. Effectiveness of Nurse Clinicians' Service Delivery, *American Journal of Public Health* 64 (1974), 604–611.

50   Greenfield S, et al. *Op. cit.*

51   Greenfield S, Anderson H, Winickoff RN, Morgan A and Komaroff AL. Nurse-Protocol Management of Low Back Pain: Outcomes, Patient Satisfaction and Efficiency of Primary Care, *Western Jounal of Medicine* 123 (1975), 350–359.

52   Spector R, McGrath P, Alpert J, Cohen P and Aikins H. Medical Care by Nurses in an Internal Medicine Clinic, *Journal of the American Medical Association* 232 (June 23, 1975), 1234–1238.

53   Runyan JW. Medical Care by Nurses, *Journal of the American Medical Association* 234 (December 15, 1975), 1118.

54   Lewis CE and Resnik BA. *Op. cit.*

55   Feldman R, et al. *Op. cit.*

56   Schwartz JL. Economic Feasibility and Patient Diagnostic Mix of Family Nurse Practitioners. *Public Health Reports* 94 (March–April 1979), 148–155.

57   O'Hara–Devereaux M, Dervin JV, Andrus LH and Judson L. Economic Effectiveness of Family Nurse Practitioner Practice in Primary Care in California. In: *The New Health Professionals.* AA Bliss and ED Cohen (eds.). Germantown, Pa.: Aspen Systems Corp., 1977, 161–170.

58   Congress of the United States. *Op. cit.*

59   Holmes GC, Livingston G, Bassett R and Mills E. *Op. cit.*

60   Division of Research in Medical Education. *Op. cit.*

61   System Sciences, Inc. *Survey and Evaluation of the Physician Extender Reimbursement Experiment. Op. cit.*

62   *Ibid.*

63   Goldfarb MG. *Op. cit.*

64   Berki S. *Op. cit.*

65   Smith KR. *Op. cit.*

66   Reinhardt UE. Parkinson's Law and the Demand for Physicians' Services (presented at the Federal Trade Commission Conference on Competition in the Health Care Sector, Washington, D.C., June 1–2, 1977).

67   Comptroller General of the United States. *Progress and Problems in Training and Use of Assistants to Primary Care Physicians.* Washington, D.C.: U.S. General Accounting Office, April 8, 1975.

68   Bicknell WJ, Walsh DC and Tanner MM. Substantial or Decorative? Physicians' Assistants and Nurse Practitioners in the United States. *The Lancet* (November 23, 1974), 1243.

69   Division of Research in Medical Education. *Op. cit.*

70   Yankauer A, Tripp S, Andrews P, et al. The Costs of Training and the Income Generation Potential of Pediatric Nurse Practitioners, *Pediatrics,* 49 (1972), 878–887.

71   Schwartz JL. *Op. cit.*

72   Schiff DW, Fraser CH and Walters HL. The Pediatric Nurse Practitioner in the Office of Pediatricians in Private Practice, *Pediatrics* 44 (July 1969), 62–68.

73   O'Hara-Devereaux, et al. *Op. cit.*

74   Draye MA and Stetson LA. The Nurse Practitioner as an Economic Reality, *Medical Group Management* 22 (1975), 24–27.

75   Yankauer A, et al. *Op. cit.*

76   Schiff DW, et al. *Op. cit.*

77   Schwartz JL. *Op. cit.*

78   Spitzer WO, et al. *Op. cit.*

79   Berki S. *Op. cit.*

80   Congress of the United States. *Op. cit.*

81   Mauksch I. The Nurse Practitioners Movement: Where Does It Go From Here? *American Journal of Public Health* 68 (November 1978), 1074–1075.

82   Sultz HA, Zielezny M and Mathews J. Highlights: Phase 2 of a Longitudinal Study of Nurse Practitioners. In: *Nursing Personnel and the Changing Health Care System,* M Millman (ed.). Cambridge: Ballinger Publishing Co., 1978.

83   Bicknell WH, et al. *Op. cit.*

84   Congress of the United States. *Op. cit.*

85   Aiken LH, Lewis CE, Craig J, Mendenhall RC, Blendon RJ and Rogers DE. The Contribution of Specialists to the Delivery of Primary Care, *New England Journal of Medicine* 300 (June 14, 1979), 1363.

86   Institute of Medicine. *Physicians and New Health Practitioners: Issues for the 1980s.* Washington, D.C.: National Academy of Sciences, May 1979.

87   Congress of the United States. *Op. cit.*

5

FRONTIERS FOR NURSING PRACTICE

Three settings neglected by nursing offer potentially exciting opportunities for professional practice in the 1980s.

Health maintenance organizations (HMOs) will receive increased national attention in the 1980s as the nation struggles to contain the escalating costs of health care. HMOs offer comprehensive health services at a predetermined cost to the consumer. Unlike fee-for-service medical practice, HMOs have every incentive to provide the best care for the lowest cost. Nurses represent a vast, and for the most part, untapped resource for HMOs. Luft, in Chapter 17, provides an overview of the organization, financing, and purposes of HMOs. Barham and Steiger examine the experiences of nurses in the country's oldest and largest HMO, and speculate about nurses' future there and elsewhere.

Like nursing homes, mental health services, particularly for the chronically mentally ill, have been a source of increasing public concern. Over the past three decades, many of the nation's mental hospitals have closed, shifting the locus of care to the community. This transition has not been a smooth one, and many shortfalls exist in the care of the mentally ill. Mechanic, in Chapter 19, examines current mental health services and identifies important roles for nurses that are currently underdeveloped.

Health care of children is an important priority for Americans. The successful treatment of health problems in young children can greatly enhance their chances of living happy and productive lives. Over the past 10 years, a number of projects have successfully demonstrated the value of placing nurses in schools for the early detection and treatment of children's health problems. Schools face major fiscal constraints in the 1980s, and one of the challenges for nursing will be to develop cost effective strategies for providing ongoing health surveillance of children. Oda, in Chapter 20, reviews the progress made in school health services in the seventies and explores strategies to maintain these services in the 1980s.

HAROLD S. LUFT

17

HEALTH MAINTENANCE ORGANIZATIONS: IMPLICATIONS FOR NURSING

Although various types of health maintenance organizations (HMOs) have been in existence for over a half century, there is currently renewed policy interest in promoting HMOs to restructure the medical care system. The primary purpose of such a restructuring is to contain medical care costs while maintaining the quality of medical care. Such HMO growth may have a significant impact on the demand for nursing services. But even though further HMOs growth and development is likely, the precise nature of that development is unpredictable. By reviewing some key aspects of HMO performance, however, it is possible to present some informed speculation about the future. The first section reviews some of the major aspects of HMO performance, especially relating to the use of nurses and other personnel. The second section presents some of the reasons for slow HMO growth in the past, and the third section outlines why their growth in the future is expected to be more rapid. The final section suggests some of the implications increased HMO growth may have for the nursing profession.

CURRENT PERFORMANCE OF HEALTH MAINTENANCE ORGANIZATIONS

An HMO is defined as an organization that assumes a contractual responsibility to provide or ensure the delivery of a stated range of health services, including physician or hospital services, to a voluntarily enrolled population in return for a fixed periodic payment with minimal copayments (or additional charges) related to utilization. The HMO also bears some or all of the risk associated with the provision of services — it does not pass this risk on to an external insurer. This definition is purposely broad to include the wide range of organizations that are generally recognized as HMO and HMO-type plans. The design of an HMO is based upon the view that by making the organization responsible for the delivery of services within a budget limited by the fixed periodic payments or capitation, strong cost-containing incentives are created. These cost-containing incentives are the basis of much of the current policy interest in HMOs.

Although every HMO has certain unique characteristics, it is important to distinguish two rather different HMO models. In the prepaid group practice model, or PGP, physicians and other health professionals practice together and their patients are primarily HMO members.* In a PGP HMO, physicians are typically paid a salary plus some bonus or profit share that depends on their own performance and that of the HMO in general.** The second major type of HMO is the individual practice association, or IPA, in which physicians practice in their own offices with a primarily non-HMO clientele and also have some HMO members for patients. The physician typically bills the HMO on a fee-for-service basis, but part of the fee is withheld. If total HMO costs, including hospital and referral services, are kept within the budget, the withheld fees are returned to the physician; otherwise, they will be used to cover the HMO deficit. Thus, the IPA physician has a financial incentive to contain the use of expensive services.***

The available evidence indicates substantially different styles of performance and effectiveness for the two types of HMOs.[1] Enrollees in PGPs receive their medical care for 10% to 40% lower cost than enrollees in conventional health insurance plans. The lower total expenditures, which includes premium, out-of-pocket cost, and out-of-plan costs, appear to be primarily the result of less hospitalization per HMO member per year. After controlling the age and sex differences among enrolled populations, PGP

---

*Some authors distinguish staff model HMOs, in which all the providers are employees of the HMO from group model HMOs, in which the providers are organized as a legally distinct body that contracts with the HMO to provide medical services. In both instances, however, nurses are likely to be employees.

**Discussions of physician payment schemes are rare in the published literature, and I have never come across any discussion of bonuses for nurses and other personnel, even if they are part of the primary care team. This is not to say, however, that such sharing arrangements do not occur either through official channels or informally.

***The federal government uses a definition of IPA HMOs that is largely based upon the contractual relation between the physicians and the HMO. Some HMOs that function effectively as PGPs are legally constituted as IPAs. This chapter will focus on the stereotypic PGP and IPA as outlined in the preceding paragraphs.

enrollees have about 30% fewer hospital days. While length of stay may be somewhat lower for PGP members, most of the hospitalization differences seems to occur through lower admission rates. Various factors may account for this lower admission rate, including a more conservative practice style by HMO physicians, increased use of "do-not-admit" or outpatient surgery, and greater aversion to hospitalization by PGP enrollees. Although the broader benefit package offered by HMOs results in their members obtaining more preventive medical services, there is little evidence that this explains the lower hospitalization rate. Measures of the process and outcome of treatment also suggest that PGPs are able to maintain low hospitalization rates without adverse effects on the quality of medical care.[2]

At the same time that hospital use is lower for PGP enrollees, the use of ambulatory services is slightly above that of people with conventional coverage. Enrollee satisfaction varies with the question being asked. PGP members are less satisfied than are conventionally covered people with their doctor–patient relationship; they have less continuity with the same provider; and they are dissatisfied with the amount of time it takes to get an appointment. On the other hand, they are far more satisfied with their financial coverage and the amount of time they have to wait in the office once they have an appointment. One measure of how enrollees balance these various aspects is the trends in enrollment among employee groups who have had an HMO option for a decade or more. In almost every instance the HMO market share has increased and in some employee groups a third to a half of the eligible people are PGP members.

Although a few IPAs date back to the early 1950s, their growth is a much more recent phenomenon and there is relatively little evidence on their performance. To date, there are no studies demonstrating lower costs for IPA enrollees. Studies of hospital use by IPA enrollees are mixed, but on average their use is lower than that of people in conventional plans, but not as low as that of PGP enrollees. Enrollees in IPAs experience the same quality of care and express similar patterns of consumer satisfaction as do people with conventional coverage, with the exception that IPA enrollees are more pleased with the financial coverage offered by their plan.

The term "health maintenance organization" suggests an emphasis on health promotion and disease prevention.* If the HMO's enrollees stay healthy, the organization does better financially, in contrast to the situation for fee-for-service providers and hospitals, who are paid for services rendered. While it is true that HMO enrollees receive more preventive checkups, immunizations, and health screenings, this is largely a reflection of their more

---

*The term was coined in the early 1970s for inclusion as part of the Nixon administration's proposals for reshaping the health care system. It was designed as an alternative to "prepaid group practice" and was broadened to encompass the IPA.

comprehensive coverage for such services. Furthermore, HMOs do not particularly seem to be at the forefront of efforts to encourage changes in life-style, although they sometimes actively promote such efforts as part of their programs.

The difference between PGPs and IPAs also have substantial implications for the use of nursing personnel. Rarely does an individual physician contracting with an IPA have more than 15% of his or her patients on a prepaid basis, and even then payment is rendered by the HMO on a fee-for-service basis. As a result, IPA physicians are not likely to change their practice styles substantially except, perhaps, by exercising more stringent controls over hospital use. The PGP HMO has several organizational features that may result in altered roles for nurses. Since the physicians practice in groups, the availability of a large number of patients in a single location may allow certain economies of scale through specialization. For instance, a large group practice may be able to hire nurses to manage patients with specific types of chronic conditions, such as diabetes, hypertension, or arthritis. Staff can be supported full time to specialize in prenatal or postnatal care. Nurses can also handle patient problems over the telephone and serve as triage coordinators. Nurses may also take on active roles in educational, counseling, and rehabilitation services. Primary care practice teams composed of physicians and nurses have been implemented in several PGPs.

These practice innovations in PGPs also occur in fee-for-service practice, but there are several reasons to believe they will be used more extensively in prepaid settings. The fact that the HMO is responsible for the provision of all covered services within a fixed budget creates strong incentives to economize. For instance, telephone triage may alleviate the need for a substantial fraction of patients to see a physician. In fee-for-service practice, handling patient problems on the telephone would mean increased personnel costs but lost office revenue. In a prepaid setting the system may easily pay for itself by allowing the providers to devote more attention to the sicker patients. Prepayment also allows an HMO to pay for certain services that are not covered in conventional plans, such as nutritional or life-style counseling, in anticipation that such programs will reduce the use of more costly medical and hospital services. Such health promotion programs are often led by nursing personnel. Primary care teams allow a physician, in concert with nursing and other personnel, to care for a larger panel of patients. This can be attractive for both fee-for-service and prepaid physicians, but physicians in independent practice with a larger than usual patient load may find it difficult to get others to share on-call arrangements. In a large group setting special arrangements can be made for on-call coverage.

The prepayment aspect of the HMO may also increase patient acceptance of an expanded role for nurses. Some patients paying fee for service may feel that if they are paying full fee, they want to be seen by a physician and not a nurse. In a prepaid system the cash transaction is eliminated and the enrollee is offered treatment by the appropriate provider, be it nurse or physician. In fact, the extra time and attention paid by the nurse to the patient's psychosocial needs may help offset the typical PGP enrollee's dissatisfaction with the physician–patient relationship.

Detailed surveys of the nursing role in various types of HMOs have not been undertaken. While there are quite a few studies of particular HMOs, it is not clear that these are representative of all HMOs or that the patterns are substantially different from those in similarly selected fee-for-service practices. However, the case studies do suggest the potential for important innovations in the role of nurses in HMOs, a point to which we will return.

One national survey of fee-for-service and prepaid group practices offers some insight into current patterns.[3] PGPs tend to use more nonphysician medical personnel (nurses, physician's assistants, nurse practitioners, and technicians) per full-time equivalent physician than do fee-for-service groups. Moreover, physicians in PGPs see fewer patients per week, indicating that for a given number of patient visits, perhaps on the order of one-third more nurses might be required. These figures might suggest that nurses in PGPs have an expanded role in patient care, yet some other data from the same study belie this inference. For instance, among three tasks — taking initial history, taking blood pressure reading, and phoning the results of tests to patients and explaining results — physicians in PGPs were significantly *less* likely than those in fee-for-service groups to delegate the first two tasks to nonphysician personnel. (No difference was observed for the third task.) Furthermore, nurses (registered nurses and licensed practical nurses) perform clerical tasks in 60% of the PGPs in contrast to 41% of the fee-for-service groups and, in those groups that have nurses doing clerical work, the average amount of time is 57% greater in PGPs. These limited data suggest that the case studies may, in fact, not be representative and that speculation on the future impact of HMOs should be treated with caution.

FACTORS LIMITING HEALTH MAINTENANCE ORGANIZATION GROWTH

One may ask why, if HMOs are so good, they still enroll only about 4% of the nation's population? This low market share nationally is the result of several factors that influence the availability of HMOs, on one hand, and the interest people have in enrolling in them, on the other hand.

HMOs are only available in certain parts of the country. In some states, such as California and Hawaii, HMOs enroll over 15% of the population, while other states, such as Nevada, Mississippi, and Vermont, have no

HMOs. This uneven distribution of plans reflects the historical opposition to HMOs from certain segments of the medical profession. Although the American Medical Association (AMA) has officially taken a neutral stand since the late 1950s, some local medical societies still vigorously oppose HMOs. Even without such opposition, HMOs are difficult and expensive to get started. The nonprofit orientation of most HMOs make it extremely difficult to obtain the initial capital required for a PGP. Moreover, there has been a severe shortage of experienced managers who can successfully administer either PGPs or IPAs. In addition, until recently most HMOs were based on a traditional PGP model, which may have been felt to be inappropriate in specific situations. Recently there has been much more innovation in the structure of HMOs, so plans are now developed from existing fee-for-service groups and networks of individual practitioners.

Even where HMOs have been established, they have often not been made available as an option for employee groups. The federal HMO Act now requires all firms with 25 or more employees to offer a qualified HMO as an option if one is available locally. Even without the mandate of the HMO Act, employers have recenly become much more aware of their payments for health insurance benefits and, in some areas, have begun to encourage or even sponsor HMO development. Employers have also begun to restructure their benefits options in ways that encourage employees to choose lower cost options, which are often HMOs. Another factor that has traditionally slowed the growth of PGPs is the resistance most people have had to giving up an existing physician–patient relationship. Thus, much of the growth of most PGPs has come from recent arrivals in an area and this naturally limits their expansion rate. With the development of IPAs and other forms of HMOs that include providers already in practice, more and more people can change their insurance plan to an HMO without changing providers. This can result in markedly higher growth rates. Finally, some people have preferred the one-on-one physician continuity offered by the independent practitioner. As physicians opt increasingly for group practice, long vacations, and reduced on-call time, the practice styles of fee-for-service and PGP physicians may become more similar and lead to greater acceptance of PGPs.

POTENTIAL FOR FUTURE HEALTH MAINTENANCE ORGANIZATION GROWTH

Some of the factors that have retarded HMO growth in the past are no longer major obstacles. More and more people know about HMOs, concern over medical care costs is increasing, and employers, in particular, are looking for alternatives to the existing system. The recent growth in HMOs, in conjunction with new training programs, is beginning to develop a pool of experienced HMO managers. Although federal grants and loans for HMO development are likely to disappear, private sources of funding are beginning to appear through Blue Cross, Blue Shield, commercial insurers, hospitals, and for-profit corporate-based HMOs.

Certain legislative changes on the horizon may have an even greater impact on encouraging HMO growth. Various bills have been introduced in Congress to alter the tax treatment of health insurance fringe benefits with the intent of encouraging consumer senstivity to premium cost differences. Most of these bills would have the effect of enhancing the attractiveness of HMOs to employed persons. Several states are currently actively encouraging their Medicaid beneficiaries to enroll in HMOs. As pressures on state budgets increase and federal support for Medicaid decreases, there is likely to be even more emphasis on HMO–Medicaid programs. Medicare beneficiaries are currently underrepresented in HMOs, partly because of long-standing ties to physicians, but also because existing Medicare rules discourage capitation payments and offer no incentives for beneficiaries to enroll in HMOs. New legislation is pending that offers capitation payments to HMOs and potential addition benefits for the elderly and disabled who join those HMOs that can contain costs.[4]

All these factors suggest continued and increased growth in both the number of HMOs and their total enrollment. More important, however, the next decade is likely to see a substantial increase in innovation by HMOs. This expectation is based upon several factors including the entry of new types of sponsors and organizations, the increased competition for enrollees, reduced regulation of the HMO industry, and increased coverage of higher cost, sicker people. Recent HMO growth has already spawned networks of fee-for-service groups and primary care practitioners. Moreover, as more new people become involved in the design of health care options, new ideas are likely to be tested. Competition in the medical care market is increasing because of legislative pressures for cost containment, an increasing supply of physicians, and a surplus of hospital beds. Federal and state regulation of the specific ways in which an HMO is structured or chooses to deliver services is likely to be reduced so that even more flexibility in organizational design will be possible. An expanded enrollment of Medicare and Medicaid beneficiaries may offer a fertile field for creative ideas concerning the provision of alternatives to expensive hospital and medical services. In particular, HMOs may expand substantially their limited emphasis of home care, hospice, and nursing home services. Most HMOs have focussed on enrolling members of employee groups and their families, much as is the case for conventional insurers. These enrollees tend to be relatively healthy and require primarily traditional medical care. If the Medicare and Medicaid programs are modified to be more attractive to HMOs, the organizations will have to respond to the different needs of a population with more serious and generally chronic health problems.

Until now, the relative lack of innovation in the use of health care personnel in HMOs has partially reflected the desire of existing HMOs to avoid censure by organized medicine. Amid charges that prepayment would result in cut-rate care, skimping, and other nefarious activities, HMO physicians sought to maintain rather traditional practice styles. The extensive substitution of nurses for physicians would surely have been used as damning evidence by the medical establishment. Although no longer vulnerable, these HMOs, like most other organizations, may have found it difficult to change "the way things are done." (Newer HMOs, without this institutional history, can be more innovative.) Finally, substantial cost savings from lower hospital care use may have blunted any further pressures to innovate. However, as the number of HMOs increases and as they begin to compete with each other, and not just with the conventional insurers, there may be additional pressure to adopt a more efficient practice style.

IMPLICATIONS FOR NURSING OF HEALTH MAINTENANCE ORGANIZATION GROWTH

The substantial growth of HMOs may have implications both for the number of nurses demanded by the medical sector and for the types of jobs they will fill. Several models have been developed to estimate the potential impact of HMO growth on the demand for nurses.[5] They indicate that a near quadrupling of HMO enrollment — from 3% to 11% of the population — would reduce the demand for nurses by about 3%, mainly because of lower hospitalization rates. Although it is not worthwhile to belabor the point, even this estimate is likely to overstate the direct effects of HMO growth.*

Let us assume that PGPs reduce hospital use by 20%. (This is somewhat less than the observed differences in order to allow for the selection into PGPs of people who are normally low users of hospital care.) Let x be the number of nurses necessary to provide inpatient care for a population with conventional coverage. Thus, the current situation is $0.03 \cdot 80x + 0.97x =$

---

*Direct effects refer to the change in practice patterns experienced by the HMO enrollees. Indirect effects of substantial HMO growth would include a competitive response by conventional providers to reduce hospital use. Such indirect effects, if they occur, could be of substantially greater importance.

700, where the first term represents the demand by the 3% of the population in PGPs at an 80% use rate, 0.97x represents the rest of the population, and 700 is the approximate number of nurses in thousands. This can be solved for x: $0.994x = 700$, and $x = 704.2$. An increase in HMO enrollment to 11% implies $0.11 \cdot 0.80x + 0.89x = 0.11 \cdot 0.80(704.2) + 0.89(704.2) = 0.987(704.2) = 688.7$ and $688.7/700 = .984$ or a 1.6% decline. Furthermore, even these estimates are generous. The lower hospital use by HMO members almost certainly occurs in those cases that require less than the average amount of nursing — minor surgery, the last few days of medical admissions, diagnostic workups, and the like. Thus, a 20% reduction in hospital days will result in less than a 20% reduction in nursing.

The Congressional Budget Office (CBO) estimates focus primarily on HMO reductions in hospital use, perhaps because ambulatory use by HMO enrollees approximates that of conventionally covered people. While the visit rates are comparable, it does appear that PGPs use more personnel — both physicians and nurses — per visit. The available data are very crude, but they suggest that PGP physicians each use 1.62 nonphysician medical personnel while the average office-based practitioner uses 1.12 such personnel.[7] The latter figure includes 0.31 FTE registered nurses and 0.17 FTE licensed practical nurses. Moreover, office-based practitioners have 90 office visits per week in contrast to 78 for PGP physicians. Combining the effects of more personnel and fewer visits per physician in PGPs, we can estimate that an average PGP might require 0.932 hr of nonphysician medical personnel per visit in contrast to 0.496 hr for all office practitioners, or a 67% increase. If PGPs use a personnel mix similar to that of office practitioners, the 0.932 hr per visit will include 0.230 hr of registered nurse time and 0.126 hr of licensed practical nurse time. Assuming an increase in HMO enrollment from 6 million to 26 million, and that each enrollee makes four visits per year, this implies 80 million additional visits to HMOs rather than to fee-for-service practitioners. This will result in about 5,500 additional registered nurses and about 3,000 additional licensed practical nurses. While a 1.2% increase is not very impressive, it would approximately offset the estimated decline in hospital-based nurses calculated above.

This exercise suggests that even marked increases in HMO enrollment are not likely to have a major impact on the total demand for nurses, although there may be some shifting from inpatient to outpatient work. However, these estimates are based upon current practice patterns and the preceding discussion suggested that the future is likely to bring substantial innovation by HMOs. Some of the innovation may occur in inpatient settings, such as through increased use of nonphysician surgical assistants, nurse anesthetists, and other alternatives to costly physician services. Even more significant changes are likely to occur in the outpatient setting. HMOs will probably increase their reliance on primary care teams, with the nurse often serving as the major provider of care, rather than as an assistant to the physician. Special treatment management programs for patients with chronic illnesses are likely to become more common. Such programs will often be staffed almost entirely by nursing personnel. HMOs have also increased their benefit coverage in certain areas such as mental health, and nurses with psychiatric training are likely to be in high demand. Additional counseling and behavioral change programs have been established by several HMOs in an attempt to foster life-style changes and primary prevention. Specially trained nurse counselors often staff such programs.

The most significant changes in personnel use are likely to result from increased enrollment in HMOs by Medicare and Medicaid beneficiaries. These people tend to have much greater needs for medical care than the employed population, many of their problems are chronic, and in many cases traditional medical intervention is insufficient. HMOs will have clear incentives to emphasize home and hospice care rather than inpatient placement. They may find that early intervention and home visits may be particularly worthwhile among high-risk people. The social support and caring role may be more important for these groups that for the typical middle-class patient.

HMOs are often either praised or criticized for providing different approaches to medical care delivery. It is true that they hospitalize their pateints less frequently and there are numerous case studies of innovative practice patterns. However, this chapter suggests that current patterns of personnel use in HMOs are rather similar to those in conventional fee-for-service practice, and even substantial expansions of the current HMO model will have little noticeable effect on nursing personnel. The implications for nurses of future HMO growth lie in the *potential* for substantial expansion of nursing roles in HMOs and a refocusing of HMO attention on non-acute care medical services. The likely growth in competition among HMOs and between HMOs conventional providers will provide the impetus for such innovation. It will be at least partly up to the nursing profession to help guide those changes.

REFERENCES

1   Luft, Harold S. *Health Maintenance Organizatuons: Dimensions of Performance*, New York: Wiley-Interscience, 1981.
2   Cunningham, Frances C. and Williamson, John W. "How Does the Quality of Health care in HMOs Compare to that in Other Settings? An Analytic Literature Review, 1958–1979." *Group Health Journal* 1:1 (Winter 1980), 4–25.

3 Held, Philip J. and Reinhardt, Uwe E. "Prepaid Medical Practices: A Summary of Findings from a Recent Survey of Group Practices in the United States—A Comparison of Fee-for-Service and Prepaid Groups." *Group Health Journal* 1:2 (Summer 1980), 4–15.

4 Trieger, Sidney, Galblum, Trudi W., and Riley, Gerald. *HMOs: Issues and Alternatives for Medicine and Medicaid.* Health Care Financing Administration, Office of Research Demonstrations, and Statistics, Washington, D.C., 1981. HHS Pub. No. (HFCA) 03107.

5 Congressional Budget Office, *Nursing Education and Training: Alternative Federal Approaches*, Washington, DC: U.S. Government Printing Office, 1978.

6 American Medical Association, *Profile of Medical Practice, 1977.* Chicago, IL, 1977

7 Held and Reinhardt, *Op. Cit.*

VIRGINIA Z. BARHAM
NANCY J. STEIGER

18

HEALTH MAINTENANCE ORGANIZATIONS AND NURSE PRACTITIONERS: THE KAISER EXPERIENCE

The Kaiser–Permanente Medical Care Program is the largest federally qualified health maintenance organization (HMO) in the nation, and serves members in Northern California, Southern California, Hawaii, Northeast Oregon, Vancouver, Washington, Denver, Cleveland, and metropolitan Washington, D.C. In total, these programs provided health care for well over 3.9 million members by the end of 1980.

Health care has been provided by the Kaiser organization since 1933 when Dr. Sidney R. Garfield organized a medical staff and established a portable hospital in the Southern California desert to provide care for a construction crew building the Los Angeles aquaduct.[1-3] Providing these services requires more than 4,000 full-time physicians and approximately 35,000 nonphysician personnel. There are 30 program-owned and operated community hospitals and 78 medical office facilities. In Denver and Dallas, where Kaiser neither owns nor operates a hospital, Kaiser Health Plan members are hospitalized in local community facilities.

Among the nonphysician personnel are nurse practitioners. Nurse practitioners are used in the Colorado, Hawaii, Ohio, and Oregon regions but the greatest use occurs in Northern and Southern California. The contributions of Kaiser nurse practitioners will be discussed as they relate to improving access, controlling costs, expanding services, and improving consumer satisfaction. Based on this discussion, speculation as to the future of the nurse practitioners at Kaiser is considered.

IMPROVING ACCESS

As it is known today, the Kaiser–Permanente Medical Care Program has six basic principles that have become known as the "genetic code." They are (1) group practice; (2) integration of facilities, combining both inpatient and out-patient facilities for maximum use of equipment as well as personnel; (3) prepayment; (4) preventive medicine, emphasizing well care and sick care; (5) voluntary enrollment, enabling those who do not like the prepaid group practice format the choice of an alternative type of plan that provides a barometer of patient satisfaction; and (6) physician responsibility, not only for patient care, but for other aspects of the program including financing, planning, allocating resources, and the training and using of nurse practitioners.

Kaiser is different from many of the newly established HMOs in its use of nurse practitioners, because the plan was established well before the nurse practitioner concept evolved in the mid-1960s. Practice patterns dominated by physicians were well established, unlike institutions such as the Harvard Community Health Plan where nursing was involved from its inception, and a nursing director and nursing staff were present on opening day.[4]

Training programs for nurse practitioners developed slowly within the Kaiser organization. The number of nurse practitioners employed increased primarily at medical centers where rapid growth in health plan membership occurred or where experimental programs were conducted. In 1971 there were only 23 nurse practitioners employed by Kaiser in California; by the end of 1980, there were approximately 357. The addition of this large group of health professionals has helped improve patients' access to care.

Much of the improved access occurred in adult medicine where there were backlogs of requests for physical examinations. After nurse practitioners were trained to conduct routine health appraisals, the workload of physicians was lessened and the waiting time for an appointment was appreciably reduced. In a 1976 survey in the Southern California region, within a 4-wk period, 103 nurse practitioners put in 9,300 hours of time on tasks that would otherwise have been done by physicians. Nurse practitioners and physicians were found to spend equivalent time for return visits, limited visits, and walk-in and short appointments. However, it took the nurse practitioner 50 min to do a complete history and physical examination while it took physicians only 30 min. There was no measure of the quality or thoroughness of the two groups.

At the Oregon region's Health Appraisal Center, nurse practitioners working with one physician, focus on providing extremely thorough one-visit, 2-hr appraisals By specializing in this way the Center is able to offer a superior health service on relatively short notice to a great many members

By 1978 when the unit was in full service the Center performed physical examinations and tests on almost 14 000 people annually [5]

Historically prepaid group practice health care programs have been able to bring medical care to isolated areas where none was available In Hawaii Kaiser operates a state-funded outreach program that makes medical care accessible to people who otherwise would have none Local residents are employed because of their knowledge of customs of the area and local geography After training, outreach workers go to health plan members homes to assess the general health status of the family and compliance with prescribed medical regimens If additional care is needed a nurse practitioner or physician comes to the home to provide the appropriate health care

As nurse practitioners continued to grow in numbers and expand their services within the Kaiser- Permanente program, accessibility of care has improved, waiting times have decreased, and services have become more comprehensive Counseling and health education have become as important and appropriate as medical care

CONTROLLING COSTS

Statistics regarding the cost-effectiveness of nurse practitioners for Kaiser are extremely limited. In fee-for-service settings, cost-effectiveness can be determined quite simply by the comparison of total revenues and expenses before and after use of nurse practitioners. Contract prepaid programs, such as Kaiser, have difficulty defining a generally acceptable model for cost-effectiveness. Since separate cost centers for physicians and nurse practitioners are not feasible with the current method of operation, precise figures for support personnel, space use, and all other costs are not available. The only readily identifiable costs are salaries and fringe benefits.

A comparison of costs of nurse practitioners *versus* physicians in the provision of outpatient care was completed in 1979, based on the first quarter statistics for 1978. Table 18-1 compares the unit cost of a physician visit and a nurse practitioner visit by department. The total unit cost was calculated by accounting for the direct cost of physicians' and nurse practitioners' time, and the cost of personnel such as clinic assistants, registered nurses, and licensed practical nurses, working directly with them, and therefore affected by their productivity (referred to as controllable costs). The total unit cost when nurse practitioners provide care is $2.45 less in medicine, $8.71 less in obstetrics/gynecology, and $0.43 in pediatrics.

TABLE 18-1 Comparison of Unit Office Visit Costs Provided by Physicians (MDs) and Nurse Practitioners (NPs) The Permanente Medical Group Quarter Ending March 31, 1978

	Cost of MD Visit		
	Medicine	Ob Gyn	Pediatrics
MD	$13.25	$12.66	$12.11
Controllable Costs	5.70	6.71	5.17
Total	$18.95	$19.37	$17.28
	Cost of NP Visit		
	Medicine	Ob Gyn	Pediatrics
NP	$ 7.82	$ 4.68	$ 7.87
Controllable Costs	8.68	5.98	9.84
Total	16.50	10.66	17.71

Savings (Loss) Per NP Visit		
Medicine	Ob Gyn	Pediatrics
$2.45	$8.71	($0.43)

Feldman, R.: Nurse Practitioners: Permanente Medical Group Regional Survey (Mimeographed Report). Oakland, Cal., Permanente Medical Group, November 1980

As indicated in Table 18–2, when the differences in unit visit costs between physicians and nurse practitioners are calculated on an annual basis for each full-time equivalent (FTE) nurse practitioner, the cost savings are impressive for medicine and obstetrics/gynecology, and modest losses were realized in pediatrics. Nurse practitioners in obstetrics/gynecology saved almost $1.5

TABLE 18.2 Nurse Practitioner Cost Annualized Figures. Calculated from the Difference in Unit Visit Costs Between Physicians (MDs) and Full-Time Equivalent Nurse Practitioners (NP FTE).

Annual Cost Savings (Loss)/NP FTE	
Department	Savings (Loss)
Medicine	$ 7,148
Ob Gyn	41,889
Pediatrics	(1,277)
Annualized Total Department Savings (Loss)	
Department	Savings (Loss)
Medicine	$ 381,004
Ob Gyn	1,461,921
Pediatrics	(26,020)
Total	$1,816,905

Feldman, R.: Nurse Practitioners: Permanente Medical Group Regional Survey (Mimeographed Report). Oakland, Cal., Permanente Medical Group, November 1980

TABLE 18-3 Productivity of Physicians (MDs) and Nurse Practitioners (NPs) in Ambulatory Care. The Permanente Medical Group, Quarter Ending March 31, 1978

	FTEs*	Visits per Quarter	Visits/ FTE	Visits/ FTE/Day
MDs				
Medicine	419.8	466,258	1,111	17.4
Ob Gyn	128.9	138,206	1,072	16.8
Pediatrics	201.4	273,256	1,357	21.2
NPs				
Medicine	53.3	38,878	729	11.4
Ob Gyn	34.9	41,961	1,202	18.8
Pediatrics	21.2	15,128	714	11.2

* Full-time equivalent

Feldman, R.: Nurse Practitioners: Permanente Medical Group Regional Survey (Mimeographed Report); Oakland, CA Permanente Medical Group, November 1980

million a year while in medicine they saved almost $400,000 a year, resulting in a total savings to Kaiser of over $1.8 million a year for all nurse practitioners even when losses in pediatrics are included.

The cost-effectiveness of nurse practitioners in the Northern California region is significant since they are responsible for 400,000 office visits per year, or 11% of all visits to medicine, obstetrics/gynecology, and pediatrics. Nurse practitioners see 23% of all outpatients in obstetrics/gynecology, 8% in medicine, and 5% in pediatrics (Table 18-3).

Pediatric nurse practitioners do not account for the level of cost savings achieved by nurse practitioners in medicine and obstetrics/gynecology. This is, in part, because pediatric nurse practitioners see fewer patients, and use more ancillary personnel. Although pediatric nurse practitioners do not save resources for the plan in terms of providing lower-cost substitutive care for physicians, they do provide additional services at minimal cost.

In the Southern California region, an elaborate computation of physician clinic time saved per nurse practitioner was devised. From May to November 1976, statistics indicated that 71.0% of physician clinic time was saved in pediatrics, 78.5% in medicine, and 66.6% in obstetrics/gynecology, for a total overall saving of 70.0% (Table 18-4).

Staff turnover is another important aspect of controlling cost. During the 1970s, the turnover rate of nurse practitioners was 15% in the Northern and Southern California regions. This relatively low figure is due, in part, to the motivation and career commitment of nurse practitioners. However, the low turnover is also due to the fact that the Kaiser–Permanente system is a major source of employment, and nurse practitioners' options for practice are limited.

HMOs like Kaiser have shown that health care is invariably less costly

TABLE 18-4 Physician (MD) Clinic Time Saved Per Nurse Practitioner (NP)

	1. No. of Nurses (entire region)	2. MD Time (in hours) that would be required to perform tasks done by all NPs in a 4-wk Period	3. MD Time that would be required to perform tasks done by each Individual NP in a 4-wk Period (Col. 2 ÷ Col. 1)	4. MDs required to perform tasks done by all NPs in a 4-wk Period (Col. 2 ÷ 120 hr by avg. MD Clinic Time in Peds, Med, 126 hr in Ob/Gyn)	5. Avg. % MD Clinic Time saved per NP (Col. 3 ÷ 120 hr MD clinic time; 126 hr in Ob/Gyn)
Pediatrics					
April 1973	19	1,452	76.0	11.5	60.5%
Nov 1973	16.75	1,436	85.7	11.4	68.0%
Sept 1974	18.5	1,643	89.0	13.0	71.0%
May 1976	31	2,645	85.0	22.0	71.0%
Medicine					
April 1973	41	2,353	57.4	18.6	45.4%
Nov 1973	39.25	2,931	74.7	23.3	59.5%
Sept 1974	41.5	3,073	74.0	24.4	59.0%
May 1976	57.25	5,395	94.2	45.0	78.5%
Ob/Gyn					
April 1973	17	836	49.2	6.6	39.0%
Nov 1973	18	1,294	72.0	10.3	57.2%
Sept 1974	16.8	1,385	82.4	11.0	65.0%
Nov 1976	15	1,261	84.0	10.0	66.6%
Total					
April 1973	77	4,641	60.3	36.8	47.8%
Nov 1973	74	5,661	76.5	45.0	61.0%
Sept 1974	76.8	6,101	79.4	48.4	63.0%
May/Nov 1976	103.25	9,301	90.0	76.0	73.0%

Kay RM: Nurse Specialist Training and Utilization Program. (Mimeographed report). Southern California Region, Kaiser-Permanente Medical Care Entities, January 1977 than sick care. The nurse practitioner program allows the significant extension of health maintenance at affordable costs. And it has been observed that patients who are cared for by nurse practitioners subsequently generate lower overall health-related costs than those cared for by physicians.[6] Lower overall costs are due in part to lower nurse practitioner salaries and in part to the use of fewer laboratory and diagnostic tests by nurse practitioners.

EXPANDING SERVICES

In addition to providing less costly care that substitutes for traditional medical services, nurse practitioners also expand the scope of services provided. Four factors have influenced nurse practitioners' potential for role expansion and the delivery of new services at Kaiser. First, there are still physicians who have a guarded acceptance of nurse practitioners and question their role within Kaiser. These attitudes stem from difficulty accepting change, reluctance to relinquish control, fear of losing contact with their patients, and doubts concerning nurse practitioners' competencies. A frequent concern voiced by physicians, particularly those in small departments, is that nurse practitioners cannot share responsibility for hospital coverage, night work in clinics, or other unpopular tasks. Some physicians prefer to hire additional physicians rather than nurse practitioners so that these duties may be shared.[7]

Second, physicians and administrators fear that expanded roles for nurses will increase their risk of malpractice suits. To date, however, there have been few malpractice claims involving nurse practitioners. The rarity of these claims is due in part to the fact the nurse practitioners are not involved with hospitalized, surgical, or seriously ill patients, and because of their excellent relationships with patients. This experience has been reassuring, and there is no evidence to indicate any trend toward an increase of malpractice suits involving nurse practitioners.[8]

Third, there has been a modification of the Nursing Practice Act within California that facilitates expansion of nurse practitioner responsibilities. Article II was modified in January, 1975, to read, "The legislature recognizes that nursing is a dynamic field, the practice of which is continually evolving to include more sophisticated patient care activities. . . . It is the legislative intent also to recognize the existence of overlapping functions between physicians and registered nurses and to permit additional sharing of functions within organized health care systems which provide for collaboration between physicians and registered nurses." Standardized procedures were required so that documented policies and procedures developed by the collaboration of physicians, nurses, and administrators would allow nurses to assume a much broader role in the delivery of health care. Such standardized procedures have been used by the nurse practitioners in defining and expanding their scope of practice.

Fourth, collective bargaining has had an impact on the roles and responsibilities of nurse practitioners at Kaiser. The California Nurses' Association is the collective bargaining agent for nursing in California. Nurse practitioners within the Northern California region have been part of the Master Contract with the California Nurses' Association since 1971. Contract language determines the definition, training, salary, and fringe benefits for nurse practitioners as it does all registered nurses within the region. Although the inclusion of the nurse practitioners in the union contract provides greater economic security, it can also hamper the development of new roles.

At Kaiser there are different types of nurse practitioners. The medical nurse practitioner is involved in health-screening procedures, conducts physical examinations, and staffs specialty units for care of patients with diabetes, obesity, and hypertension. Pediatric nurse practitioners focus primarily on well baby care, a benefit included in the Kaiser Foundation Health Plan. Working under the direction of a pediatrician, a pediatric nurse practitioner has the opportunity to follow a child's development through the early years. Pediatric nurse practitioners take medical histories, evaluate well babies, perform physical examinations for preschoolchildren, identify abnormalities, and make decisions about whether to make referrals or seek consultation. The obstetrics/gynecology nurse practitioner takes histories and performs prenatal and post-partum care in the ambulatory setting. The family nurse practitioner, the newest addition to the Kaiser system, provides primary care to children, adults, and entire families in collaboration with family practitioners.

Adult nurse practitioners have primary responsibility for conducting multiphasic examinations They also provide care through health evaluations, short appointments for acute care. and chronic disease follow-up services Adult nurse practitioners increase the accessibility of primary care services at Kaiser; conserve physician time for care of the sick patients; promote prompt appropriate screening and patient referral; establish a baseline for a health profile for each patient; and provide cost-effective quality health care

Nurse practitioners, although working more independently over time, clearly know their medical limitations and are careful to seek physician consultation when required. One major advantage of nurse practitioners is that they adhere to departmental policies more regularly than physicians, *e.g.*, in the use of drugs and monitoring side effects, recommendations for periodicity of checkups, checking on immunizations, maintaining legible records, *etc.*[9]

Since their introduction into Kaiser, nurse practitioners have continued to expand their role in diagnosis and treatment. They have become primary care providers in hypertension and diabetic clinics. Through the use of standardized procedures developed jointly with physicians, nurse practitioners also serve as primary care providers in medical short-appointment clinics where screening and treatment as well as follow-up care are provided for minor illnesses. In the Ohio region and selected California regions, nurse midwives provide exceptional continuity of care through prenatal, delivery, and postpartum stages. They teach Lamaze classes, do routine examinations and deliveries, and subsequently give instructions in child care and family planning, if requested. In most other regions served by Kaiser the obstetrics/gynecology nurse practitioners provide this care with the exception of deliveries. Pediatric nurse practitioners examine the newborn in the nursery before discharge.

The Family-Centered Prenatal Program offers parents the opportunity to leave the hospital and return home with their baby soon after delivery. If an expectant mother and her obstetrician agree that she is a candidate for the program, and both prospective parents want to pursue this option, a nurse practitioner is assigned to the family to help prepare them for the experience of going home with a baby only 6 hr old. Within 24 hrs of the discharge of mother and baby, the family is visited by a nurse practitioner. Usually these visits are made during the first 3 days, but may continue if needed. The nurse practitioner examines both mother and child, and has the opportunity to discuss breastfeeding, infant care, and a wide variety of things new parents need to know. This program has the potential to achieve major cost savings by eliminating expensive hospital days, and also meets the special needs of some parents far better than traditional postpartum hospital care.

Nurse practitioners have considerably strengthened counseling and health education services at Kaiser. Nurse practitioners are central to Kaiser's family-planning services. They hold contraceptive classes, and counsel individual patients on various birth control techniques. They also provide counseling for patients considering abortion, tubal ligation, or vasectomy. They conduct individual counseling for problems related to sex, marriage, and stress, and they teach in the Better Breathing Clubs, breast clinics, and stress management classes.

Nurse practitioners place a high priority on activities relating to health education and health promotion. This interest complements physicians' interest in complex medical problems and curative medicine. The addition of nurse practitioners to a large medical practice will almost certainly lead to an expansion of services for consumers.

IMPROVING CONSUMER SATISFACTION

Patient acceptance of care provided by nurse practitioners within Kaiser appears to be extremely good.[10,11] Ninety percent of eligible patients who were offered the opportunity elected to participate in the nurse practitioner program.

Shorter waiting times for appointments is one important factor in consumers' satisfaction with the nurse practitioner program. In a study of 2,600 patients who had been seen by a nurse practitioner for physical examinations, satisfaction with the examination appeared to be inversely related to how long the individual had to wait to get an appointment. For example, 32% of those who waited from 1 wk to 4 wk felt their physical was an excellent one as compared to 20% of the people who waited more than 4 mo.[12] Waiting time appeared to be more important to consumers than whether the examination was conducted by a nurse practitioner or physician.

Nurse practitioners also have contributed a special dimension to the health status evaluation. Whereas busy physicians often have little time to encourage patients to verbalize their health concerns, nurse practitioners are able to elicit the full range of patient concerns and questions. Questions are asked more frequently of nurse practitioners and perhaps the answers are more readily understood. Nurse practitioners often provide better patient education than physicians, primarily because of their interests and training in education, counseling, and teaching.

This emphasis on patient education has influenced attitudes of both staff and consumers about health maintenance. "There is an increased awareness of the value of well care among both patients and physicians. We're getting away from episodic, crisis-oriented sick care and directing patients into lifetime health monitoring".[13]

Collaborative practices where nurses and physicians work together has had a major positive effect upon consumer satisfaction within the Kaiser-Permanente program. Consumers increasingly define medical care in very broad terms. They want access to both the best in diagnostic and therapeutic medical care, and assistance with social adaptation to the everyday problems of living. Nurse practitioners and physicians working collaboratively can satisfy these diverse consumer expectations better than either physicians or nurses could do alone.

THE FUTURE OF THE NURSE PRACTITIONER AT KAISER

The evaluation of the use of nurse practitioners at Kaiser is approaching a critical juncture. The impending excess physician supply may be a major determinant of nurse practitioners' future in Kaiser.[14]

The role of the nurse practitioner at Kaiser was conceived of by physicians in response to the need of Kaiser Health Plan members for increased access to health care. With insufficient numbers of physicians available to meet this need, nurse practitioners were added to the program to enhance access to care at affordable costs. Now that the physician supply is more than adequate, the issue will be whether Kaiser physicians will opt to recruit physicians to replace nurse practitioners.

One of the major problems contributing to the insecure position of nurse practitioners at Kaiser is ambivalence about whether nurse practitioners should be primarily physician substitutes or whether they should maintain their nursing responsibilities as well. Although the California Nurses' Association specifically states that the nurse practitioner will continue to function as a nurse in providing direct patient care, many nurse practitioners do not have a strong identification as nurses. To some physicians, nurse practitioners assist in providing *medical* care to *physicians'* clients, thus lightening the physicians' workloads. Rather than practicing in an expanded nursing role, many nurse practitioners in the Kaiser system practice in a limited medical role.

Nurse practitioners leave themselves vulnerable to replacement by physicians by allowing themselves to be defined as physician extenders. Physicians can argue that more doctors, rather than more nurse practitioners, will be needed in the future. This contention arises from their ambivalence over the role of nurse practitioners at Kaiser, nurses' inability to substitute for physicians in hospital coverage, and the increased acuity level of caseloads carried by physicians, which result from nurse practitioners caring for commonly occurring problems. All of these factors decrease physicians' satisfaction with their practices.

Nurse practitioners have alienated many of their staff nurse colleagues by aligning themselves too closely with medicine. Nurse practitioners have also aggressively pursued increased job benefits such as higher pay, greater autonomy, personal office space, and a share of Kaiser profits, without attention to the concerns of staff nurses. This has resulted in growing antagonism between nurse practitioners and the nursing staff. Therefore, not only are nurse practitioners in a rather precarious position with regard to physicians, but they also lack the strong backing of nursing, which may be essential to their future.

Given these problems, nurse practitioners must acknowledge the threat to their survival within the Kaiser system and develop strategies for countering it. A closer alignment with nursing is essential. If nurse practitioners continue to practice as physician extenders (and certainly not all do), they will either be replaced by more physicians, or by others who can be trained to provide similar, perhaps more cost-effective service. By acknowledging their foundation in nursing, nurse practitioners can ensure for themselves a continuing role, even with a surplus of physicians.

A critical component for nurse practitioner survival in the Kaiser system in the future is to maximize their unique contributions. In this regard, there are several options nurse practitioners can pursue. The Graduate Medical Education National Advisory Committee (GMENAC) projected a surplus of physicians in most specialties, but the field of preventive medicine is a notable exception (see Chap. 14). "Comprehensive prevention, however, entails skills and efforts that are beyond the capabilities of many a good doctor".[15] Inherent in attempts at prevention are client education and self-care teaching. Draye and Pesznecker found that nearly half of all interventions made by family nurse practitioners included teaching and health promotion.[16] In order for nurse practitioners to provide these services, the value of health promotion must be acknowledged and resources made available.

Currently, however, little time is allocated in the Kaiser System for nurse practitioners to provide teaching interventions. In fact, in Kaiser surveys, nurse practitioners were evaluated by how quickly they performed histories and physicals as compared to physicians, not whether they adequately met patients' needs.[17]

Through client teaching and health promotion, nurse practitioners can make a unique contribution to patient care, a contribution that is supported by the basic philosophy of Kaiser to provide preventive medicine, emphasizing well care and sick care. Nurse practitioners will have the basis for their claim that they make a unique contribution to the Kaiser system by spending more of their time equipping their clients with the knowledge and skills to take better care of themselves and their families, to detect early signs of illness, and to more effectively manage chronic disease.

According to Healthy People, The Surgeon General's Report, more than half of the deaths in the United States are due to unhealthy behavior or inappropriate lifestyles.[18] Nurse practitioners emphasize illness prevention and health promotion, which may provide the impetus for Kaiser Health Plan patients to improve their health habits, reduce the risk of illness, and possibly increase the quality of their lives. These interventions should result in a decreased demand for care, and reduced overall costs, a further justification of the nurse practitioner role. By providing nursing services in a collaborative rather than competitive practice with physicians, nurse practitioners can counter the threat a surplus of physicians poses to their future.

Nurse practitioners do not have sufficient outcome data substantiating their particular contributions. Instead of focusing on the nature of the encounter and outcome of nurse practitioner interventions, studies to evaluate the cost-effectiveness of such interventions have focused on the length of time a nurse practitioner spends with a client and the number of clients seen in an average day, week, or month.[19-22] In addition, much of the research addresses the ability of nurse practitioners to deliver traditional medical care safely and effectively, and to be accepted by patients.[23, 24] Data on these measures of nurse practitioner effectiveness have been uniformly favorable.

The few studies that have documented outcomes of care have also been positive. Runyon, for example, studied 1,006 patients with diabetes, hypertension, or cardiac disease cared for over a 2-yr period by nurse practitioners.[25] These patients achieved significant reductions in diastolic blood pressure and blood glucose, and used 50% fewer hospital days than a control group followed in hospital outpatient clinics. Ford suggested that patient outcome measures, such as behavioral changes, health maintenance, disease prevention, use of services, and transference of problem-solving ability in self-care, deserve attention to document the impact of nurse practitioner interventions.[26] Nursing research is needed to provide such documentation.

In summary, if nurse practitioners are viewed as low-cost substitutes for physicians, their future with Kaiser is bleak. But if they can complement the focus of physicians on illness detection and treatment with a focus on health maintenance, health education, disease prevention, and self-care education, and if they can document the validity of this client-centered orientation, then nurse practitioners can look forward to a rewarding and secure future of independent and collaborative practice.

REFERENCES

1 Kaiser Annual Report. Organized Health Care Delivery Systems: A Historical Perspective. Kaiser Foundation Medical Care Program, 1978

2 Garfield SR: The delivery of medical care. Scientific American 222: 15–23, April 1970

3 Garfield S: Multiphasic health testing and medical care as a right. New Engl J Med 283:1,087–1,089, 1970

4 Bates B: Nursing in a health maintenance organization. Am J Public Health: 991–994, 1972

5 Kaiser Annual Report: Challenges of Change. Kaiser–Permanente Medical Care Program. 1979

6 Taller S: Where nurse practitioners expand good care. Patient Care 13: 184–212, 1979

7   Feldman R: Nurse Practitioners: Permanente Medical Group Regional Survey (Mimeographed Report). Oakland, CA, Permanente Medical Group, 1980

8   Ibid

9   Ibid

10   Ibid

11   Taller S, op cit

12   Kay RM: Nurse Specialists Training and Utilization Program (Mimeographed report). Southern California region, Kaiser–Permanente Medical Care Entries, Jan 1977

13   Taller S, op cit

14   US Congress, Health Program, Office of Technology Assessment: Technologies for Forecasting Physician Supply and Requirements. 1980

15   Ingelfinger FJ: Medicine: meritorious or meretricious. Science 200, No. 26: 942–946, 1978

16   Draye M, Peznecker B: Teaching activities of family nurse practitioners. Nurse Practitioner 5, No. 5: 28–33, 1980

17   Kay RM, op cit

18   Department of Health, Education & Welfare Public Service: Healthy People: The Surgeon General's Report on Health Promotion & Disease Prevention (Pub. No. 79-55071). Washington DC, US Government Printing Office, 1979

19   Henriques C, Virgademo V, Kahane M: Performance of adult health appraisal examinations utilizing nurse practitioners-physician teams and paramedical personnel. Am J Public Health 24, No. 1: 47–53, 1974

20   Levine D, Morlock L, Mushlin A, Shapiro S, Malitz F: The role of new health practitioners in a prepaid group practice: Provider differences in process and outcomes of medical care. Med Care 4, No. 4: 326–347, 1976

21   Burkett GL, Parker-Harris M, Kuhn J, Escovitz GH: A comparative study of physicians' and nurses' conceptions of the role of the nurse practitioner. Am J Public Health 68, No. 11: 1,090–1,096, 1979

22   Levine JL, Orr S, Sheatsley D, Lohr JA, Brodie B: The nurse practitioner: Role, physician utilization, patient acceptance. Nurs Res 27, No. 4: 245–254, 1978

23   Jacobs KD: Does the nurse practitioner involve the patient in his care? Nursing Outlook 28, No. 8: 501–505, 1980

24   Linn L: Patient acceptance of the family nurse practitioner. Med Care 14, No. 4: 357–364, 1976

25   Runyon J: The Memphis disease program: Comparisons in outcome and the nurse's expanded role. JAMA 213, No. 3: 264–267, 1975

26   Ford L: A nurse for all settings: The nurse practitioner. Nursing Outlook 27, No. 8: 516–521, 1979

DAVID MECHANIC

19

NURSING AND MENTAL HEALTH CARE: EXPANDING FUTURE POSSIBILITIES FOR NURSING SERVICES

The mental health field continues to be plagued by competing and conflicting models of care, by lack of adequate knowledge of cause, prevention, and treatment, and by the force of traditional practice.[1] Despite this, the care of the mentally ill has undergone a remarkable transformation, relocating the provision of treatment in large part from inpatient services to ambulatory and community settings. With federal and state support, there has been a substantial increase in access to mental health services, growing acceptability of care for psychiatric disorder, and increased respect for the needs and rights of the mentally ill. In 1955 approximately half of all episodes of mental health care were in state and county mental hospitals; 25 yr later, less than one-tenth of all such episodes were in such institutions. During this same period, the number of episodes treated in mental health facilities increased from 1.7 million to 6.4 million, most care now being provided in psychiatric outpatient settings and mental health centers.[2] The number of resident patients in mental hospitals decreased dramatically, many now living in community housing, board and care facilities, and nursing homes. These changes reflect new social attitudes, changing social policies and administrative practices, the availability of more effective psychoactive drugs, and new sources of financing for the community maintenance and treatment of the mentally ill. Despite these advances, it is clear that the mentally ill — particularly those with more severe disorders — remain a neglected population, outside the mainstream of responsible and effective treatment and rehabilitative services.

Although nursing has a long tradition in inpatient psychiatric settings, the potentials for nursing in the mental health arena remain undeveloped. Al-

343

though nursing shares these potentials with general medicine and psychiatry, psychology, and social work practice, nurses because of their numbers, types of training, and traditions are in an advantageous position to assume not only a broader role in the mental health field, but one with significant opportunities for a major leadership role. The success of the expansion of nursing roles within mental health depends substantially on reimbursement policies and institutional practices, and thus nursing as a profession must exercise leadership in implementing models of mental health care that will attract public support and the interest of financing agencies. Changes in nursing practice in specialized technical areas such as surgical and intensive care nursing on the one hand, and in the expansion of nursing roles in primary care and pediatric practice on the other, suggest possibilities. The focus of my argument, however, is that nursing may have unique opportunities in mental health practice because of the way it is structured relative to medical practice and because of the special needs of mental patients, and, in addition because it more effectively bridges the physical and social needs of mental patients than competing mental health specialties.

Traditionally, psychiatry and the care of the mentally ill has been relatively isolated from the mainstream of medical and nursing care. Before 1955 the mentally ill were largely treated in public institutions staffed predominantly by aides, while people with economic means obtained care in private hospitals or, more frequently, from psychiatrists in private office-based practice. Much of the institutional public care was custodial, and nursing roles were traditional. In subsequent years, psychotherapeutic practice increased in both public and private settings, but such care was largely directed at populations with moderate psychiatric illnesses and problems in living and not at the more chronic patients, who were increasingly released to the community. While nurses had a growing treatment role in mental health centers and psychiatric outpatient clinics, they were secondary to the growing numbers of social workers and psychologists providing psychotherapy and counseling. Nursing, of course, continued its involvement with public mental hospitals, and took up a major role in psychiatric units in voluntary hospitals.

In the 1970s there was a rapid increase in the number of psychiatric beds in voluntary general hospitals and a significant growth of psychiatric proprietary beds. The recent enlargement of the profit-oriented hospital sector in psychiatry has escaped general notice but reflects the availability of psychiatric inpatient coverage in third party insurance. Those with such insurance are increasingly treated in such facilities while the indigent are referred to public institutions. While the relocation of psychiatric care to the voluntary community hospital assists in the reestablishment of a link between general medicine and psychiatry, the shift has reflected a very traditional, if somewhat expanded, medical approach to both psychiatric nursing and psychiatric care.

Although there are some master's level psychiatric nurses, the vast majority of nurses working in inpatient psychiatric units are registered nurses with very limited mental health training. What we have seen is an adaptation to the hospital as it functions in other areas of care in contrast to the exploitation of new forms of nursing practice and responsibility. Consistent with hospital practice generally, nurses remain under the tight reign of medical authority, and are not able to effectively exercise independent judgment. Nor has nursing as a profession given consideration to what roles it might fruitfully play relative to the large numbers of mental patients increasingly found in nursing homes, board and care facilities, and in ambulatory medical care. In the discussion that follows, I examine the needs of patients and the opportunities for mental health nursing in decentralized community care facilities and in ambulatory medical care. I also consider some of the political and policy issues that inhibit the effective expansion of nursing roles.

THE CARE OF THE CHRONIC MENTAL PATIENT

Mental health policy in recent decades has resulted in large numbers of chronic mental patients in community settings. These patients have profound medical and social needs that are dealt with often in an uneven and ineffective way. The chronically mentally ill are also difficult to deal with, have profound disabilities that respond only very slowly to intervention, and often do not appreciate their own needs or efforts to help them. Such patients often require persistent, skilled efforts to deal with their psychological and medical disabilities and to bolster their self-esteem, coping capacities, and available social supports.

At present, a wide variety of personnel participate in community care programs serving such patients. Most typically, these programs are administered by professional social workers or psychologists, with baccalaureate graduates in social work and the social sciences providing much "routine" service. Although many of these workers develop significant therapeutic and supportive skills as a result of practical experience, they often lack the necessary background and training to respond effectively to the formidable problems patients have and the personal and social issues they must face. Many chronic psychotic patients in the community are on long-term psychoactive drugs. Patient failure to follow drug regimens adequately, and the adverse and unpleasant effects related to the use of these drugs require aggressive care on the one hand and careful drug monitoring on the other. With increasing evidence of the high prevalence of tardive dyskinesia and other extrapyramidal symptoms with the use of the antipsychotics, it is essential to have caretakers knowledgeable about pharmacologic issues and working cooperatively with psychiatrists to achieve a sensible and effective drug program that limits adverse effects. There is growing indication that patients on long-term drug therapies develop their own viewpoints about these drugs and their effects, and modify medical advice on the basis of such perceptions. Sophisticated drug management requires balancing an appropriate drug regimen in light of the realities of the patient's attitudes, level of understanding, and functioning.

Nurses are in a strategic position for many of the functions required in effective community care programs for chronic mental patients. They could bring to the task not only a long tradition and training in socioemotional and supportive aspects of care but also familiarity with drugs and pharmacological issues. Increasingly, nurses are being trained in supportive psychotherapy and behavioral change techniques as well, and the close association of nursing with medicine gives it considerable credibility with patients in the medication area — an essential aspect of the community care task. Nurses tend to lack, however, the organizational skills and a broad understanding of the complex range of social programs and financial entitlements that provide support for mental patients in the community. They also may not know how to effectively negotiate and integrate these for the benefit of the patient.

Similar needs for sophisticated psychiatric nursing exist in nursing homes and sheltered care facilities.[3] There are now more chronic mentally ill persons in such settings than in mental hospitals, and many such patients are not elderly. They require sophisticated drug management and monitoring, social programs of active involvement, and significant interpersonal support. Various studies suggest that in many nursing and board and care homes such patients are kept relatively inactive and given excessive medication to minimize management problems and potential incidents. A common picture is the patient, heavily drugged, eyes glued to a television set, staring into space.[4] Well-trained nurses in mental health in such settings not only could bring a more rational drug approach but would also allow for the development of an active daily regimen fitted appropriately to the capacities and needs of the individual patients. The realistic opportunities and constraints on such roles are considered later.

COMPONENTS OF PSYCHIATRIC NURSING IN COMMUNITY CARE

Nursing can play an expanded role in community mental health care that bridges the necessary medical, psychological, and social care required for effective maintenance of the chronically mentally ill.[5] While some of the necessary skills and knowledge are not currently emphasized in nursing education, neither the curricula nor necessary educational affiliations with schools of psychology or social work would be particularly difficult. Politically, the most difficult challenge would be to prepare nurses more thoroughly in psychopharmacology and to increase their competence and responsibility in prescribing. But even in the absence of legal legitimacy, nurses can play an important expanded role.

There are at least six areas of major concern in the care of the typical chronic patient. Attention should be focused on how nurses or nurse–social worker teams might acquire the competence to carry out the necessary functions of care in each of these areas.

MATERIAL WELFARE

Deinsitutionalization is only possible because of the growth of welfare legislation that funds both subsistence and medical care costs of patients. Minimally adequate funding for chronic patients depends on the knowledge and ability to take advantage of varying categorical programs at federal, state, and local levels that pay for such needs as housing, food, subsistence, and medical care. Mental health personnel familiar with how to "exploit" existing entitlements legally can do a great deal more for their patients than their inexperienced colleagues.

Patients also require assistance with many basic needs dependent on material resources or their reasonable use. At a primitive level, patients require adequate shelter and nutrition. In many communities, the chronically ill are viewed as undesirable and not only have difficulty in locating suitable housing but also are exploited economically. As communities resist new board and care facilities, halfway houses, and other housing arrangements for the chronically ill, mental health programs have often followed the line of least resistance, locating housing for patients in the most ecologically undesirable areas of cities where patients suffer high risk of victimization and other dangers and indignities. Successful community care requires not only an awareness of patients' material needs, but a knowledge of community organization and welfare arrangements that allows the effective use of public resources. This involves not only the welfare system, but planning for the location of patient residences in good proximity to needed services and other community facilities.

COPING

The adequacy of a person's functioning depends on problem-solving capacities that are acquired in the process of one's social development. What may be an ordinary situation to those with skills or otherwise adequate cultural preparation in a crisis for those who lack them. Chronic mental patients commonly lack basic skills and knowledge essential for everyday living, and the absence of such skills, or their erosion due to chronic illness, exacerbates problems of adjustment. Such deficiencies make it difficult for patients to obtain and retain employment, establish interpersonal relations, get around their community, maintain adequate living quarters, and avoid difficulties with the authorities. Moreover, because such patients are dependent, they have continuing contacts with services and official bureaucracies, and their skills in managing such relationships have important bearing on their welfare. In recent years, demonstration programs have made it evident that teaching patients such simple skills as budgeting, use of public transportation, house maintenance, and self-presentation can contribute a great deal to their effective community adjustment.[6] Nurses are in an excellent position to organize, teach, and monitor such living skills in community care programs, and to do so in a context that takes account of patients' disabilities, drug regimen, and overall physical needs.

PSYCHOLOGICAL FUNCTIONING

Improving chronic patients' psychological functioning in a direct way is both the most difficult and most uncertain aspect of care. It is well established that long-term chronic patients have major psychological difficulties, and psychotherapeutic efforts have not been impressive in modifying or ameliorating deficiencies commonly found in this population.

Psychiatric nurses are increasingly trained in psychotherapeutic methods and techniques of behavior control, and these techniques constitute part of a larger strategy of approach to the needs of the chronically impaired patient. Obviously, patients have various individual needs relative to their personalities and particular disabilities. Schizophrenic patients, for example, have difficulties with intense personal relationships and are more vulnerable in these circumstances, while chronically depressed patients are unusually susceptible to feelings of helplessness and despair in situations in which they suffer a sense of loss. Existing evidence and experience suggest that a pragmatic approach that sets tangible goals and is supportive of the patient's efforts offer more promise than diffuse psychotherapy. Perhaps the most substantial therapeutic efforts are achieved indirectly by developing networks of social support that enhance patients' coping efforts and sense of self-esteem, which are notoriously deficient.

SOCIAL SUPPORTS

It is widely believed, and increasingly substantiated, that the absence of social support makes people vulnerable to interpersonal and environmental assaults and other adversities. Often the simple knowledge that help will be available if needed gives people the confidence to cope successfully. Supports are important not only for the instrumental assistance they might provide, but also for the reinforcement and self-affirmation that come from the sympathetic and empathic interests of others.

The chronically mentally ill are particularly vulnerable because supports are commonly unavailable and such patients are very much isolated from usual community associations. These patients may either have no close relatives, or have over the course of time alienated family and significant others by their bizarre behavior and personal difficulties. Moreover, many patients have difficulty maintaining close personal relations, and such relations depend on an awareness and understanding by significant others of the problems associated with chronic illness. Effective community care requires careful attention to the development and maintenance of community and interpersonal supports. Efforts may be essential to coach the patients themselves in their roles and responsibilities, by providing information and support to relatives and friends and maintaining sympathetic but aggressive contact with patients. Chronic patients not only typically lack supports, but they are also often less likely to seek them out and maintain them, and service systems must be well organized and aggressive.

In emphasizing the importance of social supports, we must recognize the limitations of our understanding. We use the term "social support" glibly, referring to a variety of human emotions and processes. It may mean relatedness and the availability of ordinary types of assistance, or it may refer to such strong and ambivalent emotions as intimacy and love. It may involve the availability of mundane instrumental assistance and everyday social contacts, or relate to the person's sense of worth and its validation. Strong human ties inevitably involve ambivalent relations and reciprocal obligations and expectations. Thus, they are not only a source of gratification and sense of belonging but also a source of stress. We still know too little about what aspects of support are most essential for the chronic patient and under what conditions certain types of "support" may be noxious. Some patients function best isolated from intense ties and associations, and are more vulnerable as their involvements increase. Others become overdependent on others in a way that handicaps them in exercising adult responsibilities. Sensitive exploration and reappraisal, both in general and in individual cases, is what is needed, not dogma.

SUSTAINING MOTIVATION

Successful social adaptation depends on a continuing willingness to remain engaged and on a commitment to ongoing activities. Withdrawal is a natural, and often an effective, means of reducing one's sense of threat or disappointment in the short run, but if it persists it substantially handicaps the person.

Chronic patients typically have a history of failure and disappointment, and this creates an incentive to withdraw, reduce hopes and expectations, and hold back in engaging in everyday tasks. The consequence is that skills and social contacts erode, and patients have less and less confidence in their ability to perform ordinary life tasks.

It is now well understood that withdrawal and inactivity among chronic patients result in personal deterioration and an incapacity to continue or regain important social roles. The specific activities patients perform are less important than their continued involvement, contact with other people, and exposure to the expectations and constraints of social demands. Effective community care cannot tolerate inactivity, withdrawal, and apathy, and must develop a structure for patients that makes demands without overtaxing the patient's ability to conform. The appropriate role of community care is to build expectations that patients can meet but that also challenge them and contribute to their experiences of coping mastery and self-worth. Doing this well requires knowing the patient, monitoring his progress carefully, and modifying the program of care in response to feedback.

HEALTH MAINTENANCE

Chronic mental patients require not only excellent mental health care but also careful attention to their physical health needs. Poor nutrition, neglect, and other conditions associated with both serious impairment and deprived circumstances ensure the inevitability of many health problems in this population. In addition, the long-term use of high doses of powerful psychoactive drugs, often combined in irregular ways and with the use of alcohol, creates a serious potential threat to health. In addition, patients require a range of medically related services such as contraception, which is essential because many chronic patients are incapable of effective parenthood. Moreover, persons with psychiatric illness tend to have more illness in general than others in the population, and continuing monitoring and provision of medical care is desirable.[7]

Drug monitoring itself requires a thoughtful, sensitive but aggressive approach. The evidence is substantial that many chronic patients, such as schizophrenics, require continued medication if episodes of psychosis are to be minimized, and patients in crisis commonly discontinue their medication, which results in even more serious problems in functioning. The adverse effects of the antipsychotics are sufficiently unpleasant to induce patients to attempt to function without them, often resulting in problems. Only through aggressive monitoring and encouragement is it possible to achieve high levels of conformity and safety in achieving medication requirements. This must be undertaken with a good knowledge of the noxious effects of long-term drug use and a sensitive awareness of how to schedule dose and administration to achieve the least personal discomfort and danger to health consistent with the need for treatment. The utility of personnel who are sensitive to physical need and physical health and who have some appreciation of pharmacologic issues is apparent. When combined with effective psychosocial skills it offers the potential for excellent management of a difficult problem.

In sum, the ingredients of successful community care — material welfare, coping, psychological functioning, social support, sustained motivation, and health maintenance — are all consistent with nursing traditions and roles. Nurses, with appropriate training, can fill an important social need in responding effectively to the chronically impaired patient in the community as well as to those with psychological problems seen in office-based and clinic contexts. We now move on to consider the latter setting.

PSYCHOLOGICAL CARE IN AMBULATORY MEDICAL SETTINGS

Psychosocial and psychological problems are prevalent among patients in ambulatory medical care settings. Such problems may accompany or be a product of serious physical illness, or they may be the primary complaint, reported directly or expressed indirectly through vague or generalized complaints of ill health, or lack of physical well-being as typified by fatigue, insomnia, irritability, and diffuse physical discomforts. The appropriate diagnosis and management of such problems is frequently a formidable clinical challenge.

Estimates of psychosocial and psychological problems in medical practice vary widely depending on the case-finding criteria used, and, although consistently large, they have no clinical importance by themselves. The far more significant fact is that as much as three-fifths of the instances of psychiatric morbidity measured in community epidemiologic studies are managed exclusively within the general medical care sector.[8] The frequent use of psychoactive drugs in general medical practice reflects physicians' attempts to cope with such problems, but there is also disconcerting data suggesting that major psychiatric problems are not recognized or appropriately managed, sometimes resulting in suicide and other problems that possibly could be prevented.[9, 10]

The role of the physician in identifying symptoms and diagnosing disease by necessity focuses clinical appraisal narrowly, while patients tend to have much broader concepts of their physical health status, influenced by their overall sense of well-being and social functioning.[11] Thus, while physicians are trained to pursue a narrow technical approach, patients are more attuned to their total experience, their sense of vitality, and their ability to perform social roles. The unique viewpoints of physician and patient make it inevitable in part that there will be gaps in communication and understanding.[12]

Studies of psychosocial stress and patterns of response to symptoms indicate that psychological distress not only influences perceptions of health but also is an important trigger in bringing patients to the physician.[13] Studies of illness behavior and the presentation of complaints illustrate the complexity of expressions of psychosocial distress and related symptoms. In some cases, the expression of illness serves as an excuse for failure to meet social expectations or to explain failure or inadequate performance, or it may be a means for justifying release from usual obligations.[14, 15] Moreover, there are sociocultural differences in how people define symptoms, evaluate them, and respond. While some may see psychosocial problems as stigmatizing and be reluctant to admit them, others have learned elaborate psychological vocabularies to conceptualize and express their sense of distress. Still others have no conscious awareness of the link between their life problems and sense of physical discomfort, and complain of general malaise. Such patients may vigorously resist the attribution of the source of their problem to psychosocial areas, insisting that their problem is entirely physical.

How patients express their distress affects the course of their treatment. Patients who persistently complain of physical symptoms that fit no discernible disease pattern are subjected to many diagnostic, laboratory, and treatment procedures, some of which are both costly and risky. While criteria for evaluating and treating such patients are too imprecise to make definite estimates of unnecessary treatment, existing studies suggest that many patients who express psychological distress through organic symptoms are subjected to unnecessary medical and surgical interventions.[16]

It is difficult to define precisely the nature of psychosocial complaints seen in primary medical care, since the description depends substantially on the assumptions underlying the classification system. Much disagreement persists about the proper classification of psychiatric and psychosocial conditions and the appropriate boundaries between disorder and ordinary problems of everyday life. Studies of the content of primary care suggest that psychotic conditions are relatively uncommon, but a significant number of patients (perhaps as many as 10% to 15% of all patients at any time) suffer from moderate levels of depression, anxiety, and related personality disorders. In one study physicians asked to evaluate the source of such problems attributed them most frequently to marital and other domestic problems and occupational and employment difficulties—yet referrals to social services were unusual.[17] The most common forms of therapy were the prescription of psychoactive drugs and some reassurance and counseling. While general physicians see more depressed, alcoholic, and generally distressed patients than practitioners in the specialized mental health sector, the effective management of such patients remains a neglected area.

OPTIONS FOR NURSING EDUCATION

Trends in community mental health care, and the growing recognition of the importance of psychosocial problems and psychological disorders in general medical care, offer some exciting opportunities for nursing educators. There is a need for nurses working in general ambulatory settings who have the skills and sophistication to successfully monitor and manage many of the psychological problems that are presented or that are associated with chronic illness. Such a role at a simple level requires training in behavioral issues, psychological appraisal, and social psychological techniques; at a more sophisticated level it may involve training for a nursing role with increased emphasis on psychopharmacology and the use of psychoactive drugs, behavioral and other psychotherapeutic techniques, and rehabilitation skills relative to improving coping capacities and social supports. The more sophisticated role — equivalent to a "mental health nurse practitioner" — can also define a core professional role in the emerging spectrum of community care programs for the mentally ill. The full realization of such a role would include legal authority for prescribing certain commonly used psychoactive drugs.

The need for a role equivalent to a mental health nurse practitioner might involve cooperation or joint programs between existing nursing and schools of social work. Nursing education could provide the traditional emphasis on caring and familiarity with the general medical context. Social work schools could contribute relevant training in community organization and social welfare. Indeed, a master's degree combining nursing skills and social work training may be a viable option. However such programs might be organized, the fact remains that a need for this mix of services exists. Nursing offers both the potential range of skills and the social legitimacy with patients to perform this role credibly. The general training and versatility of the nurse also makes possible a combination of functions in smaller medical practices and community settings, which makes the introduction of such a new role more economically feasible.

There are a number of conditions that make the introduction of such a role promising at this time. First, the issue of psychological disorder in medical practice is receiving greater prominence, and such problems will increase with the growing numbers of aged persons and with deinstitutionalization efforts. Second, psychiatric coverage is increasing in insurance programs, providing new treatment opportunities. Third, despite the mounting interest in both the chronic psychiatric patient and the distressed patient in general practice, psychiatry as a specialty remains somewhat divorced from both populations, focusing on acute psychosis and outpatient psychiatry, with depressed patients and others seeking psychotherapy for a variety of problems in living. Although the potential client population is very large, psychiatry has made no large investment in training psychiatrists to work closely with primary care physicians. Psychiatrists tend to devote their efforts toward outpatient psychotherapy or to diagnosis and psychoactive medication, with a growing interest in biologic developments and more narrow medical roles. Moreover, psychiatry as a specialty is increasingly unattractive to young physicians deciding on residency programs, and it constitutes one of the few medical specialities in which a shortage of manpower is forecast for coming decades. Psychosocial care is increasingly left in institutional settings to psychologists and social workers, professionals quite willing to assume the challenge, while nursing has largely remained behind. Why nursing has not taken up this potential more aggressively is not my concern here. What I would emphasize, however, is its special advantages because of its traditional link with mainstream medical care, an advantage not only in relation to working with physicians but, more importantly, with patients.

An analysis by Freidson of the failure of a Family Health Maintenance Demonstration is highly suggestive.[18] In this demonstration, a social worker and nurse were included as part of a primary care team.[19] Nurses in the demonstration achieved greater legitimacy in dealing with emotional problems than the social worker. Freidson maintains that patients do not see emotional problems of everyday life to be distinct, but seeing a social worker implied a discontinuity with normal functioning. In contrast, the roles of physicians and nurse were more continuous with the routine delivery of services, and did not require the same conceptual transition in patients' conceptions of their problems. While it has been argued that such a transition in conceptualization is necessary for effective treatment, this contention remains debatable, and the fact is that patients resist if the treatment offered is divergent from their values and conceptions. While professionals from all fields can learn to be attentive to patients needs and perceptions, nursing has more immediate legitimacy with many patients than some of the other helping professions.

The opportunity for new psychiatric nursing roles may be particularly relevant in larger organizational settings for medical care such as health maintenance organizations (HMOs). Such organizations are acutely aware of the demands for medical care made by psychiatrically distressed patients and those with psychiatric disorders, and are concerned with how their needs can be met in a cost-effective way. Psychiatric patients use not only expensive psychological resources but also substantially more general outpatient, inpatient, and ancillary services. [20, 21] The traditional approach of referral to office-based psychiatrists is an extraordinarily expensive approach, and drains resources that can be effectively applied to other needs. Such organizations have been receptive to the use of nonphysicians for supportive and therapeutic roles, and innovative techniques of brief individual and group psychotherapy. In such settings psychiatrists, psychologists, social workers, and nurses play interchangeable roles to a considerable degree, although nursing has yet to exploit the potential in such organizations for an expanded mental health role.

CHALLENGES TO AN EXPANDED NURSING ROLE IN MENTAL HEALTH CARE

The success of any profession in the health field depends on its ability to achieve recognition as a reimbursable provider by such government programs as Medicare and Medicaid and by other third party insurers. The role of mental health nursing in both community and office-based practice would be immediately viable if nurses could bill for mental health services either by themselves or even through physicians. In this regard, they are not only in direct competition with physicians — some of whom might offer comparable services — but also with psychologists, social workers, and other mental health counselors. Among these competitors, only psychologists have been relatively successful in freeing themselves to some extent from medical dominance and achieving legitimacy as an alternative mental health provider.

Social workers, in contrast, have been politically less successful in achieving status as independent providers, and most social workers in mental health are employed in public and private agencies. Although these agencies may receive reimbursement for their services, social workers cannot bill independently as private practitioners. Even in the case of medical care of the chronically mentally ill, reimbursement is very restrictive and does not adequately cover the range of services necessary for an effective community care program. Such programs must depend on categorically allocated funding, and such budgets are typically inadequate and under attack. The failures of community mental health care are in large part a product of the reimbursement system and the inadequacy of funding for the types of functions I have described.

While the uncertainty of reimbursement limits the potential of expanded mental health nursing roles, the traditional versatility of nursing may facilitate the institutionalization of these roles. A major problem with the introduction of many types of physician extension is that gaining the advantage of substitution requires sufficient volume of patient demand to keep everyone relatively busy. In small medical practices, the introduction of new roles may not achieve the expected savings because physicians may not be required to provide the same volume of service as previously. To the extent that the introduction of a new professional does not result in demand to full capacity, the innovation may not be cost effective. Because nurses are more versatile than social workers or psychologists and are experienced in performing a wider range of functions, they may be more cost-effective providers in such setting as office-based practices, small HMOs, community programs, general ambulatory medical clinics, and the like.

The object of the roles proposed, however, is not to substitute for physicians, but rather to offer services that physicians fail to give or in which they have little interest or expertise. The extension of services, whether in the physician's office or in a community program, depends on the willingness of the consumer, the insurer, or a public program to pay for it.

In the HMO, where a broad range of services are prepaid, using a mental health nurse practitioner may be more cost-effective than traditional referral practices to psychiatric specialty care. Large HMOs already commonly use social workers and psychologists in providing mental health care, and in smaller units where using nonphysicians for delivering such services remains an issue ideologically and economically, nurses may provide a more continuous transition than other mental health professionals. There is a growing body of literature suggesting that attention to mental health concerns of patients results in a reduction of general medical utilization.[22] If valid, it should be an additional incentive for HMOs to expand mental health services in a controlled fashion.

The situation is somewhat different in fee-for-service, office-based practice. Here we have little incentive to reduce patient use and no clear financial mechanism to pay for the expanded services provided by the mental health nurse. In such settings, the ability of nurses to perform traditional as well as expanded roles makes them more valuable to a smaller practice, allows them to use the working day more efficiently, and involves less economic risk to the practice in adding them. Once in these settings, nurses with expanded skills can demonstrate their value.

The situation in community programs, nursing homes, board and care facilities, and the like is most precarious because such care is chronically underfunded, and without better reimbursement there is little capacity or incentive to introduce more sophisticated, and more expensive, personnel. The ability to introduce a mental health nurse practitioner is likely to depend on the size of the facility, its source of income, and the resourcefulness and progressiveness of administrative personnel. A mental health nurse practitioner, however, might be able to function effectively, even under the existing adverse conditions, if attached to a community agency contracting with a variety of smaller institutions to provide particular types of services. Here it might be possible to put together categorical funding and some contract monies to support the necessary nursing personnel, and particularly if they can substitute in some areas for more expensive psychiatric personnel.

In the long run, the future of nursing — not only in these roles but in many others — will depend on reimbursement policy, change in medical practice definitions, and court judgments. With the growing number of physicians in the United States, it is inevitable that medicine as a political and economic force will attempt to reassert its dominance, and will show less tolerance of expanded functions and growing independence of the other health professions. Whatever the potential skills and contributions of nursing to mental health care or any other new role, the functions and legitimacy of nursing will be determined politically. Demonstrations of what a well-trained mental health nurse can achieve are a form of political capital. Building these expectations and perceptions on the part of legislators and the educated public is a task for nursing as a profession and as a major political actor in the health care arena. An early step is to demonstrate that such nurse practitioners can be trained successfully and that they can perform the necessary roles equally well or better, and at less cost, than traditional mental health personnel.

REFERENCES

1   David Mechanic, *Mental Health and Social Policy* (2nd ed.) New Jersey: Prentice-Hall, Inc., 1980.

2   U.S. President's Commission on Mental Health, "Report of the Task Panel on the Nature and Scope of the Problems," Vol. I, Vol. II Appendix. (Washington, D.C.: U.S. Government Printing Office, 1978.

3   Stephen P. Segal and Uri Aviram, *The Mentally Ill in Community-Based Sheltered Care: A Study of Community Care and Social Integration.* (New York: Wiley–Interscience, 1978.)

4   Bernard A. Stotsky, *The Nursing Home and the Aged Psychiatric Patient.* N.Y.: Appleton-Century-Crofts, 1970.

5   Leonard I. Stein and Mary Ann Test, eds., *Alternatives to Mental Hospital Treatment.* (New York: Plenum, 1978).

6   Leonard Stein and Mary Ann Test, "Alternative to Mental Hospital Treatment I. Conceptual Model, Treatment Program, and Clinical Evaluation." *Archives of General Psychiatry*, 37 (1980), pp. 392–397.

7   Michael Eastwood, *The Relation Between Physical and Mental Illness* (Toronto: University of Toronto Press, 1975).

8   Darrel Regier, "The Nature and Scope of Mental Health Problems in Primary Care: Variability and Methodology," in Institute of Medicine, *Mental Health Services in General Health Care*. A Conference Report, Vol. 1. (Washington, D.C., National Academy of Sciences, 1979).

9   David Goldberg and Peter Huxley, *Mental Health in the Community: The Pathways to Psychiatric Care*. New York: Tavistock Publications, 1980.

10   George Murphy, "The Physician's Responsibility for Suicide: I, An Error of Commission; II, An Error of Omission," *Annals of Internal Medicine*, 82 (March 1975), pp. 301–304, pp. 305–309.

11   Richard Tessler and David Mechanic, "Psychological Distress and Perceived Health Status," *Journal of Health and Social Behavior*, 19 (September, 1978), pp. 254–262.

12   David Mechanic, *Medical Sociology* (2nd ed.; New York: The Free Press, 1978.)

13   Richard Tessler, David Mechanic and Margaret Dimond, "The Effect of Psychological Distress on Physician Utilization: A Prospective Study," *Journal of Health and Social Behavior*, 17 (December, 1976), pp. 353–364.

14   Stephen Cole and Robert Lejeune, "Illness and the Legitimation of Failure," *American Sociological Review*, 37 (June, 1972), pp. 347–356.

15   Mark G. Field, *Doctor and Patient in Soviet Russia* (Cambridge; Harvard University Press, 1957).

16   Pauline B. Bart, "Social Science and Vocabularies of Discomfort: What Happened to Female Hysteria?" *Journal of Health and Social Behavior*, 9 (September, 1968), pp. 188–193.

17   Paul Williams and Michael Shepard, "Psychosocial Disorders in Primary Medical Care," in David Mechanic (ed.), *Symptoms, Illness Behavior and Help-Seeking*, New York: Neale Watson Academic Publications, 1981, in press.

18   Eliot Freidson, "Specialities Without Roots: The Utilization of New Services," *Human Organization*, 18 (1959), pp. 112–116.

19   George Silver, *Family Medical Care: A Design for Health Maintenance* (Cambridge, Massachusetts: Ballinger, 1974).

20   Janet Hankin and Julianne Oktay, *Mental Disorder and Primary Medical Care: An Analytical Review of the Literature*. (Rockville, Maryland: National Institute of Mental Health Series, D, 1979, No. 5.

21   Institute of Medicine, *Mental Health Services in General Health Care*. A Conference Report, Vol. 1 (Washington, D.C., National Academy of Sciences, 1979).

22   Kenneth Jones and Thomas Vischi, "Impact of Alcohol, Drug Abuse and Mental Health Treatment on Medical Care Utilization: A Review of the Research Literature," Supplement to *Medical Care*, 17 (December, 1979) entire issue.

DOROTHY S. ODA

20

SCHOOL HEALTH SERVICES: GROWTH POTENTIAL FOR NURSING

"Children are one-third of our present and all of our future."[1] Both professionals and the public readily acknowledge that the children and youth of today are our richest human potential resource for the future and that their health deserves protection and care. There is an assumption that such a tacit understanding generates a consensus that is somehow translated into adequate services for this population. Unfortunately, such is not the case, particularly for the usually well or nearly well school-age children in America. Although schools spend $1 billion annually on school health, a critical analysis of school health services indicates there is much to be desired in its organization, delivery, and evaluation.[2–7]

The school health scene is one of curious contradictions. On the one hand, there are technologically advanced roles for nurses such as the school nurse practitioner, with primary care capabilities, and, on the other hand, the school nurse teacher or school health consultant (nurse) who stresses health education and counseling in more traditional roles. These are *seemingly* divergent school nursing developments with the school nurse practitioner moving toward the (ambulatory) sick care model and the nurse teacher or consultant emphasizing a preventive orientation. In actuality, both are directed toward *educational health maintenance*, that is, keeping the student well enough to attend school and learn to the fullest extent possible. Another apparent paradox is that some school districts are developing a variety of new health service delivery patterns while others are sharply curtailing their health services due to budget constraints and declining enrollment. However, the common goal of all school health programs is to provide the most effective services with increasingly limited resources.

The health of young students should be a national priority investment in terms of the later returns of productivity, leadership, and longevity within the populace. As in other health care delivery systems, nurses are the largest single group of health professionals in school health services. These nurses are better prepared than ever and are more effectively organized than before. Yet, there is still a critical need for school nursing to strengthen its image and its power to influence the all-important resource allocation decisions. This chapter will explore the current status of school health and school nursing as a basis for viewing the options and projections for the future of nursing in school settings.

The role of schools in child health is being actively debated. Some advocate that schools limit their involvement to health education, emergency care, maintenance of a safe and healthy environment, health evaluations for problem conditions, and services for special education. Others would opt for schools providing broad-based, comprehensive primary care services. In the final analysis, health services in schools must have an impact on the health of students as it affects their learning.

OBJECTIVES OF SCHOOL HEALTH SERVICES

School health services involve three required benefit components: *direct benefits* or averted costs (*e.g.* reduction of school absences resulting in savings of state reimbursement loss, which is calculated on attendance); *indirect benefits*, which represent the potential savings or indirect costs (*e.g.*, immunization and checks to avoid illness, time loss, hospitalization, or medical care costs); *intangible benefits*, which are based on more abstract factors (*e.g.*, psychic pain incurred from pain, suffering, and grief) and are difficult to isolate, much less measure as to costs.

School nurses have always checked the condition of students to decide whether they should or should not remain in school. Stomachaches, earaches, sore throats, injuries, and head lice are among the common problems seen daily by a school nurse and are possible bases for exclusion from school. The nurse's professional judgment and decision can directly benefit schools by the retention of students who may be inappropriately sent home. Screening and immunization activities carried out by school nurses help to prevent communicable diseases such as measles and mumps. Conditions such as scoliosis and dental caries are prevented from becoming serious problems requiring more extensive treatment. These indirect benefits save school reimbursement funds as well as health costs for the families.

At school, a school nurse practitioner can perform physical examinations and provide initial and ongoing case management of children with common illnesses and health problems, thereby saving time and costs for those without a regular medical care source. Health assessments by school nurses for special education and mainstreaming of children in regular classrooms can increase education dollars for school districts and reduce expensive home-teaching costs.

Health education is another strong service of school nurses. Usually as the only health professional located in schools, the school nurse is a rich resource for preventive health information. Some school nurses assume a specific teaching component in health areas or conduct a health careers class in high schools as part of the budgeted teaching staff.

Whatever the role or range of services (including those with intangible benefits), nursing in schools is appropriate and vital when it effectively responds to the health needs of school children and their families.

CURRENT STATUS OF SCHOOL NURSING

As a practice area, school nursing is one of the oldest specialties. It began in the 1900s when Lillian Wald placed the first nurse in a New York school.[8] It is currently estimated that there are 22,000 to 30,000 nurses, working in approximately 90,000 schools, concerned with the health of about 43 million school children in the United States.[9, 10]

A major difficulty in arriving at an accurate count of practicing school nurses is that there is more than one possible employing agency. That is, nurses providing school health services may be employed by the local school district or county (or equivalent) school department, or be members of the local public health department furnishing nursing coverage of schools. There may even be a joint school district–public health department sponsorship of services. To further complicate matters, nurses in some public health nursing agencies specialize in school nursing while others carry school duty in addition to other field service responsibilities. Therefore, the number of school nurses may vary according to the particular definition of a school nurse used or method of data collection. If a school nurse designation indicates only those who are employees of a school district or department, it can exclude public health nurses assigned to schools on a full-time or part-time basis. Many other interpretations are possible and the count is then subject to a number of variations depending upon source and interpretation.

The type and range of services provided by one school nurse as compared with another is as varied as there are practitioners of this specialty.[11, 12] The laws and regulations affecting school health services, school nurses, and school nursing practice are also factors that influence the composition of services. Kohn and others have determined in a comprehensive state-by-state survey that local boards of education have primary responsibility for conducting school health programs in 45 states; in five states this responsibility rests with local health departments. At the state level 24 education departments have primary regulatory responsibilities while 12 state health departments have primary responsibilities for school health services. Many states have more than one agency involved.[13]

The same report details some specific requirements within school health services. For example, immunization of school children is required in 47 states, and 27 states mandate screening for vision and hearing. Sixteen states require that children have physical examinations upon entrance to school and ten states require dental examinations. It is noted that a large number of communities, upon local initiative, exceed in practice their state's minimum requirements.[14] One illustration of this is the increasingly popular scoliosis screening presently being conducted in schools.

Taking into account such requirements, specific services in school health can be categorized as mandated (required by law); permissive (not required by law but recommended or customary); and optional (as time or inclination dictates). Associated with any category of services are certain tasks such as the organization and administration of the service, tracking and follow up of those children with identified needs, and the inevitable records to be kept and reports to be filed. These components create a mosaic of possible health services for every local school district and each school nurse to implement. In many school districts, school nursing service is synonymous with school health service. Nonetheless, it must be pointed out that a collection of school health *services* does not automatically constitute an organized school health *program* that systematically and comprehensively encompasses the health needs of students. Whatever the sponsorship and spectrum of services, the need is to define the goals and establish the highest standard for the services rendered in a particular community.[15]

SCHOOL NURSES AND SCHOOL NURSE PRACTITIONERS

As varied as school health programs are throughout the nation, the nurses who work in them also have a multiplicity of preparation and background. The latest available survey of state certification for school nurses (1976) indicates that 23 of the states have mandatory school nursing certification. Ten states have permissive requirements. Four states are currently developing certification requirements with 14 states indicating no plans for certification. When certification is required, the minimum requirements range from licensure as a registered nurse to combinations of specific courses, work experience, and a baccalaureate degree.[16]

The role of the school nurse has long been the topic of considerable study and debate by nurses and non-nurses.[17-19] Most findings conclude that the role is difficult to define and lacks clarity and consensus. However, these perceptions of an "ambiguous" role are largely based on sociologic role concepts espoused by such theorists as Parsons, which apply in a given system with normative patterns of performance.[20] The very question of such requisites for role analysis is raised by a researcher who nonetheless observed that "if there is a role, it seems to consist of a hodgepodge of improvisations."[21] He further concludes that school nurses do not occupy a typical nursing role and what is needed by such a nurse is optimal capacity for independent professional judgment in health matters.

These latter findings, presented as probable negative attributes, can also be interpreted as the very reasons nurses become school nurses.[22] The flexibility, independence, and variability inherent in the role can be seen as job attractions by nurses who have previously worked in a highly structured and regimented hospital. There is a surfeit of research on differing school nurse role perceptions. These discrepancies have now been identified and verified. Now, more research is needed to discern role components and determinants in school nursing so that the role variations can be categorized and evaluated with implications for service and education.

The advent of the school nurse practitioner movement in the last decade was greeted with mixed reactions by school nurses. Some nurses viewed it as a heaven-sent solution to the need for a clearer role and as a means of receiving third party reimbursement for services not heretofore rendered by nurses in a school setting (e.g., physical examinations). This was seen as a potential method of achieving a measure of economic independence from reliance on an already strained school budget. Other nurses felt highly threatened that their less visible health education and counseling skills, emphasized by nonpractitioner school nurses, would become less valued and even obsolete in comparison with diagnostic skills and equipment.

Whatever the reaction, the functioning and role of the school nurse practitioner was seen as less confusing in the view of most school nurses, school staff, and administrators. School nurse practitioners had sharper assessment skills and could actually provide care, with medical backup, for common illnesses and injuries.[23] In some ways, this appears to be a return to the very early clinical emphasis of school health services from 1900 to the 1930s, when communicable diseases and poor physical conditions were prevalent. Following this period, from the 1930s to the 1960s prevention was stressed and characterized the thrust of school health programs. These changes in school health services and school nursing are probably related more to societal and economic factors affecting family and community life rather than to developments in nursing.[24] One direct result of the nurse practitioner movement is the eventual upgrading of the assessment skills of all nurses. Some of the newer nursing assessment skills that were formerly exclusively part of practitioner preparation are now being incorporated into basic nursing education programs. This will obviously be useful to nurses in school settings who daily evaluate whether a child should or should not remain in school because of a health condition.

The use of nurse practitioners in schools is still being debated in some circles but is a past issue in others. The usual arguments against school nurse practitioner use are centered around the question of the school being used as a health care delivery site *vis-a-vis* an education setting. The duplication of services with existing sources of care and the fragmentation of total family care are other reasons often cited in opposition. Proponents point out that availability of care does not guarantee access to or use of services and primary health care could and should be provided to a school population segment *not* receiving care. Another reason given in support of school nurse practitioners is their higher level of triage and other health and development evaluation skills. Their services are also viewed as a possible source of income if and when third party reimbursement for nurses becomes widespread. Their ability to generate such partially or wholly self-supporting funds is viewed with optimism and a potential answer to diminishing education dollars for school health services.

Along with school nurse role variations, different school health services have differing priorities, emphases, and funding levels depending upon the community. It is doubtful that school nurse practitioners functioning in a fully expanded role — conducting physical examinations, making diagnoses, treating minor injuries, managing common childhood illness, and identifying children with serious clinical problems for referral — will be appropriate for all schools. However, contrary to popular notions, there are communities with school-age children who do not have a regular medical care source except in severe emergencies.[25] The school nurse practitioner may be the most logical primary health care provider for this medically underserved group.

To maintain relevancy to the needs of school children, school health services and school nurses have changed and are changing. The question is not whether changes should be made but in what direction? A nurse in a school setting constantly faces conflicting priorities of health and education demands. The isolation of most school nurses from *nursing* supervision adds to this conflict by making decisions regarding productivity an individual responsibility, and professional strength becomes a personal struggle. Whichever priority is stressed or whatever pattern of services is used, the cooperation and collaboration of both public and private interests must undergird a sound school health program.

INNOVATIVE SCHOOL HEALTH PROGRAMS

The effectiveness of health services in schools must be shown if parents, communities, and ultimately local education boards are to make decisions supporting such services. Toward this end, there are a number of programs in operation or being developed that attempt to organize their services in response to community needs. Most involve school or pediatric nurse practitioners functioning in expanded roles, but some include nonpractitioner or regular school nurses.

Cambridge, Massachusetts, reorganized its municipal ambulatory child health services in 1965 by the passage of an ordinance.[26] The goal of comprehensive and coordinated school and well child programs using existing city budgets involved administrative centralization. Previously fragmented city public health programs for children, many of whom had no primary care services, became the responsibility of the Department of Pediatrics at the Cambridge Hospital. Consolidation of the medical components of the Head Start and Follow-Through Program budgets were then possible. Only existing monies allocated to school health and well child programs were used for the reorganization. Decentralization of delivery sites took place using school health facilities in the target communities of Cambridge. The need for primary health care services and decreased dependence on the emergency ward were realized with no additional overhead costs. The pediatric nurse practitioner was viewed as primary caretakers in the system and replaced traditional school nurses when they retired.

The advantage of consolidating categorical programs with the use of existing sites for services to target communities are increased accessibility with decreased fragmentation and duplication with no additional expenditure. The need for ambulatory primary care was fulfilled with medical backup from a hospital and affiliated medical school. While Cambridge's comprehensive child health program is located on site in the school with school clinics, the appropriate pediatric nurse practitioner functioning tends to emphasize the sick care component of practice capabilities. This program underscores what many feel is the distinction between a pediatric nurse practitioner and a school nurse practitioner role, in that the former is seen to perform services in a school while the latter integrates the services within school activities.

Another program using only previously allocated funds of about $500,000 (in 1979) was developed in Gary, Indiana. In an attempt to improve attendance and test scores, the superintendent of schools established a Basic Skills Support Program, which included screening by a school nurse and further evaluation by a school nurse practitioner. In 1977, of the 20% of the kindergarten students referred for follow up, one-third had significant health problems. The program is based on the premise that there is a relationship between academic performance and health.[27] The Gary program makes optimal use of two existing levels of school nursing – initial screening and assessment by the regular school nurse and comprehensive evaluation by the school nurse practitioner.

The Posen-Robbins Program is located in the south side of Chicago. Both the communities of Posen and Robbins have a sociologically complex multicultural population. Unemployment and low-income level employment is common, and health care services are severely inadequate. School officials were instrumental in developing a nonprofit corporation, the Posen-Robbins School Health Corporation, separate from the school system with funding assistance from The Robert Wood Johnson Foundation.[28]

The two clinics in elementary schools are staffed by two pediatric nurse practitioners, six health aides, four outreach workers, and four clinic clerks. A business manager and two assistants are also employees of the health corporation. The corporation contracts with two pediatricians on a part-time basis for backup and consultation. The corporation can be reimbursed for Early Periodic Screening, Diagnosis, and Treatment (EPSDT) and Medicaid services. Families who can pay are billed for services at prevailing rates set by the Chicago Pediatric Society. No health funds exist in the school system to be reallocated. The self-supporting capability of this health corporation is a major evaluation issue. The question to be answered is whether adequate third party reimbursement funds can be generated to meet the $250,000 fixed cost budget. It was hoped initially that eventually 80% would be met with generated funds, with 20% assumed by the school district.[29] Currently, 20% of costs are being recovered. If the cost recovery goal is not met, alternative funding methods, such as a prepaid plan or supplementation by a regular school health allocation (if available), may be possibilities.

Mary Hooker Elementary School in Hartford, Connecticut, has 780 students and a health unit. Most of the children come from low income families – approximately 94% are Medicaid eligible – and more than 60% live with one parent. The school was selected as a demonstration project site because of the absence of medical service in the area. This Hartford program was the result of combined efforts of the University of Connecticut Medical School and the Hartford Board of Education with financial support provided by The Robert Wood Johnson Foundation. Comprehensive health care services are available in a 25 ft by 50 ft trailer permanently located on the school premises. The staff includes two full-time pediatric nurse practitioners, a part-time pediatrician, a part-time dentist, a dental hygienist, and several health aides.

The provision of school health service on site that includes both medical and dental components is ideal. The realities of such a program being totally self-supporting are, however, rather grim. Partial self-support at a cost of $110 per child for 10 mo of the year including support costs holds promise, especially with school budget augmentation.* The use of pediatric nurse practitioners as primary care providers with a sick care model for reimbursement raises the issue again of the degree of integration of health service and school activities.

The newest and largest of the school health programs is The Robert Wood Johnson Foundation National School Health Program with demonstration sites in four states. Questions being asked of these programs include the following:

- To what extent is access to health care for children improved by a different school health service program?
- To what extent can school nurse practitioners with the supervision of a physician provide necessary health services?
- Is the school nurse practitioner able to improve the completed referral rate and be successful in the coordination of care for children having no usual source of care?
- Can financing mechanisms be developed that enable programs to sustain themselves?

The four state programs together have 30 school nurse practitioners serving a total of over 30,000 children. Each state model differs in organizational pattern and was developed to fit particular community needs.

Colorado has three sites — rural, urban, and a private nonprofit health corporation overlayed over existing school health services. The rural site provides primary health care to a low-income, rapidly growing city of 7,000 with limited medical resources. The school nurse practitioners furnish a vital health service for increasing numbers of children in this energy boomtown. The urban site has adequate medical coverage but some children in this agricultural and heavy trucking area still lack primary care. Networking with the medical community is an important function of the school nurse practitioners in this setting. The corporation provides services on a 24-hour basis with school nurse practitioners on rotating call. Medical backup is also contracted by the corporation. Data are being collected to analyze its partial or total self-supporting capability. This corporation differs from the one at Posen-Robbins in that a regular school health service with school nurses operates in this

* Lewis J (Project Director). Personal communication, March 9, 1981.

school system but without school nurse practitioners or primary care services. Together the two types of services make up a two-level system of school health.

In some of the demonstration schools, as in New York, a different form of two-level school health service exists with a school nurse teacher (non-school nurse practitioner) and a school nurse practitioner for primary care. In actuality, with health aides it is almost a three-level system. Although not suitable for all schools or school districts, a possible model for the future may include aides and school nurses (or nurse teachers) with referrals to a school nurse practitioner for complex cases or specific specialized services. This pattern is not unlike the use of clinical nurse specialists in acute care settings. New York also passed enabling legislation to permit school nurse practitioners to write prescriptions within this program. This may well set a precedent for nurse practitioners in schools following the demonstration program period.

North Dakota, with great distances between communities, promises to provide information regarding school nurse practitioners working with medical backup as far away as 60 mi. In these closely knit small towns, the nurse practitioners (who are family nurse practitioners with additional school health preparation) tend to become health advisors to the students, their families, and other community members. They are integrated not only with the school system but with the total community. The Utah program is located in a rural area with a single family practice group as the medical backup for the school nurse practitioners. Within a conservatively oriented community, the public relations aspect of school nursing assumes considerable significance. The nurses are finding that knowledge and skills of community organization and development are necessary if their work is to be well understood and supported. They are learning that the interface of school and community can be an area of strong influence on their practice.

The purpose of the National School Health Program and its comprehensive evaluation is to garner the interest of a wider audience for school health and to provide information for possible replication of the programs. Aside from descriptions of model programs, a wide range of formative as well as summative evaluation data should prove helpful to those with school health concerns and interests.

SCHOOL HEALTH FINANCING ISSUES

Economic competition for the public education dollar is a reality that must be faced. Shrinking resources plague virtually every public service or organization. Proving cost-effectiveness, defined by Quade as "a technique designed to assist a decision maker in identifying a preferred choice among possible alternatives," may no longer be deemed adequate.[30] Cost–benefit analysis, which consists of "identifying all the benefits that will accrue from the program of interest and converting them into equivalent dollars in the year they will accrue," may be increasingly demanded.[31]

In school health, direct benefits based on prevention are not easy to measure accurately. The indirect benefits are even more difficult to assess, and the intangible are practically impossible to calculate as cause and effect due to school nursing. If the education financial pie is to be divided according to calculable cost–benefit dollars, school health services will be faced with a monumental evaluation task. However, the demonstration of school health service cost effectiveness is essential for school nursing to remain viable as well as to grow. Systematic means to do this have not been a consistent priority of school nurses until hard budget choices began to affect their positions in large numbers. It is not uncommon now to read of the *threatened* elimination of school nursing staff. This experience of threatened layoff is, unfortunately, also commonly shared by teachers as well as other school support staff. The need now is to move toward more creative and consistent funding for school health services.

Inadequate third party reimbursement for nursing services can be a stumbling block for advocates of a partially or totally self-supporting school health program. This problem plagues the nursing profession as a whole and is a major deterrent to independent nursing practice. Limited reimbursement is available for specific services from federal resources such as EPSDT and Medicaid. What is sought by school nurses and school nurse practitioners is payment for preventive services, such as health education, counseling, and follow-up care. Reimbursement by private as well as public funds would enhance the ability of the school nurse and school nurse practitioner to generate at least part of their own funding without allocation or reallocation of the education dollar—a frequent point of contention. Total reliance on sharing the increasingly stringent school budget diminishes the future of school nursing.

Increased service without increased funding or the same service with less funding is a familiar process in school health. A number of health services in schools are instituted to meet mandates (such as vision and hearing screening and immunization checks). Other services are the consequences of a regulation, such as mainstreaming of handicapped students who need hyperalimentation or nasogastric tube feeding. Yet, associated funds for such services are noticeably inadequate. Consequently, the responsibilities (not to mention the related record keeping), are added to the already overburdened school nurse, who then must rearrange her priorities usually to the consternation of the school staff accustomed to her previous schedule. The constant extension of services without reduction of other responsibilities or augmention of staff results in tremendous role strain and frustration for the school nurse. This in turn contributes to decreased nurse visibility and further role ambiguity for others in the school, with consequences at budget planning time.

Many schools spend less than 1% of their budget on health services. The best school-based primary care units vary in cost from $30 to $150 per child per year, which is highly cost-effective from the standpoint of public health care but more than most school health programs now spend.[32] Without increased categorical funding or third party reimbursement, school-based primary care cannot expand, particularly in view of a steadily declining school enrollment. Pooling of various sources is probably the only realistic method of supporting anything but minimal school health services. This creative fiscal management would presuppose linkages between school health services and hospitals, private or group practices, medical schools, and child health projects in public health departments.

Current funding sources used by schools include the Elementary and Secondary Education Act (ESEA) — Title I, Migrant Education, Child Development, Comprehensive Employment and Training Act (CETA), Title XIX–EPSDT, and Medicaid. Questions to be resolved are whether schools should be the actual sponsor and provider of comprehensive primary health care services as well as be eligible for a provider number (as a nonhealth facility). Some schools have, in fact, been granted provider numbers for certain services such as screening and Head Start health services. An alternative is to organize services under the auspices of an established provider such as a health department, hospital, or a health center on site at a school.

The reimbursement of certain preventive health services by nurses remains an even more difficult issue. Health education and counseling are important services of traditional nurses and nurse practitioners in schools. Yet, except where nurses take the place of a teacher, no direct reimbursement or cost saving for individual service appears feasible.

Parental and public support are basic factors essential to any school health program funding. The low priority of child health in public policy is a significant weakness in the promotion of child health support and expansion.[33] At the local level, consumer activism is increasingly apparent in many health care systems and community services. In schools, parents and guardians are becoming involved in matters affecting the health and well-being of their children. The mass media frequently report instances of parents demanding safety precautions for hazardous conditions in the school environment — from traffic problems, waste material hazards, and building dangers, to earthquake dangers.

When school staff layoffs have been threatened, concerned parents have joined teacher and nurse picket lines in protest. In a number of cases, community groups joined forces to reverse decisions to eliminate school nursing staff.[34] Parent dissatisfaction and advocacy can be a powerful political force when public funds are involved. Inadequate school health services appear to be meeting with parental discontent with shifting economic and social factors affecting the quality of family life.[35] This community energy can provide moral and financial support to programs that demonstrate effectiveness in meeting health care needs in schools.

Recent federal legislation has placed certain new demands on schools and provided some increased funding. Public Law 94-142, The Education of All Handicapped Children Act of 1975, has enabled children with disabling conditions to be mainstreamed in the regular classroom or in the least restrictive environment. However, inherent in this process is the presence of children who need special health care techniques. Teachers now have children in their classes with needs with which they are unaccustomed and unprepared to deal. A school nurse, the only regular health professional in the school, is a logical resource for the child, family, and teacher.

Nurses, teachers, school administrators, parents, and community groups must work together to form effective child health interest coalitions to influence public policy decisions and fiscal allocations.

SUMMARY, IMPLICATIONS, AND PROJECTIONS

School health services and school nursing will undoubtedly continue to experience gains and losses as in the past. As the political climate changes, support from many quarters can be expected to ebb and flow. The certainty is that nurses and the schools they work in are committed to offering the best available health services within their perceptions of feasibility — some schools' services are admittedly at a minimum level, other schools are reorganizing existing resources, and still others are expanding their programs.

Newer influences such as active parental involvement will probably continue to grow and have an impact on school health programs. Changing needs will require adaptation of services to maintain relevance. A critical need will be for school health services and school nursing to demonstrate effectiveness with valid supporting data. It will no longer be adequate or acceptable to function without evaluation of the outcome of service on a *collective* basis. Anecdotal records of individual cases, while interesting, will not suffice. Statistical analyses, epidemiologic studies, comparative research, and program evaluations will need to be implemented based on accepted planning and research models.

The potential for widespread use of professional nurses in schools is high with respect to need, setting, and professional preparation fit. The actualization of this potential will be contingent largely upon the ability of the school health services and school nurses themselves to demonstrate their worth and compete for the educational budget allocation. The competition for limited resources is and will be increasing. However, undeniably, the health needs of school children are also increasing, and parents, particularly the single and working ones, will need to recognize along with school officials that health problems do affect learning and, ultimately, the family and the school. One example of this multiple effect is school absence due to common illnesses — caretakers must lose work time and incur costs of outside medical care while schools lose attendance reimbursement. Studies have shown that well-prepared nurses can reduce this time loss by skillful evaluation and by identification of high-risk pupils.[36-38]

A common myth is that most children have a regular medical care source. In fact, in the mid 1970s, approximately one-third, or 15 million, of the over 45 million school-age children did not have medical care except for severe emergency situations.[39] While no available data are accurately predictive, the 70,000 surplus of physicians forecast within 10 yr in a report by the Graduate Medical Education National Advisory Committee (GMENAC) will not necessarily ensure a solution to the problem of child health care access.[40] Higher family mobility together with increased specialization in the medical profession combine to blur the traditional role of a family doctor. Once children reach school age, the school has the most constant contact with them.[41] To better meet child health needs, the schools are considered by many health care professionals an appropriate site for primary health care.[42-45]

The impact of a physician surplus may be increased resistance to the use of school nurse practitioners based on the notion of duplication of services and competition for patients. However, a recent national report indicated that a review of innovative programs using nurse practitioners revealed no evidence to date that expanded school-based health services will reduce appropriate encounters with pediatricians, but a strong likelihood exists that inappropriate encounters may be reduced.[46]

SCHOOL NURSE PREPARATION AND PRACTICE

The school nurse *versus* the school nurse practitioner debate will probably continue for some time. It is a necessary growth process with change that some conflict and controversy take place. For practical purposes, it need not be an adversary or even competitive situation; that is, the two approaches should be viewed as differing but not necessarily opposing. Like so many nursing skills, what are initially considered expanded skills later become basic. This occurred with blood pressure measurement and venipuncture. Therefore, it would be a logical supposition that some level of assessment skills will eventually become an integral part of all school nurses' repertoire of competencies.

The number of school nurse practitioners will, in all probability, grow with the current 16 school nurse practitioner programs available in the United States.[47] Concurrently, practicing regular school nurses will be upgrading their knowledge and skills through workshops and continuing education courses in areas such as health and development history assessment. There is little doubt that as school nurse practitioners become more available and better known to school officials, they will be used increasingly at some level of expanded nursing practice. For example, rural or inner-city areas with critical need for primary health care services can have them functioning in fully expanded roles diagnosing, treating, and prescribing with medical backup for common illnesses and injuries. Other communities with adequate medical and other health care services available and used may have school nurse practitioners for certain expanded functions such as sports physical examinations, comprehensive physicals, psychosocial and cognitive evaluations, and identification of learning problems.

School nurses without practitioner skills will continue to do health and development histories for special education with their level of skills being improved with kits such as the Family Assessment Tool as well as with courses.[48] The preventive aspects long carried out by all school nurses, such as health education, health counseling, follow-up, and networking of care for children with identified problems, will remain significant components of school nursing.

School nurses will also incorporate newer aspects of health consumerism such as Project Health PACT (Participative and Assertive Consumer Training) or Nurses' Model Self-Care, which are aimed toward increasing peoples' awareness and astuteness of being participative health consumers with responsibility for their own health.[49, 50]

An important component of school nursing practice not always recognized is role definition and promotion. Working in a school setting is like no other area in nursing practice. The nurse with a medically-oriented background functions in an educationally-oriented setting with differing priorities, emphasis, and operational systems. Health services in schools are, for the most part, elective and they must be actively promoted.[51] Most nurses new to the school setting experience a form of culture shock, and a period of adjustment is needed. A pediatric or family nurse practitioner is not instantly synonymous with a school nurse practitioner simply because she is located in a school. Therefore, a school health component, either as an addition or postgraduate course, is necessary for proper functioning as well as for reduction of role conflict and confusion. From a knowledge and skill standpoint, the pediatric or family nurse practitioner would also benefit from increased concentration on adolescence, learning disabilities, sports medicine, and school adjustment problems.

In all likelihood the number of nurses working in the nation's schools will not be increased significantly in the future unless federal legislation requiring and funding health components is enacted. This outlook could change if nurses receive third party reimbursement for a broad range of preventive and maintenance services and schools become providers. School-based primary health care services are appropriate, if not essential, developments for certain communities and target populations.

In spite of frequent threats of cuts, school nursing staffs have remained remarkably stable *on an average* nationally. A recent limited survey indicated that while some school districts have reduced their nursing personnel, others have expanded theirs.[52] The headlines, however, are made by large scale elimination (real or threatened) of school nursing staff, while maintenance or increases in staff go unheralded. Obviously, there is always the possibility of severe reductions in education budgets that will negatively affect the number of nurses, teachers, and all other school staff members.

The nature of school nursing practice may change over time as school nurses are replaced by school nurse practitioners in many places. There will not be drastic changeovers of complete nursing staff, but the pattern will continue to be replacement by attrition. As the expanded role is better understood and accepted, school districts may elect to more fully use the skills of the school nurse practitioner. Unquestionably, all nurses in schools must be able to document what their services are and what effect they have on their clients individually and collectively. No longer will activity logs, case examples, and time schedules suffice for accountability. Service outcomes will be essential data.

PATTERNS OF DELIVERY

Just as each district differs in its educational philosophy and goal, virtually every school district in the nation has unique health care needs. Some rural schools may have a major need for comprehensive primary health care services but have a lack of available medical resources. Some urban schools may best be served with a cadre of health technicians for routine work, with referrals to professional school nurses or school nurse practitioners functioning as a team. A health corporation may be most appropriate for one community and integrated municipal and school-child health services more workable in another. A contract service with a nursing consultant group may even be a possibility for certain public or private schools. A variety of service patterns can enrich school health services as a whole with adaptability to local needs.

FINANCIAL SUPPORT

Ideally, school health services should be more reliant on health dollars rather than education dollars for assurance of the continuity and longevity of the programs. The problem is, of course, to locate federal, state, and even private sources in sufficient quantity to adequately support the program. Creativity and ingenuity are required to generate funding for supportive services in schools. One small California school district is considering the establishment of a private foundation to accept contributions for programs such as music, library, athletics, and nursing services, which it may no longer be able to support.[53]

Reimbursement for nursing services remains an issue and its positive resolution may mean the difference between nurses being able to provide more, or less, *preventive* health services. The area of financing school health services will continue to be a difficult one for nurses and school administrators as resources become increasingly limited. Unified efforts are needed for the ever necessary power of political persuasion. Bureaucracies are notoriously slow machineries and complex in nature, and nurses will need to become active in the school and educational political arena.

The concept of collective bargaining is a controversy raging in the nursing profession today. It has even more meaning for school nurses who do not have parallel striking power. Many school nurses feel that professional nursing organizations have not been helpful to them, and have become affiliated solely with teacher unions that have materially assisted them to maintain their positions and increase salaries. It will behoove nursing organizations to become more responsive to school nurses and for school nurses to become more closely allied with their own professional group for a stronger identity.

RESEARCH

Earlier studies in the area of school nursing have largely been focused on role perceptions and identification of services. Later studies moved to the more pragmatic aspects of selected populations such as teenage pregnancy or high-risk absence groups There is a paucity of research in program evaluation or service outcomes that can assist in program planning or demonstrating cost-effectiveness to influence policy or financial decision making.

Risk-taking (for school nurses) research is needed in school health. Nurses generally maintain that a professional background is necessary for high quality care. This needs validation by studies with well-controlled variables comparing selected services rendered by professionals and nonprofessionals. There is a possibility that results will be favorable for the paraprofessional. Nurses must be willing to risk such a finding if it will benefit the care of children. For example, if such a conclusion is reached, nurses can then concentrate on areas that clearly and unquestionably require professional preparation (*e.g.*, comprehensive health evaluation follow up, health counseling, and health education). Cost-efficiency and cost savings are a reality in public services. One illustration of this process geared to reorganization of services for efficiency is the use of health technicians for routine screening to enable school nurses to conduct health and development histories for special education or school nurse practitioners to perform physical examinations.

Evaluation research is a paramount need in school health, and little is now available in the literature.[54-56] Research methodologies must be rigorous and the findings couched in the language of the audience, whether they are school administrators, fiscal officials, legislators, or community groups. One school nurse or even one school district may not be able to undertake such studies. One possible method to be considered is a joint venture with interested public or private school systems and public health agencies collaborating with available university resources such as schools of public health, nursing, dentistry, and medicine.

A most pressing need in school nursing, and the best potential for its growth, is for activist school nurses with political sensitivity who can persuasively demonstrate their worth and effectiveness. This group of nurses must be unified in their efforts, with strong organizational support to make themselves professionally known and valued. School nursing of the future will require nursing entrepreneurs who have a good measure of interpersonal, management, political, and research skills to enhance their clinical competencies. Support and pressure for school, child, and youth health services need a broad public power base for impact at the local, state, and federal levels.

The health needs of school children will not diminish without adequate care services, and school nurses are prepared to provide the needed services. There is one basic yet ultimate question that is posed to everyone in school health: Should schools deliver health services? The most compelling reply came from a New Jersey school nurse who said, "Show me the school system anywhere which doesn't have children with handicapping conditions, neurological deficiencies, cardiovascular problems, hypertension, sickle cell anemia, VD, drug abuse, alcohol abuse, or pregnancy, and I'll show you the school system that can get out of the health business."[57]

REFERENCES

1   Select Panel for the Promotion of Child Health. *Better Health for Our Children: A National Strategy.* Volume I, Report to the United States Congress and the Secretary of Health and Human Services. Washington, DC: Government Printing Office, 1981.

2   The Robert Wood Johnson Foundation, *School Health Services Special Report* Number One. Princeton, New Jersey: The Foundation, 1979.

3   Lynch, A., "There is No Health in School Health," *Journal of School Health* 49:410–413, 1977.

4   Gilman, S., and Nader, P.R., "Measuring the Effectiveness of a School Health Program: Methods and Preliminary Analysis," *Journal of School Health* 49:486–492, 1980.

5   Kenney, J.B., "The Role and Responsibility of Schools in Affecting Dental Health Status—a Potential Yet Unrealized," *Journal of Public Health Dentistry* 39:262–267, 1979.

6   Allanson, J.F., "School Nursing Services—Some Current Justifications and Cost–Benefit Implications," *Journal of School Health* 48:603–607, 1978.

7   Howell, K.A., and Martin, J.E., "An Evaluation Model for School Health Services," *Journal of School Health* 48:433–442, 1978.

8   Wald, L., *The House on Henry Street*. New York: Holt and Co., 1915.

9   The Robert Wood Johnson Foundation. *op. cit.*

10 United States Department of Health, Education, and Welfare. Office of Child Affairs. *Survey of School Health Services: Methodological Note*. Washington, D.C., Office of Child Affairs, 1978.

11 Igoe, J., "What is School Nursing? A Plea for More Standardized Roles," *Maternal Child Nursing* 5:307–311, 1980a.

12 Leong, S., "School Nursing is What the School Nurse Makes It," *Journal of School Health* 49:479, 1979.

13 Kohn, M.A., et al., *School Health Services and Nurse Practitioners: A Survey of State Laws* Washington, D.C.: Center for Law and Social Policy, 1979.

14 *Ibid.*

15 Nader, P.R. *Options for School Health*. Germantown, Maryland: Aspen Systems Corporation, 1978.

16 Castle, A.S., and Jerrick, S.J., *School Health in America: A Survey of State School Health Programs*. Kent, Ohio: American School Health Association, 1976.

17 Greenhill, E.D., "Perceptions of the School Nurse's Role," *Journal of School Health* 49:368–371, 1979.

18 Hawkins, N.G., "Is There a School Nurse Role?" *American Journal of Nursing* 7:744–751, 1971.

19 Forbes, O., "The Role and Functions of the School Nurse as Perceived by 115 Public School Teachers from Three Selected Counties," *Journal of School Health* 37:101–106, 1967.

20 Parsons, T., and Shils, E.A., (eds). *Toward a General Theory of Action*. Cambridge, Massachusetts: Howard University Press, 1951. Chapter 4.

21 Hawkins, N.G., *op. cit.*

22 Oda, D.S., "The Nature of Nursing in Schools: A Study of a Coordinate Work Role." Unpublished doctoral dissertation. University of California, San Francisco, 1973.

23 Hilman, N.A., and McAtee, P.R., "The School Nurse Practitioner and her Practice: A Study of Traditional and Expanded Health Care Responsibilities for Nurses in Elementary Schools." *Journal of School Health* 43:431–441, 1973.

24 Igoe, J.B., "Changing Patterns in School Health and School Nursing," *Nursing Outlook* 28:486–491, 1980b.

25 Silver, N.K., et al., "The School Nurse Practitioner: Providing Improved Health Care to Children," *Pediatrics* 58:580–584, 1976.

26 Porter, P.J. "The Cambridge Story," *American Journal of Public Health* 71:86–88, Supplement January, 1981.

27 The Robert Wood Johnson Foundation, *op. cit.*

28 Cronin, G., and Young, W.M., "Posen-Robbins: A Model School Health Care Project," *Nurse Practitioner* 2:22–25, 1977.

29 Cronin, J. and Young, W.M. *400 Navels: The Future of School Health in America.* Bloomington, Indiana. Phi Delta Kappa, 1979.

30 Quade, E.S., "Introduction and Overview" in T. Goldin (ed.) *Cost/Effectiveness Analysis.* New York: Praeger, 1967.

31 Bootman, J.L., et al., "Cost-Benefit Analysis: A Research Tool for Evaluating Innovative Health Programs," *Evaluation and the Health Professions* 2:129–154, 1979.

32 Select Panel for the Promotion of Child Health *op. cit.* p. 249.

33 Foltz, A. *Uncertainties of Federal Child Health Policies: Impact in Two States* DHEW Pub. No. (PHS) 78–3190, Washington, DC: National Center for Health Services Research, 1978.

34 Oda, D.S. "The Making of a School Nurse" *Journal of School Health* 49:539, 1979.

35 Igoe, J.B., 1980b, *op. cit.*

36 Hilmar, N.S., and McAtee, P.R. *op. cit.*

37 Basco, D., et al., "Epidemiological Analysis of School Populations as a Basis for Change in School Nursing Practice," *American Journal of Public Health* 62:491–497, 1972.

38 Tuthill, R.W., et al., "Evaluating a School Health Program Focused on High Absence Pupils: A Research Design," *American Journal of Public Health* 62:40–42, 1972.

39 Silver, H.K., et al., *op. cit.*

40 News and Reports. "The GMENAC Report" *Nursing Outlook* 28:715, 717, 718, 1980.

41 Martin, E.W., and Richmond, J.B., "An Historical Perspective," *Journal of School Health* 50:244–245, 1980.

42 Nader, P.R. "The School Health Service: Making Primary Care Effective," *Pediatric Clinics of North America* 21:57–73, 1974.

43 Igoe, J.B., "School-based Health Service," *Journal of School Health* 49:291–292, 1979.

44 Cook, D.E., "The Role of Primary Health Care in Schools," *Journal of School Health* 49:183–184, 1979.

45 Newton, J. "Primary Health Care in a School Setting," *Journal of School Health* 49:54, 1979.

46 Select Panel for the Promotion of Child Health. *op. cit.*, p. 250

47 Igoe, J.B., 1980b, *op. cit.*

48 Holt, S.J., and Robinson, T.M., "The School Nurse's Family Assessment Tool," *American Journal of Nursing* 79:950–953, 1979.

49 Igoe, J.B., 1980b, *op. cit.*

50   Baldi, S., et al. *For Your Health: A Model for Self Care.* South Laguna, California: Nurses Model Health, 1980.

51   Oda, D.S. "Increasing School Nurse Role Effectiveness," *American Journal of Public Health* 64:591–595, 1974.

52   Oda, D.S. "School Nursing: Current Observations and Future Projections," *Journal of School Health* 49:437–439, 1979.

53   "Foundation Considered for School Programs," *Oakland Tribune,* March 11, 1981. Oakland, California.

54   Brink, S.G., et al., "Nurses and Nurse Practitioners in Schools," *Journal of School Health* 51:7–10, 1981.

55   Oda, D.S., et al., "School Nursing and Dental Referrals," *Journal of School Health* 50:393–396, 1980.

56   McAtee, P.A., "Nurse Practitioners in Our Schools? An Assessment of Their Expanded Role Compared with School Nurses," *Clinical Pediatrics* 13:360–362, 1974.

57   The Robert Wood Johnson Foundation, *op. cit.* p. 7.

PART 6

STRATEGIES FOR INCREASING NURSES' AUTONOMY

Nurses have been slow to explore strategies used by other occupational groups to improve their economic and general welfare. Part VI explores several of these strategies in detail: collective bargaining, supplemental nursing service agencies, state legislative action, and antitrust litigation. The purpose of this section is to begin to educate nurses about the benefits and liabilities of these strategies to achieve needed change.

In Chapter 21, Cleland provides an overview of the issues relating to nurses' economic and general welfare and the control of nursing practice. Cleland discusses collective bargaining, the use of contract mechanisms, and negotiations to achieve greater professional autonomy and more appropriate economic remuneration.

Prescott, in Chapter 22, reports preliminary findings from the first national study of supplemental agency employment of nurses. The rapid growth of supplemental agencies has raised concern, but Prescott also carefully analyzes the potential of these agencies to break hospitals' monopsonistic control of the nurse labor market. Supplemental agencies have introduced an important new factor into nurse employment that must be carefully analyzed by nursing in the coming decade. In fact, nurses may want to act swiftly to gain control of this rapidly growing enterprise.

In Chapter 23, Latanich and Schultheiss, two lawyers employed by the Federal Trade Commission, provide a detailed analysis of antitrust litigation and its potential to improve competition in health care. Enabling legislation and third party insurance policy are also considered. An executive summary precedes the paper for readers who wish an orientation to the topic. Since the issues are complex, the paper is necessarily detailed. However, it provides a comprehensive analysis of litigation as a strategy for change and is highly recommended for all readers.

VIRGINIA CLELAND

21

NURSES' ECONOMICS AND THE CONTROL OF NURSING PRACTICE

Nursing is at a crossroad. Through research, demonstration, and experience, nurses have developed knowledge about nursing care and its delivery, but they are unable to implement change because of nursing's lack of autonomy in major practice settings. Federal and state laws and regulations have changed the rules governing the health care system, and nursing has lost power in the practice setting. Nursing will not be granted greater autonomy over its practice. Rather, nurses must assume greater decision-making authority within their scope of practice. Demands cannot be made nor the decision-making authority accepted without professional risk; however, inaction is the greater risk and the choices are clear.

THE PROBLEM

There is dissatisfaction among nurses employed in service institutions and agencies. Levels of nurse dissatisfaction with employment are reflected in turnover rates and scarcity of job applicants. The associated problems have prompted special studies by the National Commission on Nursing of the American Hospital Association (AHA), the Robert Wood Johnson Foundation, and the Institute of Medicine of the National Academy of Sciences. While these studies are yet to be published, I predict their conclusions will show that the rights of nurses have been substantially and continuously violated by employing institutions. Claire Fagin identified nurses' rights as the following:

1   The right to find dignity in self-expression and self-enhancement through the use of our special abilities and educational background.

2   The right to recognition for our contribution through the provision of an environment for its practice, and proper professional economic rewards.

3   The right to a work environment which will minimize physical and emotional stress and health risks.

4   The right to control what is professional practice within the limits of the law.

5   The right to set standards for excellence in nursing.

6   The right to participate in policy making affecting nursing.

7   The right to social and political action in behalf of nursing and health care.[1]

In that paper Fagin defined a right as a "just claim to anything to which one is entitled such as power or privilege. A 'right' is that which one may properly demand or claim as just, moral, or legal. A close synonym to right is prerogative."[2]

Nurses find in their employment a lack of opportunity to contribute, directly or indirectly, to goal setting and program development. Often, staff nurses are forced to absorb activities delegated by other departments and are permitted to practice nursing only if there is surplus time. They may be forced to accept assignments for which they are unprepared or overprepared. They carry heavy responsibility without commensurate authority. Routinely, staff nurses must accept supervision from nurse managers whose employment goals are more closely aligned with institutional management than the accountability of nursing to the public.

Great numbers of nurses are employed in service institutions with little or no opportunity for promotion. With the great increase in the numbers of part-time nurses, it is not uncommon for a head nurse to be responsible for 30 to 60 employees. A span of control of this size is incomprehensible in any other field, yet a nurse will accept the position to be on the day shift, have weekends free, and because it represents a promotion. The newly appointed head nurse may suffer an actual loss of income due to elimination of overtime pay and holiday or shift differentials. Sibson, an authority in the field of compensation, has recommended that a supervisor's pay level should be at least two levels higher than the grade of the highest-rated job supervised, 15% higher than the straight-time earnings of highest paid subordinate, or 25% higher than the average gross pay of all subordinates.[3] If a shift differential is paid at all (commonly $0.50 to $0.75 per hour in nonunionized nursing settings), it is small and ineffective in terms of encouraging staff members to elect to work the less popular shifts.[4, 5]

The practice of treating all registered nurses as equivalent by not recognizing previous experience or previous education has tended to create an employment model with little differentiation and almost complete substitutability. If a unit needs another registered nurse and one is not available, a licensed practical nurse is sent to the unit; if an licensed practical nurse is not available, a nursing assistant may be assigned. Nurses in such employment settings lose their sense of self-worth. They come to realize that management views them only as "hands and feet" and to not show up for work makes little difference. Absenteeism rates are suspected to closely parallel the nurse's self-esteem. Where workers lack identity as valued employees, absenteeism rates climb.

Many nurses are electing to work for temporary nurse employment agencies. If the only decision a staff nurse is permitted to make is related to whether or not she works, then the temporary agencies permit many options in relation to that decision. When personal plans change, the nurse can increase or decrease the amount of employment on very short notice.

Between 1972 and 1977 there was a 25% increase in the number of registered nurses, with the total reaching 1,409,434.[6] Since only 3% of the greatly increased pool of nurses were seeking employment, this reflects an enormous increase in demand. The same study reported that in 1976 70% of registered nurses were employed in nursing, 4.4% of registered nurses were employed outside of nursing, and 3% were engaged in job changes (total 77.4%). This compares very favorably with the employment of men over 18 yr of age (78%) and greatly exceeds that of women in general (47%). With such a high proportion of nurses already employed, any major shift in employment patterns must come from decreasing the proportion of part-time employees in favor of larger proportions of full-time workers. A 1979 study of 510 registered nurses in Michigan found that 40% of the part-time nurses have no children under the age of 18.[7] Large numbers of nurses are working part time not because they have young children, but as a means of coping with a highly stressful work environment and the problems of combining work and home responsibilities. Income levels are so low that nurses opt for part-time work rather than pay for the substitute household services full-time employment would require.

Since 1974, with the enactment of the National Health Planning and Resources Act, hospitals have faced increased pressure to bring under control the great inflation of health care costs. While cost containment is an institutional byword, hospital administrators appease physicians' demands because they admit all patients and enable the hospital to maintain the bed occupancy level necessary for fiscal solvency. I believe that the National Health Planning Resources Act and the search for a means to control inflation in the health care sector have together had the effect of reducing nursing's power base within hospitals. Because nurses are such a large employee category in the institution, major attention has been directed, by institutional collusion,

TABLE 21-1 Average Monthly Salaries for a Staff Nurse — All Institutions

	1974	1975	1976	1977	1978	1979
Current dollars	$758	806	867	912	983	1041
1974 dollars	$758	739	751	742	743	707

University of Texas at Galveston National Survey of Hospital and Medical School Salaries.

at holding the line on nurse's salaries. As the rate of inflation has increased, nurses' salaries have fallen significantly. Conley in an article on the Consumer Price Index showed the effect of inflation on staff nurse salaries.[8]

The responses of nurses to salaries that have not kept pace with inflation have been (1) to leave hospital employment, (2) to seek employment with temporary agencies, (3) to engage in job hopping, (4) to increase absenteeism, and (5) to work part time instead of full time. All of these effects combined have had disastrous effects upon productivity in the employment setting and upon job satisfaction of the individual nurse.

In a provocative chapter on "The Market for Registered Nurses," Paul Feldstein in his book *Health Care Economics* presents an interesting account of the effects of the federal Nurse Training Act (NTA).[9] He suggests that nursing leaders made the choice to subsidize educational programs instead of students at the entry levels of nursing to enable the profession to move its education programs into the mainstream of general education, an important professional goal. An eventual result was that NTA-subsidized nursing education enabled hospitals to hire nurses for entry level positions at falsely reduced pay levels. Feldstein makes a strong case that an increase in nurse wages is much cheaper for the public than subsidy of nursing education.

Feldstein reports that market elasticity in nursing has been estimated by various economists as 0.5 to 1.5; that is, a 1% increase in salaries will produce a 1% increase in nurse participation in the work force. With 74.4% of all registered nurses currently employed, I believe that elasticity is actually lower, because influences of the women's movement and inflation have already brought inactive nurses into the work force. The last several years in Michigan have been ones with high general unemployment and severe depression because of the struggling automobile industry. Simultaneously, this has been the first time in nursing history that a general economic depression has not been associated with fully staffed nursing departments. The obvious explanation is that the nurses were already employed.

Subsidy of nursing education should be limited to research training and graduate nursing education as has been common in other fields of graduate education. At entry level of practice, the emphasis should be upon the availability of student loans and attractive salaries, career potentials, and defensible compensation models that promote individual investment in self-commitment and professional commitment.

With the decreasing supply of 18 yr olds and the increasing career options available to women, the need for nurses cannot be met just by recruiting increased numbers of young women into nursing. Rather the need must be met by (1) recruiting more men into nursing, which will be dependent upon the availability of improved salaries for registered nurses and increased potential for higher salaries through career advancement and (2) increasing the productivity of all nurses. Productivity requires increasing the proportion of nurses who elect to work full time instead of part time; decreasing the use of nurses for non-nursing activities; decreasing job turnover and absenteeism; decreasing the employment of licensed practical nurses and nursing assistants who require considerable on-the-job training and supervision by nurses and who have many hours per shift of poor-use potential. To produce such changes in use will require salary increases of 20% to 30%. Lesser increases, because of poor market elasticity in nursing, will merely increase health care costs.

The changes nursing departments must make to be able to improve productivity and quality of care require that nursing be given greatly increased control over nursing practice. The American Nurses' Association's (ANA) Commission on Nursing Services has outlined 20 characteristics of a professional nursing department, as follows:

Characteristics of a Professional Climate of Administration and Practice in a Nursing Department

1   The department has sufficient autonomy and budgetary control to be able to assume accountability for the quality of nursing practice and the outcomes of nursing care.
2   There exists in the department a system of direct communication with the board of trustees and mechanisms for shared governance, including either (1) contracted agreements or bylaws approved by the board of trustees or (2) rules and regulations to provide for clinical privileges and accountability to the governing body and to the patient.
3   Planning of program and of budget reflects variable levels of patient needs and requisite levels of staff competence.
4   Institutional policies administered by the nursing department assure shared responsibility between the institution and the individual nurse for development and maintenance of competence of the practitioners.
5   Support is given to experiments in staff utilization that have likelihood of improving the quality of care and of containing costs.
6   The compensation system for nurses recognizes educational preparation, prior professional experience and level of clinical competence, as well as length of service.
7   Nursing policies and practices are congruent with the ANA Code for Nurses, ANA Standards for Nursing Services, ANA Standards of Nursing Practice, the state nursing practice act, the standards of the voluntary accrediting body appro-

priate to the agency and the requirements of the regulatory body appropriate to the agency.

8   Administrators are appointed whose preparation and practice are consistent with the roles, responsibilities, and qualifications for nursing administrators identified by the ANA Commission on Nursing Services.

9   Practicing nurses have individual accountability for the care of each patient/ client.

10   Provision is made for nurse-to-nurse consultation within the facility and between agencies or institutions.

11   An evaluation program assesses practitioner performance and administrative effectiveness, as well as patient outcomes.

12   Nurses receive administrative support in the role of patient advocate.

13   Staff and administrative support are provided for nursing studies and research.

14   Nursing administration and staff activities result in a sense of accomplishment and commitment to professional practice.

15   A joint practice committee promotes collegial relationships between physicians and nurses.

16   Effective around-the-clock support services are available so that nurses are not doing the work of other departments of the organization.

17   Nursing administration participates fully, by title and actions, in top level administrative decision making and with the governing body.

18   A nursing management information system and other resources are used to develop and manage planning, budgeting and monitoring quality of nursing care.

19   Nurses effectively recommend decisions on admission, placement, and discharge of patients.

20   A plan is in operation to maintain and enhance the competence of nurses through promotion strategies, scholarship resources and continuing education programming in order to meet the increasingly complex needs of patients and requirements of high technologies.[10]

The foregoing list provides a well-developed outline of what is needed, and can provide a legitimate set of goals for nursing management and staff to achieve. These goals, along with the definition of the nature and scope of nursing practice contained in *Nursing: A Social Policy Statement*, provide nurses, the public, and hospital boards with professionally, publicly, and economically defensible goals.[11] It is time for the profession to confront directly the issue of control of nursing practice by nurses.

ALTERNATIVES

It is unlikely that significantly higher salaries for nurses can be achieved except through the formation of collectivities of nurses and the use of contract law. Three possible general strategies will be described.

CONTRACTING CORPORATIONS

It would be possible under contract law for nurses to band together and form partnerships or corporations to contract with health service institutions for providing nurses services in specific areas or for the institution as a whole. Nurses could be members with profit-sharing rights or employees of nurse-controlled corporations. There has been considerable growth of this mechanism within medicine, and we have seen physician corporations contract to provide services for emergency, laboratory, radiologic, orthopaedic, urologic divisions, and others. Sometimes these contracts are limited to physician services but they may include all employees in the service area.

The power of this mechanism is that it frees the principals to be as creative and imaginative as possible in the development of contracts for the provision of professional services. It carries economic risk as well as opportunity for significant economic gain and professional freedom. Economic risk provides an empirical screen for the cost-effectiveness of staffing strategies.

Contracting by a group to provide services is a method that should be encouraged so that nursing as a profession can gain experience in its advantages and disadvantages. It is not a method that is ready to be used extensively by the masses of nurses today.

The use of temporary nursing services agencies is another example of a contracting mechanism. Aiken, Blendon and Rogers report that there are over 3,000 such agencies now operating in the United States.[12] The costs to health service agencies are high but are offset by the ability to hire additional staff only when needed and the ability to keep beds in use that could not otherwise be staffed. The nurse, through agency contracting, has been able to trade unwanted fringe benefits (often duplicative of those provided the family through the spouse's employment) for a considerably higher hourly rate. It is not uncommon to find registries offering hourly rates of twice the rate (without fringe benefits) offered by health service agencies in the same area. There have been many questions raised by the opponents of temporary agencies about the quality and continuity of nursing care provided but in fairness it must be acknowledged that these same questions remain unanswered in most institutional nursing services.

COLLECTIVE BARGAINING

The Health Amendments added to the National Labor Relations Act (NLRA) in 1974 have made it possible for nurses employed in private nonprofit health service institutions to engage in collective bargaining. Many more nurses are now turning to this legal process to improve the economics of their employment and to gain more control over the conditions under which they practice nursing. Feldman and Lee have reported that in 1977, just 3 yr after the coverage of nurses under the NLRA was expanded, 29% of all hospital nurses worked under collective bargaining agreements. This compares to less than 10% of registered nurses in nongovernmental hospitals in 1969.[13, 14] More nurses have been organized in governmental hospitals because before 1974 there were public sector labor laws in many of the states.

The historical roots of the distrust many nurses have for collective bargaining lies in a belief that strikes are unprofessional at best and repugnant at worst. The NLRA requires that where a health service institution is involved, the union must give 10 days notice of an intention to strike in order that mediation services can be used in an attempt to resolve the conflict. This 10-day period is sufficiently long to enable a hospital to stop admitting new patients, discharge most patients (average stay is about 7 days), and transfer remaining patients to other facilities. The fact that hospitals do not choose to do these things in the face of a strike indicates that the issue is economics and not quality of care.

Since 1945 the ANA has supported collective bargaining efforts by nurses. In recent years this support reflects about 10% to 12% of the association's budget. These monies are used for legal, educational, consultative, and public relations support. The activities relating to unit organizing, certifying, and negotiating are developed and supported by the state nurses' association (SNA), if that state chooses to support a collective-bargaining program. In general, in the states that have a liberal labor philosophy, there is a relatively active collective bargaining program in the SNA. By and large, SNAs do not choose their targets; instead they wait for nurses in an agency to request services. Usually it takes several months before a local group can achieve sufficiently high ANA membership level for the SNA officials to be able to defend expending association funds in the organizing activity. This requirement is easier to meet in small public health agencies, but these contracts have little economic effect beyond that agency.

In contrast, other well-established unions can come into a state, select the most politically meaningful target, put organizers in the field and charge the new nurse members nothing until that union has won the election and negotiated a contract. It is surprising that outside unions do not already represent the majority of nurses.

Richard Miller has provided a good overview of what is happening in hospital collective bargaining.[15] Nursing has used hierarchical relationships, self-effacing dedication, and selfless devotion to duty as a pathway to professionalism. As the numbers of diploma nurses in the work force decreases, gone too will be the passive obedience to administrative authority common today. The change will make unionization easier.[16]

The major unions making significant incursions among nurses include Service Employees International Union (SEIU), American Federation of State, County, and Municipal Employees (AFSME), District 1199 (health service workers) of the Retail, Wholesale and Department Store Workers Union. These unions have made their greatest inroads with nonprofessional hospital workers but have also shown increasing success with nurses. There are regional patterns with these unions but, in general, SEIU is stronger in the private sector and AFSCME in the public sector. Since 1977 District 1199 has led a separate division solely for registered nurses. The American Federation of Teachers has established a division for nurses, and has been putting significant resources into its organizing activities among nurses.

If the ANA fails to expand its collective bargaining activities and merely stands by while nurses are organized by other groups, the association must be prepared to lose over half its members. Staff nurses who are organized by other unions will not be willing to simultaneously support ANA. Such a loss of membership could not be sustained economically and the organization remain as it is today. As importantly, ANA would cease to be entitled to speak for nurses and nursing in governmental affairs. When ANA can no longer speak as the largest organization of nurses, it will lose its effectiveness in Washington. SNAs that choose not to offer collective bargaining to its members could be placed in receivership for its collective bargaining function. These services might then be offered by the national organization on a special capitation basis that could support a system of regional offices for collective bargaining activities. The collective bargaining function of ANA cannot be conducted as in the past and remain competitive in the field of labor relations. ANA cannot survive economically or politically without a much stronger collective-bargaining program.

COMBINING A SHARED GOVERNANCE MODEL AND COLLECTIVE BARGAINING

For professional nurses to be able to support collective action wholeheartedly, a new model is needed. A major conflict pertaining to collective bargaining within the ANA pertains to the negotiation of practice issues relating to patient care and staffing standards and the occasional dichotomy between professional values and local bargaining unit goals.

The executive committee of the AHA has stated, "The staffing of a hospital must be an objective process and should not be controlled by a group with special interest. . . . Nurses as an organized group are not legally responsible for patient care. Only management has the responsibility to determine the number of employees, their qualifications, and their assignment within the institution so as to be consistent with the best patient care, the most effective utilization of personnel."[17]

Such a policy position leaves the individually licensed nurses legally accountable for the nursing care they provide but with no control over the quantity or quality of staffing nor any protection from the demands by the institution or medical staff for engaging in activities outside the scope of nursing practice. There has also been a willingness of institutional administrators to "buy-off" patient care demands with economic counterproposals that may place the nurse negotiators in an untenable position with the rest of the union members. To limit negotiations to wages and hours leaves the bargaining unit helpless to improve professional practice.

The shared governance model shown in Figure 21-1 is a modification and refinement of one published earlier, and includes changes to accommodate the profession's movement in the areas of entry into practice and certification.[18]

The institutional structure shown on the left suggests the nursing structure within a health service institution. Power and authority are delegated downward from the board of trustees. There has been extensive documentation that bureaucratic organizations promote efficient allocation of resources and coordination of activities, but do not accommodate well the contributions of professionals and scientists.[19] There is a strong tendency for patterns of communication to extend downward with little opportunity for contributions of the staff to move upward through the line managers. Initiative and creativity may be stifled by line administrators who have spent years obtaining their respective positions and who may view change as personally risky or inherently undesirable.

The structure on the right in the diagram reflects a traditional union organization (local bargaining unit). With unionization, all registered nurses are divided into two groups: supervisors and nonsupervisors. Under the NLRA, supervisors do not include the coordinating type of leaders of which there seem to be many in nursing structures. Rather a supervisor is clearly defined as one "having authority . . . to hire, transfer, suspend, lay-off, recall, promote, discharge, assign, reward, or discipline. . . . or to effectively recommend such action."[20]

What is unique in the structure proposed here is the categorization of nurses within the local bargaining unit. I believe that this is needed to resolve many of the conflicts inherent in collective bargaining in nursing. This is patterned after academic and medical governance models, which channel the professional power that derives from individual expertise. The staff designations by nursing practice levels permits distinctions to be made in the negotiation of salaries; it also permits election by broad categories to governance positions. In universities these categories include instructor, assistant profes-

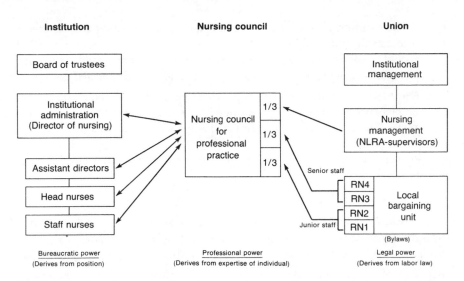

| Institution | Nursing council | Union |

FIGURE 21-1. Schema for interdependence of professional practice policy making and collective bargaining.

sor, associate professor, and professor. In medical staff organizations the categories of courtesy, associate, active, and consulting medical staff are common.

A brief description of the nursing practice levels is shown here. All personnel are assumed to be legally licensed to practice in the state in which employed.

- *Registered nurse 1 (RN1)* is an associate degree or diploma graduate with less than 1 yr experience, or a baccalaureate graduate receiving orientation, or a nurse without recent applicable experience in nursing practice. An RN1 must function under the direct supervision of a more experienced nurse.

- *Registered nurse 2 (RN2)* is a graduate from an associate degree or a diploma program who has had at least 1 year of applicable experience within the last 5 yr. The RN2 may also be a graduate of a baccalaureate degree program who has completed orientation. Essential responsibilities consist of planning and organizing patient care congruent with the current medical therapy plan.

- *Registered nurse 3 (RN3)* is a graduate of an accredited baccalaureate nursing program, who has 1 yr related experience and who demonstrates ability to practice professional nursing in a clinical area. A nurse graduated from an associate degree or diploma program with 3 yr to 5 yr applicable experience within the last 5 yr may occasionally qualify, but this is not an expected level of performance. Nurses certified by ANA at less than the advanced levels would normally be included here. This nurse has responsibility and authority for planning, providing, and evaluating care for a specific group of patients and is expected to have understanding and skill in the use of teaching and learning theories, team leadership, and evaluation of work performance of others. An RN3 would be able to engage in effective group teaching and could carry out a home assessment, by telephone or in person, of a discharged patient.

- *Registered nurse 4 (RN4)* holds a master's degree with a major in nursing and has had at least 3 yr applicable experience within the last 5 yr. This nurse has a comprehensive understanding of mental health, concepts, community nursing, family dynamics, and teaching and learning theories, in addition to demonstrated competence in an area of clinical practice.

These classifications are an abbreviated version of a system negotiated into the contract at City of Hope Hospital in Duarte, California. Thus, this categorization was accepted by the local bargaining unit and by the personnel department of that institution. In negotiated contracts RN1s might not be included in the bargaining unit until after the probationary period has passed.

These practice levels of nurses (herein referred to as RN2, RN3, and RN4) are in the process of being fully described by the ANA. These levels, defined by education, experience, and competency, must be incorporated into collective bargaining contracts in order to provide a system of upward mobility that rewards nurses differentially at various competency levels. Staffing requirements as defined by patient needs, professional standards, and accreditation requirements should determine the numbers of nurses required at various practice levels by an institution or agency. Third party reimbursement could then be tied into these service requirements and related costs of staff. It is unreasonable to expect that all persons providing direct patient care services be paid at the same scale. It is unreasonable and it does not work. Wages must be increased at the professional–practice leadership levels to provide incentives for nurses to seek advanced preparation.

All registered nurse practice levels can be accommodated in the same collective bargaining unit providing the basic framework of practice levels has been incorporated into the institution's nursing personnel framework. Separate job descriptions are needed for each level. All institutions will provide these levels when accreditation or reimbursement standards require a portion of staff at the senior competency levels.

The bylaws of the local bargaining units could provide for election of representatives to the nursing council. Since bylaws of local bargaining units are approved by SNAs, the local bargaining unit would have to comply if this were ANA's policy. The distribution of one-third of council members from nursing management, one-third from RN4 and RN3 (senior staff) levels, and one-third from RN2 and RN1 (junior staff) levels permits a proportional distribution that can accommodate the smallest group within the institution. The total size of the nursing council would be somewhat dependent upon the size of the institution. Management representatives could be elected by the management group or be appointed by the director of nursing, or could serve by nature of their institutional positions.

The third portion of the model is the nursing council. The local bargaining unit's bylaws would guarantee the process by which individuals are elected to the council. The nursing council would determine nursing practice policy and would function outside the jurisdiction of the union contract. As a university council establishes academic policy, and a medical staff organization its medical policy, here the nursing council formulates nursing practice policy. University councils and medical staff organizations have to operate within the financial constraints of the parent institution and likewise, here, the nursing council.

Using this type of model can resolve many of the profession's problems with the concept of collective bargaining. The union can negotiate freely in the area of hours, wages, and general conditions of work. Work load can be defined by the nursing council, with the union reserving the right to file a grievance for members who believe their workloads are inappropriate. The grievance procedure guarantees the process of the review but the standard is developed by the nursing council or the profession.

The nursing council would have its own set of bylaws that would specify its standing committees. It is best for the bylaws of the nursing council to be approved by the board of trustees of the institution or agency in order that compatibility with major corporation goals to be ensured. A member of the local bargaining unit or a member of management could be appointed to a specific committee because of special interest or competence, even though he does not serve on the nursing council. Some examples of possible standing committees might be staffing (long range planning, staffing standards); personnel (recruitment, absenteeism, turnover, promotions, search committee); staff development (orientation, inservice education, continuing education, academic study, travel monies); quality assurance (practice standards, performance evaluation, patient advocacy); and joint practice (multiprofessional concerns). The costs of the nursing council are legitimate institutional costs.

Once a policy has been approved by the nursing council but falls within the purview of the bargaining contract, either management or the staff council can bring the item to the negotiating table. Because the policy has been extensively discussed and developed in the nursing council in a non-adversarial manner, it is usually possible to negotiate the item into the contract without difficulty. For example, travel would be handled as a policy in the nursing council. The policy that evolved could be folded into the union contract and, at that time, the main item for negotiation would be the amount of travel monies available for professional development. Travel time for union purposes is commonly negotiated as "released time with pay" for selected union officers with the bargaining unit responsible for related travel costs.

CONCLUSION

Within any health service institution it would be possible to implement a shared governance model without collective bargaining. Many institutions voluntarily have incorporated into their personnel practices some of the most significant innovations of labor relations. These include the use of a grievance procedure to guarantee due process, defined and graduated disciplinary processes, open personnel files, and the posting of position vacancies, to name but a few. Participative management has also been heralded as an advance but, in fact, those invited to participate are selected by management.

Shared governance, without collective bargaining, can greatly improve the nature of the work environment. The process, however, incorporated into bylaws developed by the staff and approved by institutional administration and by the board of trustees, is dependent upon administrative acceptance. Shared governance alone can have no effect on the economic welfare of nurses.

Shared governance in combination with collective bargaining can provide advantages from both options. Labor law and a signed contract provide individual nurses with significant legal protections. The negotiation process, while adversarial in nature, would permit the development of compensation packages based upon nursing practice levels and responsive to the technologic changes within health services.

The nursing council would provide a balanced forum for developing staffing models, job descriptions, evaluative standards, and staff development programs that are responsive to professional values and needed institutional changes.

Collective bargaining alone, without an independent nursing council, too often will be patterned after industrial models and will protect the *status quo*. The ANA is publicly committed to levels of practice incorporating 2-yr associate nurses, 4-yr professional nurses, 6-yr clinical specialist nurses, and 8-yr nurse researchers. The levels can be cost-effective, but it will be essential to relate practice levels and compensation to provide the necessary economic incentives to reward nurses who invest in preparation for advanced practice. Without such incentives, nursing departments cannot recruit the personnel needed. Federal subsidies at the undergraduate level have had deleterious effects upon salaries and, in any case, are not likely to be forthcoming.

With a model that combines shared governance and collective bargaining, nurses can unite in support of a greatly expanded thrust to organize nurses in their places of employment. Clearly, the alternative is non-nursing unions and a politically and economically crippled professional organization. If that were to happen, nurses would continue to be denied their professional rights.

REFERENCES

1 Fagin C: Nurses' rights. Am J Nurs 75: 82–85, 1975

2 Ibid, p 84

3 Sibson RE: Compensation, p. 179. New York, American Management Association, 1974.

4 Cleland V, Smith J, McHugh N: Inducements for nursing employment. Nurs Res 22: 414–422, 1973

5 Cleland V: Characteristics of Employed Nurses in West Michigan Health Service Area. Detroit, College of Nursing, Wayne State University, 1979

6 Roth A, Graham D, Schmittling G: National Sample Survey of Registered Nurses (HRP 0900603). Kansas City, American Nurses' Association, Technical Information Service, 1977

7 Cleland V, 1979, op cit

8 Conley P: Uses of CPI. Issues. National Council of State Boards of Nursing, Inc. 2, No. 1: 3, 1981

9 Feldstein PJ: Health Care Economics, pp. 357–379. New York, John Wiley & Sons, 1979

10 Commission on Nursing Services: Characteristics of a professional climate of administration and practice in a nursing department. American Nurse 13, 1981

11 Congress for Nursing Practice: Nursing – A Social Policy Statement. Kansas City, American Nurses' Association, 1980

12 Aiken LH, Blendon RJ, Rogers DE: The shortage of hospital nurses: A new perspective. Am J Nurs 81: 1,612–1,618, 1981

13 Feldman R, Lee L: Hospital Employees' Wages and Labor Union Organization, Final Report. Washington, DC, National Center for Health Services Research, US Department of Health and Human Services, Nov 1980

14 US Bureau of Labor Statistics: Industry Wage Survey: Hospitals, March 1969 (Bulletin No. 1688), pp 219–221. Washington, DC, US Government Printing Office, 1971

15 Miller RU: Hospitals. In Somers GG: Collective Bargaining: Contemporary American Experience, pp 373–433. Madison, WI, Industrial Relations Research Association, 1979

16 Ibid, p 404

17 Ibid, p 421

18 Cleland V: Shared governance in a professional model of collective bargaining. Journal of Nursing Administration 8: 39–43, 1978

19 Kast FE, Rosenzweig JE: Organization and Management, pp. 498–526. New York, McGraw-Hill, 1970

20 US National Labor Relations Act (as amended). Washington, DC, US Government Printing Office, 1974

PATRICIA A. PRESCOTT

22

SUPPLEMENTAL AGENCY EMPLOYMENT OF NURSES

The relatively recent and rapid growth of for-profit temporary or supplemental agencies as a source of registered nurse staff for hospitals is a major change in nurse employment. To put this change into perspective, it may be useful to examine historical patterns of nurse employment and mechanisms by which hospitals have traditionally met staffing needs.

Before the Depression most graduate nurses worked as private duty nurses employed directly by clients, and generally cared for the patient within the home. Hospitals during this period relied heavily on student nurse manpower. The number of graduate nurses in hospitals was small, and they worked either as teachers, supervisors of students, or as private duty nurses employed by a particular client. Hospitals had a large, virtually free source of nurse manpower, and the number of hospitals operating schools increased dramatically between 1900 and 1929, creating a serious surplus of nurses.[1] At the end of the 1920s approximately 75% of registered nurses worked as private entrepreneurs. The surplus of nurses created competitive conditions for these private duty nurses who began to work through commercial registries, which can be seen as the forerunner of the for-profit personnel agencies of today.

In the 1920s the commercial agencies began to dominate hospital and physician lists of private duty nurses. As Wagner noted, "These registries often extracted large fees from nurses, and if disagreement arose, dropped rebellious nurses from their roles. Once black balled, a nurse found it difficult to obtain customers and could be forced to seek a different career."[2]

The economics of the Depression, the surplus of nurses, the subsequent closing of many hospital schools of nursing, and the consequent growing need of hospitals for an inexpensive, stable labor force to replace students combined to produce the collapse of private duty nursing. By the end of World War II the majority of nurses, for the first time, were employed by hospitals. The freedoms associated with independent practice were replaced by regimentation, division of labor, and intense supervision of nursing practice.[3]

With the demise of private duty registries, hospitals increasingly had to depend on their own nurses to meet staffing needs, and often prevailed upon them to work overtime, double shifts, and so forth. Some hospitals developed hospital-run "float pools" and continued to supplement existing staff with private duty nurses.

These two major means of supplementing staffing — hospital-run pools and commercial registries — differ from today's temporary personnel services in a number of ways. First, private duty registries were predominantly brokers matching patient, physician, or institution requests for services with nurses willing to provide that service for a fee. The brokerage fee was charged to the nurse, rather than to the hospital, as is the case today, and the nurses functioned as private entrepreneurs rather than as employees. Currently, nurses working for temporary personnel services are employees of the service, which is a for-profit business firm independent of the hospitals using the nursing services. Hospitals are charged a fee for use of the nurses, who on a *per diem* basis generally work without the fringe benefits associated with employee status, such as sick time, vacation time, retirement plans, and so forth.

Hospital-run pools also differ from contemporary personnel services. While in both cases nurses work primarily on a *per diem* basis and "float" to the area of greatest staffing need, the nurse in the hospital pool is a hospital employee in much the same sense as permanent full-time staff members. Until recently, hospital float nurses were subject to most of the same conditions of employment as full-time staff. Now, however, some hospitals have developed two types of pools, one a *per diem* pool that operates much like a temporary service agency (where nurses are paid on an hours-worked basis, fringe benefits are not available, and nurses are not required to rotate shifts or to work a minimum number of hours or specified days), and one in which the usual conditions of employment are in effect with the nurses differing from permanent staff members only in the sense that they float.

In summary, today's temporary personnel agencies are similar to earlier commercial registries and hospital float pools in that they use nurses on a *per diem* basis largely to supplement hospitals' permanent staffs. However, they differ from hospital pools in that they are independent, and they differ from registries in that the nurse is an employee of the agency, and in that the hospital or user of the service is charged the brokerage fee. Further, while some of the earlier registries were for-profit concerns, most were connected in some way with nursing, that is, run by nursing organizations or by individual nurses. Today, the temporary personnel agencies are owned and operated by diverse groups, very few of which are related to nursing. The absence of professional control by nurses, as well as the absence of any regulatory or licensing body, leaves the contemporary personnel service free to operate primarily in regard to market factors, which promotes intense competition in many urban areas.

The current form of temporary service employment of nurses is relatively new, and little is known about the consequences of this employment option for nurses or for hospitals. Interesting questions surround the emergence of temporary service agencies as major suppliers of nursing personnel for hospitals. For example, what factors account for the current development of temporary agencies in hospital staffing? And what are some of the implications of continued growth of this form of nurse employment for hospitals, the nursing profession, and the practice of nursing as we now know it? The remainder of this paper will consider these questions, and will include data, where available, from the ongoing study, *Temporary Service Agencies, Nurses, and Hospitals.**

DEVELOPMENT OF TEMPORARY SERVICE EMPLOYMENT

RELATIONSHIP TO NURSE SUPPLY

It has been suggested that the growth of temporary service agencies is a direct result of a nurse shortage.[4] While the rise of agency employment is undoubtedly related to the growing inability of hospitals to fill nursing positions, explaining the rise in temporary service employment of nurses purely in terms of an economic shortage — that is, an inadequate supply of registered nurse manpower relative to the demand for registered nurse services — is not convincing for a number of reasons.

First, there is considerable debate regarding whether a shortage of nurses even exists.[5] The American Hospital Association (AHA) reports about 100,000 vacant registered nurse positions nationally. The AHA and the American Nurses Association (ANA) have taken the position that the inability to fill these positions is due primarily to an inadequate supply of registered nurses.[6, 7] On the other hand, the Nixon, Ford, and Carter administrations and numerous economists have argued that the aggregate supply of registered nurses is adequate.[8–12]

Temporary Service Agencies, Nurses and Hospitals (3-yr research grant No. NU00819. Principal Investigator Patricia A. Prescott, RN, Ph.D, funded by Division of Nursing, HRA, PHS, July 1, 1980

The issue of whether or not an economically defined nursing shortage exists is complex and controversial. Some of the arguments used to support the claims of a nursing shortage include (1) increasing demand due to technologic advances and increases in patient acuity requiring more nurses; (2) the leveling off or decline in nursing school enrollments; (3) and the exodus of nurses from nursing, including those leaving the work force and those dropping their licenses and leaving the profession.[13]

Those who argue that there is no economic shortage of nurses suggest that existing vacancies are largely an artifact of improperly functioning market conditions; that the number of nurses and the ratio of nurses to population are at all-time highs that meet or exceed projected needs for nurses; that the increases in demand for nurses may be to some degree offset by a 17% decline in the number of hospital beds over the past 10 yrs; and, more recently, that hospital vacancies are due not to supply inadequacies but to the low pay, poor working conditions, and lack of autonomy, authority, and respect for nurses' contributions to both patient care and hospital management that characterize nurse employment in hospitals today.[14-20] Those favoring this explanation suggest that hospitals are not satisfying and rewarding places for many nurses to work, and that the inability of hospitals to fill positions may be more a matter of nurses not being willing to work in hospitals than of an inadequate number of registered nurses in the labor force.

The debate about the existence of a nursing shortage continues unresolved, partially because the issue is both political and economic, and partially because people use the term "shortage" in a variety of ways that are at variance with the economic meaning of the term. Regardless of the outcome of the debate over the adequacy of the registered nurse supply, all employers of nurses — hospitals, temporary service agencies, and others — are competing for the same aggregate supply. Whether that supply is judged to be adequate or not, some nurse employers, such as hospitals and nursing homes, are having difficulty recruiting and retaining registered nurses while temporary service agencies are growing and employing increasing numbers of nurses.

In California, for example, hospitals are reporting steadily increasing vacancies in staff nurse positions. Since 1977 hospital vacancies have increased from 8,300 to 10,000, despite 5,000 new graduates entering the work force each year. Further, only 55% of registered nurses licensed in California are active in nursing.[21] Against this background, temporary service agencies have proliferated and use of temporary service nurses by California hospitals has steadily increased; 53% more hospitals reported using agencies in 1979 than in 1977.[22]

The major reasons a shortage in the nurse supply does not adequately explain the rise of temporary service agencies are that (1) evidence of an economic shortage is at best inconclusive and, (2) whether the nurse supply is adequate or not, temporary service employment of nurses appears to be on the increase at the same time that hospital vacancies are steadily growing, indicating that the rise of temporary service agencies may be explained in part by the number of nurses leaving hospitals for agency employment. To understand why nurses unwilling to work for hospitals may be willing to work for temporary service agencies, it is instructive to compare the characteristics of agency and hospital employment.

RELATIONSHIP TO CONTROL OVER CONDITIONS OF EMPLOYMENT

Before the development of temporary service agencies, nurses wishing to work in hospitals did so largely in terms of the employment conditions defined by hospitals. Nurses were, and still are, commonly expected to rotate shifts, to work some percentage of weekends and holidays, to work overtime or double shifts if necessary, and to float from one unit to another based on hospital need. In general, decisions about hours of work, days off, shift rotation, and floating have been made by the hospital or nursing administrators, and staff nurses were expected to adapt to the needs of the hospital staffing system. Just a few years ago, it was not uncommon for a nurse to have different days off every week, multiple changes in shifts within a short time period, frequent requests for overtime or double shifts, expectations of working three out of four weekends, and assignment to any unit in need of additional assistance. Individual requests for changes in scheduling or exemption from the rules often were viewed as disruptive to planning or unfair to others, and variations from the established schedule were allowed only if a nurse could find another nurse willing to trade hours, days, shifts, or weekends.

The rigidity of these conditions has moderated in recent years. Some far-sighted directors of nursing have instituted flexible scheduling options and have recognized the undesirability of frequent shift changes. Despite these advances, the general conditions of nurse employment have been, and in many hospitals still are, characterized by hospital domination and inflexibility.

Temporary service agencies have altered this situation dramatically. Now nurses, rather than hospitals or agencies, can control many of the basic conditions of their employment. They are free to define for themselves if, how, when, and where they will work. When an agency has a request for service that matches a nurse's work availability, the agency calls the nurse to work. The nurse is free to accept or reject the call, and no sanctions are applied if the nurse chooses not to work.

Two studies conducted in 1979, and reported elsewhere in more detail, indicated that the single most important reasons nurses chose agency employment over hospital employment was freedom to control basic working

TABLE 22-1 Shifts Worked by Type of Nurse—Temporary Service Agency and Hospital Staff Nurses

Shift Worked	Type of Nurse	
	Temporary Service	Hospital Staff
Days	31% (N = 30)	25% (N = 27)
Evenings	33% (N = 32)	33% (N = 36)
Nights	11% (N = 11)	15% (N = 16)
Mixture of Shifts	25% (N = 25)	28% (N = 31)
Totals	100% (N = 98)	100% (N = 110)

$X^2 = 1.27$ with 3 degrees of freedom, $p = 0.73$

conditions.[23-25] The response of many nursing administrators to the flexible scheduling options available to nurses from temporary service agencies has been that "somebody has got to work the 'off' shifts and days; they can't all work eight to four, Monday through Friday." Clearly, some shifts and days are more desirable than others, and some nurses are only willing to work these preferred days and hours. Nevertheless, data from the preliminary survey of 200 staff and temporary service nurses reported in Table 22-1 indicated that there were no significant differences in the distribution of shifts worked by the sample of agency and staff nurses. As seen in Table 22-1, agency nurses worked as many evening and night shifts as did staff nurses, which dispells the notion, at least for this sample, that agency nurses work predominantly the preferred day shift. While it is inappropriate to generalize beyond this sample, anecdotal information suggests that many agency nurses prefer evening and night shifts due to family, educational, and other responsibilities. The important difference between the temporary service nurses working evenings and nights and staff nurses working these shifts, is that the choice of shift for the temporary service nurse was made by the nurse, not by the hospital or by the agency.

RELATIONSHIP TO ROLES OF TEMPORARY SERVICE NURSES

Another group of factors that may in part account for the rise of temporary service employment relates to how agency nurses are used in hospitals. While there are exceptions, especially on evening and night shifts, agency nurses generally are assigned to direct patient care rather than to supervisory or charge nurse roles. This type of assignment results from the short-term nature of the nurses' tenure in the hospital and their lack of familiarity with rules, routines, staff members, and patients. Several nurses interviewed as part of the 1979 studies indicated that despite the short duration of their contact with specific patients, they preferred this direct care role, which freed them from "nursing the system" and allowed them to focus exclusively on patient care. While data regarding the use of agency nurses are limited, it appears that agency nurses are not allowed or expected to assume some aspects of the traditional nursing role in hospitals. In particular, they are not held responsible for system maintenance functions such as supervising the work of others, enforcing hospital rules and regulations, mediating interpersonal or interdepartmental disputes, processing paper work, attending meetings, and conducting the organizational work of hospitals. As "outsiders," they are freed from many of the non–patient care and managerial functions that have been negatively associated with job satisfaction among hospital-employed nurses.[26, 27]

Several agency nurses interviewed had created situations that minimized the potentially negative aspects of being an organizational outsider while enabling them simultaneously to retain their separateness from the hospital. One nurse worked the day shift, Monday through Friday, on the same unit where she had previously worked as a hospital employee. Another nurse worked three evenings a week, always on the same type of unit, in the three hospitals close to her home. In each situation, the nurse knew the staff members, the routines, and the types of patients. These nurses felt they were sufficiently integrated into the units where they worked to provide high-quality nursing care while maintaining enough separateness to free them from system maintenance responsibilities and to preserve control over the conditions of their employment.

Whether agency employment has a positive or negative effect on how nurses practice in the hospital seems to depend in part on how the status of outsider is defined. When the agency nurse is known to those in the system, that status of outsider from the perspective of the individual nurse may be more positive than negative. On the other hand, the condition of organizational outsider has potentially negative consequences also. Some agency nurses and hospital staff members have indicated that agency nurses are often used in a nursing aide capacity because of unfamiliarity with or distrust of their abilities.[28] This underutilization of agency nurses in some situations has created resentment among nurses who have to carry a heavier load to "cover" the agency nurse. In sum, when agency nurses have some degree of familiarity with permanent staff members and the hospital, the condition of organizational outsider provides them with more control over basic employment conditions and with more freedom from system maintenance responsibilities than is enjoyed by many hospital staff nurses. Since both system maintenance activities and lack of control over working conditions have been negatively associated with job satisfaction among hospital-employed nurses, it would appear that the rise of temporary service employment can be attributed partially to these factors.

It has been suggested that the rise of temporary service employment of nurses cannot be explained solely, or even primarily, in terms of a shortage of nurses. Clearly, hospitals have been unable to meet all of their staffing needs, and agencies have responded to this unmet need by providing a service. In this sense, the growth of agencies is related to the staffing difficulties experienced by the hospitals. While the source of hospital staffing difficulties — that is, a supply shortage or an unwillingness of nurses to work in hospitals — remains hotly debated, it is clear that agencies offer nurses more control over basic conditions of employment and less responsibility for system maintenance activities than do hospitals. Further, while hospitals continue to report growing numbers of vacant positions, agency employment appears to be on the increase, suggesting that some of the major factors contributing to the rise of temporary services are the favorable conditions of employment they offer. Interestingly, some hospitals wanting to compete with, or discontinue their use of, temporary service agencies have recently created float or *per diem* pools with many of the same flexible hour options currently available through agency employment.

RELATIONSHIP TO ECONOMIC FACTORS

Another set of factors contributing to the rise of agency employment of nurses is economic in nature. Some of the economic factors relate to the wages and benefits available to the individual nurse, while others relate to cost considerations for the hospital.

First, regarding the individual nurse, both the wages and the benefits offered by agencies differ from those offered by hospitals. In general, fringe benefits such as health, life, and malpractice insurance, sick leave, vacation time, and retirement programs usually associated with hospital employment are not offered by temporary service agencies. However, the absence of fringe benefits does not seem to detract from the desirability or agency employment for many nurses.[29] This is particularly true for the young, mobile nurse who does not intend to remain employed in one setting long enough to qualify for benefits such as retirement, for the married nurse who has benefit coverage through a spouse's employment, and for the nurse who is supplementing a primary job where basic benefits are provided. The majority of the temporary service nurses interviewed as part of the 1979 studies indicated that fringe benefits, with the exception of health insurance, were of less importance than were salary and the ability to control basic conditions of employment.[30]

The wages paid by temporary service agencies appear to vary substantially by geographic region. However, data on temporary service wages are spotty. Information from two major cities indicated that the wages paid by temporary service agencies were comparable to, or slightly higher than, the starting salaries paid by hospitals. In 1978 registered nurses' salaries for five agencies in the Boston area were reported to be between $11,000 and $13,750 for 50 wk of work.[31] The average full-time staff salary for nurses working in standard metropolitan statistical areas in 1977 was $12,000 and four of the five Boston agency providers offered salaries in the $11,000 range in 1978.[32] For the Denver area, agency salaries were 6% to 9% higher than the beginning level hourly wage paid by hospitals in 1979. However, since agency-employed nurses did not receive fringe benefits, which frequently account for approximately 20% of total salary, and since agencies did not offer graded salary increases for experience or education, the total salary for an agency nurse was actually less than that paid by hospitals.

In the absence of national data on temporary service wages, we do not know to what extent the situation in Boston and Denver is generalizable. Information from at least one major eastern city indicates that agencies are offering hourly salaries 200% to 300% higher than competing hospitals.[33] This situation, difficult to understand in economic terms, may be a result of hospital efforts to defeat collective bargaining on the part of the local nurses' association. While this situation may be unique, in areas where agencies are numerous and highly competitive, or in areas where hospitals have organized to oppose organizing activities of nurses, it is reasonable to suspect that hourly salaries offered by agencies will exceed hospital starting salaries and will rise more rapidly than hospital salaries in response to competition from newly emerging agencies attempting to capture a share of the nurse market. What remains to be seen is whether agencies will exert a large and positive effect on raising nursing salaries.

Other economic considerations that may account for the rise of temporary service agencies relate to the costs of such services to hospitals. Temporary service agencies have claimed that agency usage is a cost-effective method for hospitals to supplement staff. They argue it is less expensive to use agency services than it is to staff for more than 65% to 75% occupancy.[34, 35] The assumed cost saving to the hospital derives from not having to pay for fringe benefits and recruiting and orienting costs, not having to maintain float pools, and staffing for a lower total percent of occupancy than possible when the hospital must cover occupancy fluctuations with its own employees.

Most likely, some of these claims can be substantiated for some hospitals, under some conditions, and at some level of agency usage. Unfortunately, studies conducted by disinterested parties addressing the conditions under which agency usage may be cost-effective have not appeared in the literature. In situations where hospitals are paying agencies 30% or more above the hourly cost of a permanent employee, and are using agency nurses on a regular basis to fill full-time positions, the cost savings to the hospital would seem highly questionable, compared with the cost of a permanent employee. Some hospitals have indicated that while agency usage is substantially more costly to the hospital, agencies allow the hospital to keep beds open and hence are seen as vital to the hospital's income-generating ability. The issue of whether or not agency usage is cost-effective for the hospital would seem to depend on the types of usage, the extent of usage, the per hour costs, and the consequences of not using agency nurses for the income-generating ability of the hospital.

The rise of temporary service agencies as a new type of nurse employment is undoubtedly the result of a number of political, economic, and practice factors. In particular, the growth of temporary service agencies appears to be related to the inability of hospitals to fill nursing positions, the conditions of practice and employment in hospitals, and a number of economic factors such as a higher hourly wage for the nurse and claimed cost savings for the hospital.

EXTENT OF HOSPITAL USE OF AGENCY EMPLOYED NURSES

Several studies of agency use by hospitals have been reported. White reports that usage in California in 1978 was 60%, and that it is increasing, especially in Southern California where use of agency nurses had increased 57% over that reported in 1977.[36, 37] Boyer indicates that approximately 20% of the 495 acute care, extended care, and home and public health agencies in Pennsylvania surveyed by the Pennsylvania Nurses Association reported some use of temporary service nurses in 1978.[38] A 1978 survey of city and suburban Chicago-area hospitals conducted by the Chicago Hospital Council indicated an overall use of 58%, with between 71% and 78% of city hospitals and 35% to 44% of suburban hospitals using temporary service agencies.[39]

A survey of hospitals to determine the extent of temporary service usage nationwide is underway as a part of the work of the ongoing study, *Temporary Service Agencies, Nurses, and Hospitals.* The population of eligible hospitals ($N = 4,256$) was stratified by bed size and geographic region. A disproportionate stratified random sample of 858 nonfederal, Joint Commission on Accreditation of Hospitals (JCAH)-accredited, AHA-member, short-term general hospitals was drawn.* The overall response rate to the mailed survey

*A 10% sample of hospitals with less than 100 beds, a 15% sample of hospitals with 100 to 199 beds, a 25% sample of hospitals with 200 to 399 beds, and a 50% sample of hospitals with 400 or more beds were randomly drawn.

TABLE 22-2 Percent of Temporary Service Usage by Bed Size and Geographic Region for Hospitals Completing Survey Questionnaire (N = 469)

Bed Size	Geographic Region				
	West	Midwest	South	North East	Totals
Under 100	39.1% N = 23	13.6% N = 22	11.5% N = 26	18.2% N = 11	N = 82
100– 199	58.8% N = 17	04.2% N = 24	25.0% N = 32	35.7% N = 14	N = 87
200– 399	59.2% N = 27	35.0% N = 40	27.3% N = 44	24.3% N = 37	N = 148
400 and over	70.6% N = 17	42.9% N = 56	32.5% N = 43	44.4% N = 36	N = 152
Totals	N = 84	N = 142	N = 145	N = 98	N = 469

was 58% (N = 469).† Of the 389 survey nonrespondents, 381 responded to a telephone follow-up regarding whether or not they used temporary service agencies. Thus, the usage status was obtained for 99% of the sample of 858 hospitals. Four of the eight nonrespondents refused to tell us if they used temporary service agencies, and four questionnaires were returned from closed or ineligible hospitals.

While the analysis of data from this survey is not yet complete, preliminary analysis indicates that 39.5% of all hospitals in the sample used temporary service nurses.

Table 22-2 illustrates hospital use of temporary service nurses by bed size and geographic region for survey responders, and Table 22-3 provides the same information for those hospitals that did not complete the mailed survey but did respond to the telephone follow-up regarding whether or not they used temporary service nurses.

The telephone survey of nonresponders was conducted state by state. That is, all calls to nonresponders in a given state were placed consecutively. The impression of the telephone surveyors was that, within geographic regions and within states in each region, there are pockets of users and nonusers. Thus, while the regional user rate for survey responders from hospitals of 400 plus beds in the West was 71%, there were some western com-

†The low response rate is due in part to the passive—and in some cases active—resistence to this study by some hospital associations. Some directors of nursing informed us that they had been told not to complete the questionnaire by their hospital administrators, and some hospital associations sent letters to their constituent members recommending that they not participate in the study. The ability of hospital associations to impede studies of nursing raises interesting issues about the ownership of information about nursing. It may be the case that large numbers of directors of nursing to whom the questionnaire was sent were not interested in participating in the study. However, given the amount of interest and concern directors of nursing have expressed over temporary service agencies, this explanation seems unlikely, suggesting that many directors of nursing were not free to respond to this nursing study.

TABLE 22-3 Percent of Temporary Service Usage by Bed Size and Geographic Region for Hospitals Not Returning Survey Questionnaire* (N = 381)

Bed Size	West	Midwest	South	North East	Totals
		Geographic Region			
Under 100	33.3% N = 12	27.8% N = 18	25.9% N = 27	16.7% N = 6	N = 63
100–199	71.4% N = 14	40.0% N = 20	29.4% N = 34	14.3% N = 14	N = 82
200–399	77.8% N = 18	20.0% N = 25	35.0% N = 40	44.1% N = 34	N = 17
400 and over	90.0% N = 10	69.2% N = 39	61.5% N = 39	61.3% N = 31	N = 119
Totals	N = 54	N = 102	N = 140	N = 85	N = 381

* All nonrespondents as of June 15, 1981, were contacted by phone and asked whether or not they used agency nurses. Four respondents refused to respond to the telephone survey.

munities where the user rate was zero and some where the percent of users exceeded the regional average. Additional within-region analysis will be needed to specify the geographic distribution of temporary service users and nonusers. However, as the majority of large hospitals are likely to be found in urban areas, and as agency usage generally increases with hospital bed size, it is likely that large urban areas will have higher agency usage than will small suburban and rural areas.

Data from this disproportionate stratified random sample have not yet been weighted for generalization to the population of hospitals. However, 39.5% of responder and nonresponder sample hospitals report using temporary services, demonstrating that hospital usage of temporary service nurses is both substantial and widespread.

GROWTH IN TEMPORARY SERVICE EMPLOYMENT

The economic and political implications of continued growth in the use of temporary service nurses to staff hospitals depend, to a large degree, on the type and extent of agency usage. Further, whether these implications are positive or negative depends largely on one's perspective. One potential economic consequence of growing agency usage is higher nursing wages, which is likely to be viewed as positive by nurses and negative by the hospitals having to pay those wages.

Growth in temporary service employment may lead to substantial increases in nurses' salaries by increasing the competition among employers for the available supply. If the argument advanced by Yett that hospitals have exerted a monopsonistic or oligopsonistic* control over the nurse market is correct, or even partially correct, then agencies as a new source of competition could break this control, allowing salaries to rise to their true market value.[40]

Yett has suggested that private duty nursing registries could replace or supplement nurse collective bargaining efforts to increase hospital wages.

> If the market were allowed to establish the fees, private duty earnings would rise and nurses would be attracted into this field from the inactive pool and from hospital general duty. Hospital nurse salaries would rise and the number of equilibrium vacancies would decline. When the equilibrium was finally reached, salaries in both sectors would be higher.[41]

Further, Yett indicates that registries might serve as placement agencies for hospital and private duty nurses. This relationship describes the function that temporary services are now serving for many hospitals. What Yett projects as the potential impact of nurse registries seems equally applicable for temporary services, in effect making them bargaining agents for hospital nurses.

A second and closely related consequence of temporary service employment of nurses may be on the collective bargaining efforts of nurses' associations and unions wishing to represent nurses. In at least one major city, hospitals are paying 300% more for agency nurses than they are paying their own employees. This action appears to be an effort to dilute the active organizing efforts of nurses in that city. Large-scale reliance on agency nurses would, at least in the short run, tend to decrease the potential threat of any organized job action on the part of permanent nurse employees, and to decrease the effect of their efforts to increase wages through collective bargaining contracts. Despite this potentially negative effect on wages in the short run, long-run results of agency growth would seem to favor increasing nursing wages by decreasing the oligopsonistic control of the nurse market currently enjoyed by hospitals in many areas.

Substantial increase in the supply of workers generally has a negative effect on demand for services and hence on wages. The predicted increases in nurses' wages due to increased competition among employers could be dampened if temporary service employers draw substantial numbers of nurses from the inactive pool, thereby increasing the aggregate supply of working nurses and decreasing the demand for nursing services. Temporary service employment may be particularly attractive to inactive nurses, especially

---

*Monopsonistic and oligopsonistic refer to market situations in which one or each of a few *buyers* (in this case, hospitals) exerts a disproportionate influence on the market (*i.e.*, employment of nurses).

those with young children and those wanting to work sporadically. While it is possible that continued growth in agency employment could draw from the inactive pool, substantial change in that group seems unlikely.

Johnson notes that 46% of the inactive nurses in 1977 were over 60 yr old, employed in another field, or not seeking to return to nursing. He adds,

> This leaves at the very most, 54 percent or approximately 228,000 individuals who could conceivably be tapped for employment. But over 100,000 of this latter group are under 40 and have children under 18 years age. There is a continuous stream of individuals returning to the work force from this group, and it is presumed that many more would return if conditions were right. This leaves residual group of probably not more than 30 percent of the original 423,000 who would be genuine candidates for recruitment efforts.[42]

It is likely that substantially higher wages will be needed to induce this group back to work in order to offset the cost of child care and homemaker services, costs that Aiken and Blendon note are rising faster than nurses' salaries.[43] While a substantial increase in nurse supply could dampen wage increases, it appears unlikely that temporary service employment of nurses from the inactive pool will negatively affect wages, both because a large portion of that group is not available to recruitment and because substantially higher nurse wages will probably be needed to induce those who are potentially available back into active employment. Thus, the major economic implication of continued agency growth would seem to be higher nursing wages.

Noneconomic implications of growing agency usage relate to political considerations, such as who will control nursing in hospitals. Changes in the current balance of power over nursing in hospitals could be positive or negative depending both on how these changes evolve and one's perspective on the desirability of the current situation. Hospitals, like all complex organizations, control the work behavior of their members or employees by application of positive reinforcement (salary, promotions, raises, and so forth) and negative reinforcement (disciplinary actions, such as probation and termination of employment). Orientation and other socializing processes are used to teach employees the rules, and evaluation processes are employed to ensure adherence.

Hospital regulation of nursing practice and control over employee behavior is currently maintained through a hierarchically organized line of authority, emanating from hospital administration and proceeding through various levels of nursing administration to the staff nurse. The administrative authority is based on rights and responsibilities associated with a position in an organization. From an organizational perspective, the nurse employed by a temporary service is not subject to this authority in the same way as a hospital nurse, since the agency nurse is not a hospital employee with organizationally defined rights and responsibilities. Power to regulate the agency nurse's performance largely resides with the agency and the individual nurse.

Much of the tension between agencies as employers and hospitals as users of temporary service nurses centers on the issue of accountability. Many nursing organizations, including groups of nursing administrators, state nurses' associations, and the ANA, have attempted to address this issue by establishing standards for temporary service usage.[44] However, fixing responsibility for adherence to these standards remains problematic, as hospitals have minimal power to ensure agency compliance with standards, and many temporary service agencies have not developed orientation, evaluation, and other systems to regulate employee behavior.

A large measure of control over nursing theoretically transfers from the hospital to the agency when substantial numbers of agency nurses are used on a regular basis to staff permanent, unfilled positions. However, because few agencies have developed systems to regulate employee behavior, in a sense the temporary service nurse falls through the cracks of organizational accountability systems. Of course, the hospital, as a user of the agency service, can negotiate with the agency for control over various aspects of nursing practice. Some hospitals have refused to use agencies that do not adequately screen the credentials of nurses or do not provide at least some orientation for nurses they send to the hospital. Nevertheless, large-scale use of agency nurses could tip the balance of power over nursing away from hospitals, potentially dismantling nurses services as we know them today, and increasingly forcing hospitals to negotiate with nurses and agencies over conditions they previously controlled.

While it is likely that large-scale employment of temporary nurses in hospitals will decrease the authority of the nursing department, the impact of this change on nursing practice is less clear. On the one hand, agency employment may free nurses from system maintenance activities, thereby freeing them to nurse patients rather than hospitals. On the other hand, cutting the nurse loose from the system of hospital accountability and not providing another system could lead to a situation where the only control over the quality of care delivered would be the professional values and competencies of the individual nurse.

Claims have been made that agency nurses adversely affect the quality and continuity of care delivered in hospitals.[45] These claims are difficult to evaluate, since no systematic studies of the influence of agency nurses on quality of patient care have been located. Further, in many acute care settings, patient length of stay is extremely short. Care is episodic and tertiary, rather than ongoing and primary. Continuity, in the sense of the same person providing care during a hospitalization, is frequently not realized even when temporary nurses are not used. In these settings, the use of temporary service nurses would not appear to have negative consequences for continuity of care. Their use in other settings, such as those using primary nursing, might be more problematic if there is insufficient opportunity for the primary nurse's plan to be communicated to an agency nurse.

It would appear that negative effects on quality and continuity of care are most likely to occur when an agency nurse is introduced into a new setting for a short period without adequate orientation to the patients and the setting. While this situation certainly does occur, our interviews suggest that many agency nurses work consistently in only one clinical area (such as pediatrics) or only in a small number of hospitals. They frequently work the same shifts and the same days of the week. Agency nurses working in this manner become familiar with hospital routines and policies and generally develop positive relationships with permanent staff members. Within a relatively short period of time, they become oriented to the hospital and are less likely to provide poor quality care because of insufficient information. The potential implications of agency nurses for quality and continuity of patient care would depend on the individual nurse and the way the nurse works within the hospital.

Other consequences of the growing use of agency nurses in hospitals will depend on the type of role assumed by temporary services and the order that is negotiated among agencies, nurses, and hospitals. Where the agency is motivated primarily by profit-maximizing considerations, or the hospital is a large user and hence very dependent on the agency to "keep beds open," organizational attention by either the hospital or the agency to the quality of patient care is likely to be minimal, leaving the burden for maintaining some standard of care with individual nurses. This situation would seem to place both the individual nurse and the hospital in potential jeopardy — the nurse because she is left to function without an organizational support system, and the hospital because it is held accountable for quality of care by accrediting and regulating bodies.

Where agencies are motivated by both economic and quality-of-care considerations, and where systems of professional nursing accountability are developed, it is possible that agencies could have a substantial impact on nursing practice. Such agencies could become a vehicle for establishing a professional line of nursing authority independent of the administrative authority of hospitals and similar to the professional line of physician authority. In this situation, the temporary service would function much like private professional corporations, negotiating to provide a specified set of nursing services, similar to the physician corporation that provides medical care in the Kaiser System and in emergency departments of many hospitals. From the perspective of the nursing profession, the desirability of developing a line of authority independent of hospitals would depend largely on who controls the temporary service. Nurse-owned or nurse-controlled agencies would seem to have potential for establishing professional standards of care and systems of accountability to ensure the quality of care delivered, thus providing an avenue for nursing to exert more control over the practice of nursing in hospitals. On the other hand, business or nonprofessional ownership has shown little concern with issues or standards of professional nursing practice, and it is unlikely that agencies with such ownership would exercise their potential influence over them.

It is difficult to predict whether temporary service employment of nurses will continue to expand. Many directors of nursing responding to the hospital survey indicated that they were taking steps to decrease, or altogether discontinue, their use of agency nurses. If hospitals develop flexible staffing options and compete favorably with agencies in terms of working conditions and salaries, the growth of agencies and their potential impact on nursing services in hospitals may be minimal. On the other hand, if agency employment of nurses continues to expand, it is likely that nursing wages will increase as the competition for the available nurse supply increases, thereby decreasing the monopsonistic control of hospitals.

The potential impact of growing agency employment of nurses on the quality of care, the accountability of nurses, and the control of nursing practice in hospitals is less clear and depends to a large degree on who controls the temporary service agencies and the order negotiated among hospitals, agencies, and nurses. In the situation where agencies are concerned with quality of care, accountability, and professional nursing practice, agency employment has the potential of giving nurses more control over nursing practice than is currently found in many hospitals, where nursing is controlled largely by administrative and physician authority. However, agencies concerned primarily with maximizing profits are likely to have little impact on nursing practice, making their impact more probably on nursing wages.

REFERENCES

1   Wagner D: The proletarianization of nursing in the United States, 1932-1946. International Journal of Health Services 10, No. 2, 271–290, 1980

2   Ibid

3   Ibid

4   Young JP, Giovannetti P, Lewison D, Thomas M: Factors Affecting Nurse Staffing in Acute Care Hospitals: A Review and Critique, 59–68. (DHEW Pub. No. (HRA) 81–10). Washington DC, US Department of Health and Human Services, 1981

5   Aiken L, Blendon R: The national nurse shortage. National Journal 13, No. 21: 948–953, May 23, 1981

6   Recruitment, Retention Become Key Goals in Hospitals Quest For More Nurses. Federation of American Hospitals Review: 12–16, April-May 1980

7   Ibid, p 17–19

8   Second Report to the Congress Nursing Training Act of 1975. Report of the Secretary of Health, Education and Welfare on the Supply and Distribution and Requirements for Nurses, pp. 1–184. (DHEW Pub. No. (HRA) 79-45). March 15, 1979

9   Yett DE: The supply of nurses: An economist's view. Hospital Progress 46: 89–103, Feb 1965

10 Yett DE: Application of alternative labor market models to the data on nursing: Results and Policy Implications. In Yett DE: An Economic Analysis of the Nurse Shortage. Lexington, Ma, Lexington Books, 1975

11 Deane RT: Comparative Analysis of Four Manpower Nursing Requirements Models (DHEW Pub. No. (HRA) 79-9). Washington DC, US Department of Health, Education and Welfare, Jan 1979

12 The Supply of Health Manpower: 1970 Profile And Projections to 1990. (DHEW Publication No. (HRA) 75-38). Washington DC, Health Manpower References, US Department of Health, Education and Welfare, 1974

13 Fagin CM: The shortage of nurses in the United States. Journal of Public Health Policy 1, No. 4: 293–311, Dec 1980

14 Deane RT, op cit

15 Yett DE, 1965, op cit

16 The Supply of Health Manpower, op cit

17 A crisis in health care: The nurse shortage. STAT 2, No. 2: 82–95, 1980

18 Wandelt M: Conditions Associated With Registered Nurse Employment in Texas. Austin, University of Texas, 1981

19 Weissman C, Alexander C, Chase G: Job satisfaction among hospital nurses. Health Services Res 15, No. 4: 341–364, Winter 1980

20 Demkovich LE: The nurses shortage – Do we need to train more or just put them to work? National Journal 13: 837–840, May 9, 1981

21 White CH, and Morse LE: *Hospital Fact Book*, 5th ed, p 72. California Hospital Association, 1980

22 Ibid

23 Prescott PA, Langford TL: Supplemental agency nurses and hospital staff nurses: What are the differences? Nursing and Health Care 2, No. 4: 200–206, 1981

24 Langford TL, Prescott PA: Hospitals and supplemental nursing agencies: An uneasy balance. Journal of Nursing Administration 9, No. 11: 16–20, 1979

25 Prescott PA, Langford TL: Supplemental nursing service: Boon or bane? Am J Nurs: 2140–2144, Dec 1979

26 Munson F, Heda S: Service unit management and nurses' satisfaction. Health Serv Res 128–142, Summer 1976

27 Wandelt M, op cit

28 Langford TL, Prescott PA, op cit

29 Cleland V, Smith J, McHugh N: Inducement for nursing employment. Nurs. Res 22, No. 5: 414–422, 1973

30 Prescott, PA, Langford TL, op cit

31 Emery LA: Comparison of suppliers of private duty and temporary staff nurses. Nurs Forum 18, No. 4: 321–332, 1979

32 Roth A, Graham D, Schmittling G: National Sample Survey of Registered Nurses (1977): A Report on the Nurse Population and Factors Affecting Their Supply. Washington, DC, National Technical Information Service, US Dept. of Commerce, 1977

33 Personal Communication. Pennsylvania Nurses Association, 1981

34 Dickstein G: How to Solve Your Staffing Problems. Nursing Homes 26:18–20, 1977

35 Jett M: Use of temporary nursing personnel as cost control measure. Hospital Topics: 48–50, July-Aug 1977

36 Mahan PB, White CH: A Study of the Recruitment of Registered Nurses by California Hospitals and Nursing Homes. California Hospital Association, Aug 1978

37 Ibid

38 Boyer CM: The use of supplemental nurses: Why, where, how? Journal of Nursing Administration 9, No. 3: 56–60, 1979

39 Utilization of Nurse Registry Services by Chicago Metropolitan Area Hospitals. Chicago, IL. Chicago Hospital Council, Nov 1978

40 Yett DE, 1975, op cit

41 Yctt DE, 1975, op cit

42 Johnson W: Supply and demand for registered nurses, Part 2. Nursing and Health Care 73–79, Sept 1980

43 Aiken L, Blendon R, p 951

44 Guidelines for Use of Supplemental Nursing Services (Pub. No. NS-25 3M 12/79). American Nurses Association, 1979

TERRY S. LATANICH
PATRICIA SCHULTHEISS

23

COMPETITION AND HEALTH MANPOWER ISSUES

EXECUTIVE SUMMARY

The federal antitrust laws are enforced on three levels. The Department of Justice and the Federal Trade Commission (FTC) have responsibility for enforcing these laws on the federal level. State attorneys general can also enforce the antitrust laws. Finally, some of the federal antitrust laws are enforceable by private litigants.

Application of the antitrust laws to the professions is of relatively recent origin. While it is still uncertain exactly how these laws will be applied in the health field, it appears that the courts may apply the antitrust laws somewhat differently to conduct in the health field than to conduct in other commercial and business contexts.

There are three main areas in which the antitrust laws come to bear in efforts to increase the autonomy of nonphysician providers. In each area, the extent to which application of the antitrust and consumer protection laws can stimulate meaningful competition varies.

The most significant limitation to increased independence and autonomy for nurse practitioners and, to a lesser extent, nurse midwives is state licensing law. Although some restrictions on the permissible scope of practice of health professionals are generally recognized as necessary to protect the public's health and safety, nursing groups frequently complain that state law does not permit them to practice to the full extent of their training and ability and that it is anticompetitive for physicians and physician groups to advocate more restrictive nurse practice acts.

Advocacy of restrictive state practice acts is in most cases immune from the application of the antitrust laws. The United States Supreme Court has

419

held that the antitrust laws were not intended by Congress to reach conduct protected by the First Amendment's protections of speech, association, and petitioning of government. This exemption from the antitrust laws is very broad. For example, even when the advocacy is intended to eliminate competition, such efforts to influence governmental bodies do not violate the antitrust laws. Moreover, where lobbying efforts include the use of misrepresentations, the exemption still applies. Although this exemption is broad, it is not absolute. If advocacy activities were not genuinely intended to influence a public entity to take official action, but rather were intended to intimidate the persons complained of in the communications, such activities are probably not immune from the antitrust laws.

Although the effect of the restrictions on scope of practice may be anticompetitive, state laws and regulations defining permissible scope of practice are probably exempt from the antitrust laws under what is known as the *state action doctrine*. If an antitrust suit challenging these restrictions is brought, in order to be successful it must demonstrate either that the conduct challenged is not actively supervised by the state or that the state legislature did not contemplate that the action complained of would occur.

There is also the potential for scrutiny of these regulations through the FTC Act and the possibility for economic analysis in the form of studies comparing the performance of physicians with their nonphysician counterparts in terms of cost and quality.

Reimbursement policies also can have a major impact on consumer demand for nurse practitioner and nurse midwife services. The denial of reimbursement to these providers can have serious anticompetitive results. Reimbursement policies, however, can be extremely difficult to challenge. If the reimbursement policies do not result from acts of boycott, coercion, or intimidation, they are probably immune from scrutiny. Individual insurers usually can make an independent decision to deny reimbursement to any provider without incurring antitrust liability. There may be some latitude for challenging refusals to reimburse, however, where it can be demonstrated that the insurer is controlled by physicain groups or where groups of physicians coerce the insurer into adopting policies that deny reimbursement to the physicians' competitors.

Another potential obstacle to challenging reimbursement policies is state law. Some states have laws that appear to restrict which providers' services can and cannot be reimbursed. Other states have begun to enact laws that mandate reimbursement for specified categories of providers and these laws may provide another vehicle for challenging denials of reimbursement.

The last major obstacle faced by expanded duty nurses is the inability of these providers to gain access to health care facilities. Hospital privileges enable a practitioner not employed by an institution to use that hospital's facilities. No cases challenging the denial of privileges to a nonphysician provider on antitrust grounds have been successful to date. Only rarely will future lawsuits challenging denials of privileges on antitrust grounds be successful. It will probably only be in those instances where an anticompetitive purpose can be demonstrated, or where it can be shown that the hospital delegated its decision-making authority to the medical staff and that medical staff acted arbitrarily, that privileges decisions will be reachable on antitrust grounds.

INTRODUCTION

In many respects, health manpower questions have been the forgotten stepchild of those who advocate competition as the best means for regulating the health services market.[1] Antitrust and consumer protection enforcement have focussed primarily on attempts by physicians and physician organizations to interfere with efforts by health insurers to control costs, prevent other physicians from working with innovative health care providers such as health maintenance organizations (HMOs), fix prices through devices such as relative value fee schedules, or restrain the flow of price information through bans on advertising.[2-5] Questions concerning competition between physicians and nonphysician health provider groups have received far less attention, although, as we will discuss below, some landmark reforms have been achieved through cases brought by private litigants. While the elimination of anticompetitive practices that limit the autonomy and independence of nonphysician health providers might yield significant benefits for the public in terms of increased access to care and decreased costs, some of the hurdles encountered in bringing competition to the manpower market through the antitrust laws may prove to be insurmountable. Thus, in some areas, the most successful means to effect needed reforms may be through legislation.

The independence and autonomy of any health care provider group is essentially determined by three factors: (1) the permissible scope of practice for that group contained in state licensing laws; (2) the ability of that group to secure access to necessary health facilities, such as hospitals; and (3) the ability of that group to obtain reimbursement from private and governmental third party payers. We will discuss each of these factors, explain how the antitrust and consumer protection laws have been applied in each and point out some avenues for addressing these problems other than through traditional antitrust enforcement.

Understanding how the antitrust and consumer protection laws can be used to reform health manpower policies requires some familiarity with the basic federal antitrust and consumer protection laws that are applicable to health manpower questions, as well as a general understanding of how these laws have come to be applied to the professions. Generally speaking, the federal laws governing competition among health professionals are the Sherman Antitrust Act and the FTC Act.[6,7] Under Section 1 of the Sherman Act, "[e]very contract, combination. . . or conspiracy, in restraint of trade or commerce among the several States . . . is declared to be illegal." Section 2 of the Sherman Act prohibits monopolization, attempts to monopolize, and combinations and conspiracies to monopolize trade or commerce. The proscriptions of the FTC Act are equally broad; Section 5 prohibits "unfair methods of competition . . . and unfair or deceptive acts or practices in or affecting commerce." As we will discuss below, while the two laws are somewhat similar, the extent to which each law may be used in addressing health manpower questions may be different. While the Sherman Act can be enforced by private litigants, it appears that the FTC Act can only be enforced by the FTC. Numerous states, however, have laws similar to the FTC Act that may be enforceable by private parties.

Although the Sherman Act dates back to 1890 and the FTC Act to 1914, the application of these laws to the professions, and in particular the health professions, is of relatively recent origin. It was not until the *Goldfarb v. Virginia State Bar* decision in 1975 that the Supreme Court made it clear that the learned professions such as medicine and law were subject to the antitrust laws.[8] *Goldfarb* is an important case in understanding how the antitrust laws are applied to the professions today. First, it definitively resolved that the antitrust laws apply to the professions. It also gave birth, however, to the notion that the antitrust laws should apply somewhat differently to the professions than they do to other lines of commerce or business.[9]

In *National Society of Professional Engineers v. United States*, the Supreme Court followed its approach in *Goldfarb* and applied the antitrust laws to a ban on competitive bidding by engineers who were members of the society.[10,11] The Supreme Court analyzed the ban on competitive bidding and found this restraint to be an anticompetitive agreement in violation of the Sherman Act. The Court, however, apparently based its decision on a "rule of reason" approach rather than what is termed a "*per se*" approach. This approach looks at whether the restraint being challenged serves to promote or unreasonably inhibit competition. The Court stated that conduct that may be anticompetitive in a business setting may actually help to promote competition in professional services. Thus, courts must analyze the unique nature of a particular profession to determine whether conduct that would otherwise be prohibited in a business context will survive antitrust scrutiny when found in the professions.[12]

The difference between the rule of reason and the *per se* standards for determining antitrust liability is important to understand. Some conduct, such as price fixing and group boycotts, has been found to almost always harm or destroy competition. Conduct of this type is normally considered to be a *per se* violation of the antitrust laws. The label "*per se*" is important, because a litigant alleging this violation need only show that the conduct in question was engaged in—direct proof of the purpose or effect of the conduct does not need to be shown. Under the rule of reason, however, proof of anticompetitive purpose or effect must be shown.

These Supreme Court decisions have laid the foundation for lower courts to analyze antitrust challenges involving the professions under the rule of reason. For example, in *Arizona v. Maricopa County Medical Society*, a federal court of appeals required that the rule of reason be used to review the setting of maximum fees by physician members of a foundation for medical care.[13,14] The court seemed to proceed from the assumption that in a business context price fixing of this nature would be held to be a *per se* violation of the antitrust laws. The court's decision in this case is currently pending before the Supreme Court, which may clarify whether the antitrust laws will be applied differently to the professions than to other lines of business or commerce.

Bearing in mind these principles, we turn now to the specific limitations to increased autonomy for the nursing profession, beginning with the state licensing laws that define the permissible scope of practice for the nursing profession, and in particular, nurse practitioners.

PERMISSIBLE SCOPE OF PRACTICE

The most significant limitation to increased independence and autonomy for nurse practitioners and to a lesser extent nurse midwives, is state licensing law.[15] Some restrictions on the permissible scope of practice of health professionals are generally recognized as necessary to protect the public's health and safety. In every state, the permissible scope of nursing practice is detailed either in a statutory practice act, or through regulations promulgated by the state medical board, nursing board, or both.[16–18]

One of the most common complaints heard from the nursing profession, particularly from nurse practitioners, is that state law does not permit them to practice to the full extent of their training and ability.[19] From the perspective of the nonlawyer, it may be difficult to understand why it is not a violation of the antitrust laws for physicians to attempt to control the extent of duties a nurse practitioner may perform independently. These efforts range from testimony and lobbying by physician organizations during consideration of amendments to nursing and medical practice acts that would permit the performance of expanded duties by nurse practitioners, to the situation where concurrence by the boards of both medicine and nursing is required before expanded practice is permitted. As we explain below, however, advocacy of restrictive practice acts for nurse practitioners or other provider groups by physician groups is not in most instances a violation of the antitrust laws. Moreover, it is likely that virtually all of the state laws and regulations defining permissible scope of practice of nurse practitioners are exempt from the antitrust laws. Thus, while it may be true that unduly restrictive practice acts are anticompetitive, they do not, in most instances, violate the antitrust laws.

ADVOCACY OF RESTRICTIVE STATE LAWS

As federal law enforcers, we frequently receive complaints from nurse practitioners and other nonphysician health care providers about the anticompetitive nature of certain activities of physicians and physician groups. These complaints frequently concern the advocacy of legislation or regulatory changes that would prohibit the nonphysician providers from practicing independently or that would narrow the scope of practice of already independent practitioners. These provider groups express concern that because of the deference normally shown by state legislatures to physicians on health-related questions, physicians are able to achieve anticompetitive outcomes in legislative settings. Thus, we are frequently asked why certain efforts by physicians to impose restrictive practice acts on their potential competitors do not violate the antitrust laws.

As a general rule, activities undertaken to influence governmental decisions are exempt from the antitrust laws. This exemption, known as the *Noerr-Pennington doctrine*, is based on the finding that the Sherman Act was not intended by Congress to reach conduct protected by the First Amendment's protections of speech, association, and petitioning of government.[20] It is a broad exemption and does not depend upon the motives of the person seeking governmental action. Even when the advocacy, testimony, or lobbying is intended to eliminate competition, joint efforts to influence governmental bodies do not violate the antitrust laws. Nor is the exemption affected if the lobbying effort includes the use of misrepresentations, misleading statements, or distorted information. The courts have determined that the antitrust laws were not intended to remedy such conduct.[21]

The exemption is somewhat narrower when the activities in question are directed at judicial or administrative decision making, as opposed to legislative action. In 1972 the Supreme Court ruled that activities that effectively denied competitors access to the administrative and judicial processes were not protected from antitrust scrutiny.[22] The Court also noted that conduct that might be tolerated in the legislative arena was unacceptable in an adjudicatory proceeding, and thus conduct involving bribery, fraud, or perjury was not immune from antitrust scrutiny. While these activities might well be subject to prosecution if employed to influence the legislative process, they would not give rise to antitrust liability.

In *Feminist Women's Health Center v. Mohammad,* a federal appellate court held that the Noerr-Pennington doctrine did not apply to nongovernmental bodies that had been granted some authority under state law to monitor the quality of care delivered in the state.[23] An abortion clinic sued several obstetricians and gynecologists who were members of the local hospital's gynecology and obstetrics staff, alleging that the physicians attempted to monopolize the market for abortion services. The Center complained that the defendants attempted to coerce the clinic's physicians into severing their association with the clinic by various means, including communications to the state board of medical examiners, the local medical society, and the head of the residency program of the local hospital. The communications requesting the state board of medical examiners to investigate possible violations of the medical practice act were held immune under the Noerr-Pennington doctrine absent proof of a sham. Whether conduct is a sham depends on whether it was genuinely intended to influence a public entity to take official action or whether it was intended merely to chill otherwise proper conduct by the parties complained of in the communications.[24] The court also held, however, that although the medical society and the medical staff play some role in the regulation of the quality of medical care provided, this role did not make them public regulatory bodies.[25] Thus, the joint advocacy activities directed at the local medical society and the hospital staff were not immune under the Noerr-Pennington doctrine.[26]

In most cases, advocacy by physician groups urging state legislatures or regulatory bodies to adopt restrictive practice acts or to implement restrictive practice regulations for nonphysicians does not violate the antitrust laws. Even where economic concerns form the basis for legislative advocacy the conduct remains exempt.

STATE LAWS AND REGULATIONS

As a general rule, state statutes and regulations defining the permissible scope of medical and nursing practice are exempt from the antitrust laws under the state action doctrine. The state action doctrine is perhaps the most significant limiting factor in bringing "competition" to health manpower decision making through the antitrust laws. This doctrine was first enunciated by the Supreme Court in its 1943 decision in *Parker v. Brown.*[27] The Court in *Parker* found that the Sherman Act applies only to the conduct of private parties, not to conduct engaged in by the states.[28]

Since *Parker* the courts have struggled to define which state regulatory schemes are immune from the antitrust laws as state action. While we will not trace that development here, it is accurate to say that considerable confusion and controversy remain over the full scope and desirability of this exemption from the Sherman Act.[29] Recent cases have begun to clarify the test for determining whether a state regulatory scheme and private conduct consistent with that scheme are exempt from the Sherman Act. First, the conduct must be actively supervised by the state.[30] Second, where anticompetitive conduct has been engaged in by a subordinate state entity, such as a state licensing board, to be protected the actions of the state agency must be pursuant to a clearly articulated state policy to displace competition with regulation or monopoly public services.[31] In essence, this second prong of the test for state action requires that the state legislature have contemplated that the state agency would or might engage in the specific conduct at issue before immunity will be conferred.

In applying the state action doctrine to the state practice acts for the medical and nursing professions, it is extremely difficult, if not impossible, to argue that immunity does not attach. The first prong of the test, active state supervision, will likely be very difficult to contest. The state boards of medicine and nursing in every state actively supervise the practice of those professions.[32] There may be, however, situations where the state board is the same as the state society, and it can be argued that the state's authority has been delegated to a private party. In such an instance it could be argued that no adequate state supervision exists.

If antitrust challenges are to avoid conflict with the state action doctrine they likely must do so on the second prong — the lack of a clearly articulated state policy to displace competition with regulation. In those states where restrictions on expanded nursing practice are specified in state statutes, there is obviously an articulated state policy. In those states where the legislature has delegated to the state boards of medicine and nursing the responsibility to determine the scope of permissible practice, an argument can be made that the antitrust laws can be used to scrutinize the actions of the boards. Where the state legislature has delegated authority to a state board to define the scope of permissible practice, it is clear that the legislature contemplated that regulations would be adopted. What is not clear, however, is what the state legislature must contemplate to achieve immunity from the antitrust laws. For example, most states currently permit nurse midwives to manage routine pregnancies. If, in a state that requires that regulations defining the scope of expanded nursing practice be concurred in by the board of medicine, the state board of medicine were to define the management of all pregnancies as the exclusive domain of physicians, can it be said that the legislature contemplated the medical board's activities? The determinative question concerning immunity is whether the legislature must contemplate the action taken by the subordinate state agency (*i.e.*, adopting regulations defining the scope of practice for physicians) or contemplate the specific result of the action (*i.e.*, adopting a regulation which excludes qualified competitors). Unfortunately, prior court decisions interpreting the state action doctrine provide little, if any, guidance on this question.

It is possible that the antitrust laws can be used in situations where it can be demonstrated that the effect of the actions of a board is inconsistent with the intent of the state legislature. In a recent case involving the accounting profession, the Department of Justice challenged a regulation prohibiting competitive bidding by accountants, which had been imposed by the Texas State Board of Public Accountancy.[33] The Board had enacted the regulation pursuant to a general delegation of authority from the Texas legislature to promulgate regulations to maintain "high standards of integrity" in the profession. A federal appellate court upheld the district court's finding that the ban on competitive bidding was not contemplated by the Texas legislature and thus was not immunized by the state action doctrine.[34]

At least in this instance, the court was willing to look behind the justification offered by the state board. Thus, it is possible that in a situation where the state has authorized expanded nursing practice, and the medical board in that state passes regulations seemingly in conflict with the pronouncements of the state legislature in authorizing expanded nursing practice, the antitrust laws can be used to scrutinize the actions of the medical board.

Carefully designed and litigated private antitrust suits have the potential to avoid conflict with the state action doctrine and bring the antitrust laws to bear on the actions of medical boards in drafting scope of practice regulations. In essence, the joint decision by the members of the medical board to promulgate restrictive regulations or regulatory actions taken by the board in concert with private groups would have to be challenged as agreements in restraint of trade. Suits of this type will face an uphill battle to establish liability for the actions of medical boards.

Another possibility for reform of scope of practice laws and regulations is that of FTC intervention under the FTC Act. Section 5 of the FTC Act prohibits "unfair or deceptive acts or practices."[35] The FTC has argued that the state action doctrine does not apply to the "unfair act or practice" standard of the FTC Act where it can establish that state laws cause substantial injury to consumers, and are contrary to public policy.[36] The FTC's "unfair act or practice" authority, which is the basis for the FTC's consumer protection activities, parallels the aims of the antitrust laws in many respects, but focusses directly on the harm to consumers rather than the harm to competition, which is the focus of the antitrust laws. The Commission's authority to preempt state action, however, remains judicially untested.[37]

Even assuming that the FTC's authority to preempt state laws that are immune from Sherman Act scrutiny were upheld by the courts, it is not clear whether the Commission could, or would, employ that authority. Two factors bear directly on the ability of the Commission to exercise this authority: the difficulty of proving that the laws result in substantial injury to consumers; and pending Congressional initiatives to remove authority from the Commission to investigate state-licensed professionals.

An example of the difficult evidentiary burden the Commission carries in these matters is best demonstrated by an example from the optical market. In some states opticians are permitted by law to duplicate existing eyeglass lenses without a written prescription. In others, however, the duplication of lenses is defined in the optometric practice act as the practice of optometry. In order to determine whether the restrictions resulted in "substantial consumer injury," the FTC must analyze whether the state regulation generates offsetting benefits, such as improved quality of care.[38] An evaluation of the quality of care justification requires that the level of comparative quality between the competing provider groups be measured, a task seldom, if ever, undertaken in the health literature.

The FTC staff did, in fact, conduct a cost-quality study on this issue. The data showed that this scope of practice restriction increased consumer costs and may actually have led to an overall reduction in the quality of care available in the community.[39] Yet, in one area of performance (involving approximately 5% of all cases), the evidence showed wholly unacceptable performance by the opticians in terms of the quality of the delivered services. The question thus arises, can it be said that the regulation results in substantial consumer injury? In this instance, the Commission did not reach the question of whether the unfairness standard had been satisfied.[40] To date, the Commission has not passed on whether it believes it can balance cost against quality of services, even when the increase in quality attending restrictive state laws occurs only in a limited number of cases.

The FTC currently has pending several initiatives that seek to examine state scope of practice restrictions. These investigations focus on state laws and board regulations governing the practices of dental auxiliaries, denturists, and opticians. Even if the FTC does not (or can not) employ Section 5 of the FTC Act to challenge state laws that might be found to be "unfair acts or practices" within the meaning of Section 5, it appears that the FTC is inclined to gather information, prepare reports, and conduct landmark studies on scope of practice issues, and to use these studies as a vehicle to urge states to reform their laws in those instances where it is demonstrated that they are unduly restrictive.[41] Moreover, where such studies are conducted by the FTC, they may well be used by private litigants to bolster arguments that regulations promulgated by medical boards are anticompetitive, and not contemplated by the state legislatures in question.

The question of whether the Commission will be permitted to continue to explore scope of practice issues is clouded by pending congressional legislation designed to prevent the Commission from preempting state laws and regulations. During the consideration of the FTC Improvements Act of 1980, an amendment offered by Senators McClure and Melcher that would have eliminated Commission jurisdiction over all state-regulated professions was narrowly defeated in the Senate by a vote of 47 to 45.[42] This bill would not only have prevented the FTC from preempting state law, it would also have prevented the FTC from even conducting economic studies on these questions or bringing suit against professionals for wholly private conduct such as price fixing or deceptive advertising. Similar legislation was introduced into the House of Representatives during the First Session of the 97th Congress.[43]

SUMMARY

The limitations to employing the Sherman Act and the FTC Act to reform unduly restrictive state scope of practice laws or board regulations are considerable. There is some hope, however, that they may not be insurmountable. Through the FTC Act there is the potential for scrutiny of these regulations and hope for economic analysis in the form of studies comparing the performance of physicians with their nonphysician counterparts in terms of cost and quality.

The greatest potential for action, however, remains with private litigants. Immunity from the antitrust laws does not exist where state boards have acted outside the contemplation of their state legislatures. Where actions of medical boards have the effect of restricting the scope of practice of their competitors, inroads may be made into those actions through the antitrust laws by fashioning suits that challenge those actions as being outside the contemplation of the legislature. While such suits may succeed in avoiding the state action defense, proof will still be required that an unreasonable restraint of trade exists.

ABILITY OF NONPHYSICIAN PROVIDERS TO SECURE THIRD PARTY REIMBURSEMENT

Reimbursement policies can have a major impact on consumer demand for nurse practitioner and nurse midwife services. If third party insurers pay for physician services, but cover only a fraction or none of nurse practitioner or nurse midwife services, consumers will have an obvious disincentive to select these providers. The failure of health insurers to reimburse nurse practitioners and nurse midwives can have serious anticompetitive results.

Within the general rubric of "denial of reimbursement" are several distinct forms of denial that may have anticompetitive impacts: (1) refusals by health insurers to reimburse nonphysician providers for performing services that, even if performed by physicians, would not be reimbursed; (2) refusals by insurers to reimburse nonphysician providers for services that would be reimbursed if provided by physicians; and (3) requirements imposed by law or the insurer's internal policy that require nonphysician providers to bill their services through physicians or that require prior physician referral or determination of medical necessity. Each of these situations poses different competitive questions, and brings into play unique problems with the antitrust laws.

NONREIMBURSABLE SERVICES

Nurse practitioners and other nonphysician providers frequently encounter refusals by some health insurers to provide reimbursement for specific forms of treatment or care. Perhaps the most common examples are policies that do not cover nervous or mental disorders. An example in the nursing field can be found in the refusal of many health insurers to reimburse directly for the practice of educating and counseling patients concerning good nutrition and preventive health care.[44] Patient counseling and education, however, are major components of the care provided by nurse practitioners and nurse midwives. This fact, therefore, may be used either to deny reimbursement or to reimburse at lower levels for these practitioners' services.[45] Even though reimbursement policies of this type may have a severe impact on nonphysician providers, this problem is one that is difficult to redress under the Sherman Act or the FTC Act, because of the immunity from these laws created by the McCarran-Ferguson Act.[46] As we discuss below, the McCarran-Ferguson Act, which was enacted in 1945, exempts the "business of insurance" from the Sherman and FTC Acts to the extent that it is regulated by state law and does not involve acts of "boycott, coercion, or intimidation."[47] In *St. Paul Fire & Marine Insurance Co. v. Barry*, the Supreme Court discussed the concept of boycott as the term is used generally and in the McCarran-Ferguson Act in particular.[48] The Court stated that "[t]he generic concept of boycott refers to a method of pressuring a party with whom one has a dispute by withholding, or enlisting others to withhold, patronage or services from the target."[49] While we believe that *Barry* stands for the proposition that any boycott that violates the Sherman Act is not protected by the McCarran-Ferguson Act, at least one court has decided differently.[50]

The evidence necessary to establish a boycott is not always obvious. Although individuals have the right independently to refuse to deal with another, "it takes only a little additional action to make refusals to deal a part of a contract, combination, or conspiracy to boycott" and as such a violation of Section 1 of the Sherman Act.[51]

Although the McCarran-Ferguson Act was passed to cure problems not directly related to the questions we are addressing, its effect is to insulate from antitrust scrutiny, in most instances, insurers' decisions about which risks to insure. Congress' purpose in enacting the McCarran-Ferguson Act was a limited one. As the Supreme Court stated in *Group Life & Health Insurance Co. v. Royal Drug:* "[w]hile the power of the States to tax and regulate insurance companies was reaffirmed, the McCarran–Ferguson Act also established that the insurance industry would no longer have a blanket exemption from the antitrust laws."[52, 53]

The threshold issue in determining whether the McCarran–Ferguson Act exemption from the antitrust laws immunizes the insurers' decisions not to insure certain risks (and, in effect, certain professional services) is whether that conduct constitutes the "business of insurance." The Court in *Royal Drug* held that the spreading and underwriting of a policyholder's risk are the primary elements of an insurance contract and are clearly the business of insurance.[54] Thus, insurers' decisions concerning which services to reimburse would almost certainly come within the meaning of the business of insurance. For example, the decision by an insurer whether to provide mental health benefits significantly affects the cost of providing coverage, and would probably be held to constitute the business of insurance.[55]

Even absent the immunity conferred by the McCarran-Ferguson Act, the refusal by an individual insurer, or indeed each of the insurers in a market, to reimburse for specific health care services would not, in most instances, violate either the Sherman Act or the FTC Act. To establish an antitrust violation would require a showing of an illegal conspiracy to restrain trade. The unilateral decision by a health insurer not to reimburse for services irrespective of what type of health care provider delivers those services typically does not involve the use of a boycott or conspiracy. While the decision by an insurer not to cover a service offered by a nonphysician provider group may competitively injure that provider group, and may well constitute a cost-ineffective policy, that decision likely cannot be reached through antitrust enforcement.

There may be some latitude, however, for private parties to challenge the refusal by a private insurer or a Blue Shield plan to cover certain risks. For example, if a group of physicians threatened to withdraw from participating status in a health insurance plan unless an insurer agreed not to reimburse for routine physical examinations, whether performed by physicians or nurse practitioners, the conduct of both the insurer (if it accedes) and the group of physicians might be actionable under the antitrust laws as a boycott.[56] If it can be shown that competing insurers have jointly agreed not to cover certain services, liability may also exist. These situations are unlikely to occur very often. More likely is the use of subtle coercive tactics by one provider group to "encourage" an insurer or Blue Shield plan to insure a risk and cover specified services, but only when provided by that provider group. We discuss this issue later.

An area for inquiry that has not been explored in the cases to date concerns the refusal of Blue Shield plans to cover certain specified risks. As we discuss in the following section, one court has viewed the actions of medically controlled prepayment plans, like some Blue Shield plans, as conspiracies by competitors, because of the extent to which the boards of directors of some Blue Shield plans are dominated by representatives of the physician community. If a prepayment plan such as a Blue Shield plan is controlled by physician representatives and it can be shown that the refusal to cover a certain risk has a disproportionate impact on a nonphysician provider group, it could be argued that antitrust liability exists. For example, if a Blue Shield plan adopted a policy that it would not cover out-of-hospital births whether performed by a nurse midwife or a physician, such a policy would likely discriminate against the midwives because of their inability, in many instances, to gain access to hospitals, resulting in a greater portion of their practice being deliveries at home or at birthing centers.

An anticompetitive impact from a seemingly neutral policy might be used to establish that the actions of the board constituted a boycott. If a boycott were proved, the conduct would not be immunized from the antitrust laws under the McCarran–Ferguson Act. Numerous defenses could, of course, be advanced to demonstrate that the restraint of trade was a reasonable one.

DISCRIMINATION BETWEEN PROVIDERS FOR REIMBURSED SERVICES

A common practice of health insurers that has an adverse impact on nonphysician health providers concerns the refusal by some private insurers, Blue Shield plans, and increasingly by self-insuring employers to reimburse nonphysician providers for services that would be reimbursed had they been provided by physicians. An example in the field of nursing is the refusal of some insurers to reimburse for the services of a nurse midwife in managing prenatal care and delivery, while providing reimbursement to an obstetrician for performing comparable services.

UNILATERAL REFUSALS TO DEAL. In evaluating the antitrust liability for the decision of an insurer to reimburse only one of several competing health care providers for performing a covered service, it is important to focus on the conduct of each party separately. The first situation is where a private health insurer or a self-insuring employer acts unilaterally and decides not to reimburse nonphysicians. Under a doctrine known in the antitrust field as the *Colgate doctrine*, businesses generally have the right, acting unilaterally, to refuse to deal with whomever they wish.[57] As we discuss below, even where the refusal to deal with a potential customer may be harmful to that customer, the law imposes no legal duty to deal.[58]

The impact of this doctrine can best be seen through an example. Suppose in a small town with a single dominant employer, that employer decided to self-insure and reimburse employees only when covered services were provided by a physician. As a practical matter, the employer's decision would likely have a devastating competitive impact on nonphysician providers. It would be highly unusual behavior for a significant number of consumers to forego insurance coverage and select the uncovered provider.

This right to refuse to deal will likely make it difficult, if not impossible, to challenge unilateral determinations by private insurers or self-insurers not to reimburse nonphysician providers. Where an independent insurance company or a self-insuring employer has made a business determination that it will not provide reimbursement for nonphysicians, no antitrust liability will be found unless it can be demonstrated that the insurer's decision was coerced by competitors of the nonphysician providers or that the insurance company was a participant in a conspiracy to restrain trade.

The liability of medically controlled prepayment plans would theoretically be the same as any private insurer, but for the physician involvement in its governance. That is, a decision by a Blue Shield plan to reimburse physicians but not competing nonphysician providers would, if viewed as unilateral, be safe from antitrust challenge. In one court of appeals decision, however, two Blue Shield plans were not treated as single entities. Rather, because the board of directors of these plans included a substantial percentage of physicians or representatives of the organized medical community in the area served by the plans, the court viewed each of the plans as a combination of competing health providers. The case we refer to, *Virginia Academy of Clinical Psychologists v. Blue Shield of Virginia*, provides an excellent example to illustrate this point.[59]

Under Virginia law, both psychologists and psychiatrists are licensed to perform psychotherapy. Before 1972 the Blue Shield plans had directly reimbursed psychologists for psychotherapy services. After 1972 reimbursement was only made in those instances where billing was made through a physician. In 1973 the State of Virginia passed a nondiscrimination law that prohibited any insurer from failing to reimburse for the services of psychologists, podiatrists, chiropractors, and optometrists where those services would be reimbursed if provided by a physician.[60] The Blue Shield plans opted not to comply with the law and to reimburse psychologists only when their services were billed through a physician.[61] The court found that the refusal of Blue Shield to reimburse psychologists directly violated the Sherman Act. The court in essence found that the physicians on the Blue Shield Board of Directors had conspired to restrict their competition.[62] The court was not clear, however, on precisely how the Blue Shield directors had run afoul of the antitrust laws. For example, the court did not specifically address what composition of the board of directors, if any, would have negated a finding of a conspiracy among the directors, not did it indicate if the actions of the Board would have violated the antitrust laws if Virginia had only licensed psychologists but not adopted a nondiscrimination law.

The ability of insurers to refuse to reimburse nonphysician providers points out an important distinction between a "competitive" health care system created through enforcement of the antitrust laws and the type of system that can be created through legislative action. In several states laws have been enacted that require health insurers to reimburse specified providers if the insurer decides to insure against a specific risk. Generally termed freedom of choice laws, these statutes require that health insurers not discriminate in coverage against psychologists, podiatrists, chiropractors, optometrists, or other specified providers.[63] Freedom of choice laws redress inequality of treatment by insurance carriers and enable nonphysician providers to compete meaningfully in a market dominated by insurance. Where a state has enacted a law of this type, the refusal of an insurer to reimburse nonphysicians covered by the law likely becomes grounds for suit, even where the conduct would not constitute an antitrust violation. Thus, even in those instances where the antitrust laws cannot be used to rectify anticompetitive practices in the health manpower market, there may be alternative legislative strategies that can be employed to reach the desired goal.

The FTC has conducted an investigation of the composition of Blue Shield boards and other physician-organized medical service prepayment plans. This inquiry focused on situations in which physician-organized prepayment plans should be viewed not as single entities acting unilaterally in the decisions they make, but rather as a collection of competitors making joint decisions. Last year the FTC solicited comment on a proposal to issue an antitrust rule defining the situations in which physician control of Blue Shield plans would constitute a violation of the FTC Act.[64] Subsequently, the FTC withdrew that proposal and has determined to proceed on a case-by-case basis. The Commission has issued a policy statement explaining the circumstances in which provider control of health insurance plans raises antitrust questions. The FTC's statement draws some very important distinctions between various types of prepayment plans. The FTC's policy statement notes that if a plan has a majority of physician members who are elected in their individual capacities, antitrust liability may be different than if the medical society elected those members — the distinction between the two settings being the extent to which the actions of those physicians can be viewed as actions taken on behalf of all or most physicians.[65]

Other questions are raised with physician-sponsored health plans such as individual practice association (IPA) type HMOs. Under the rule of reason analysis discussed above, conduct that on balance is procompetitive, or at least not unreasonably anticompetitive, does not violate the antitrust laws. Thus, where a group of physicians integrate their practices to become in effect a single competing entity, conduct that might otherwise be viewed as restraining trade may well serve to create a new, procompetitive health care delivery entity.[66] The FTC's policy statement addresses these and numerous other subtle legal questions on which antitrust liability may hinge. It is likely that the Commission's statement will serve to focus this debate in the years to come.

Even in those situations where it can be argued that a Blue Shield plan has boycotted nonphysician providers, there may be other obstacles to successfully employing the antitrust laws. For example, in some states the law explicitly limits the provider groups that can be reimbursed by a Blue Shield plan. For example, under the Iowa law enabling the creation of Blue Shield plans, reimbursement plans can be established "whereby medical and surgical service may be provided at the expense of [the insurers] by duly licensed physicians and surgeons, dentists, podiatrists, osteopathic physicians, or osteopathic physicians and surgeons."[67] In a recent case a federal court found that the refusal of the Blue Shield plan in question to reimburse chiropractors was consistent with Iowa law, and was immune from scrutiny under the state action doctrine.[68] The court found that the state control over numerous aspects of insurance regulation satisfied the state supervision standard of the state action doctrine, and thus the refusal of Blue Shield to reimburse chiropractors was immune from the antitrust laws.[69]

Even absent the state action immunity found by the court, it is not clear that the refusal by Blue Shield to reimburse chiropractors would have violated the antitrust laws on the facts in this case. That determination would necessarily hinge on an evaluation under the rule of reason of the conduct of all parties in reaching the decision not to reimburse. What is important to bear in mind is that a legislative strategy to modify the Blue Shield enabling legislation or to secure passage of a freedom of choice law could avoid the result reached by the court. While the trend is toward the enactment of freedom of choice statutes, a number of states have enabling statutes for Blue Shield plans similar to the one found in Iowa.

CONCERTED REFUSALS TO DEAL. The foregoing discussion raised the issue of antitrust liability for entities acting alone in making decisions not to reimburse nonphysician providers. A different set of questions arises where an insurer or Blue Shield plan acts jointly with other persons to effect such a result. It is well settled that where an insurer engages in joint action with other parties that can be characterized as a boycott, that conduct can be reached under the antitrust laws, notwithstanding the McCarran-Ferguson Act's limited antitrust immunity.[70] The importance of establishing that coercive conduct or a boycott has been employed by third parties to influence insurers can best be seen by comparing two recent cases.

In *Virginia Academy*, a case discussed earlier, the plantiff psychologists sued the medical society representing psychiatrists (the Neuropsychiatric Society of Virginia or NSV) in addition to Blue Shield. In reaching its decision not to reimburse psychologists, the Blue Shield plans had actively consulted with NSV.[71] The court found that NSV had not conspired with Blue Shield to restrain trade. The court specifically held that it was not illegal for NSV to advance proposals for reimbursement policies to Blue Shield. Without a showing that NSV had taken steps to coerce Blue Shield's decision, the court found no basis for imposing liability. The court's treatment of NSV has significant implications. In those situations where an insurer receives data, views, or other input from individual physicians, or physician organizations, and where the substance of those data and views is to encourage the insurer not to reimburse nonphysician providers, it is likely that this conduct will not violate the antitrust laws.

This situation can be contrasted with a recent case brought by the FTC against the Michigan State Medical Society.[72] In that case, the FTC argued that the state medical society had attempted to coerce the local Blue Shield plan into making changes in its reimbursement policies. An administrative law judge found that the Medical Society, which had collected proxies from its members to collectively withdraw from participating status in Blue Shield if acceptable changes in reimbursement policy were not obtained, had engaged in an illegal group boycott.[73]

Thus, the cases seem to indicate that a physician organization's coercive private action to induce anticompetitive reimbursement policies may be subject to a successful antitrust action. Where the conduct in question is limited to pure advocacy as in *Virginia Academy*, it is doubtful that an antitrust violation exists. Under the First Amendment's protection of free speech, medical societies have a protected right to advocate policies affecting their economic interests.[74] So long as they do not go beyond advocacy, their conduct is protected. The more difficult issue is determining what conduct beyond simple advocacy will constitute an unlawful restraint of trade.

SUMMARY

The legal concepts that bear on antitrust liability for denials of reimbursement are numerous and interrelated. The state action doctrine, the McCarran-Ferguson Act, the distinctions between unilateral and joint action, and the rule of reason all bear on liability. Our discussion was designed to point out avenues for approaching these problems and show how legislative advocacy can be coupled with antitrust actions to achieve reform.

ACCESS TO HEALTH CARE FACILITIES
FOR NONPHYSICIAN PROVIDERS

For some nonphysician health care providers access to health care facilities may not be crucial to their ability to practice their profession, while for others access to facilities is a critical element in their ability to enjoy a full practice. For example, family nurse practitioners could probably enjoy full and successful practices using their skills without access to hospitals. Nurse midwives' practices, on the other hand, can and do suffer substantially when they are denied hospital privileges. Out-of-hospital deliveries, and particularly home births, are not acceptable to many who might otherwise seek the services of a nurse midwife.

Simply stated, hospital privileges enable a practitioner not employed by the institution to use hospital facilities. The term "hospital privileges," however, is used loosely to refer to a variety of situations.[75] In the context of physicians, hospital privileges are generally understood to mean the ability to admit patients to, and treat them in, the hospital.[76] In discussions of nonphysicians, however, hospital privileges may, and often do, denote something less than the entire range of prerogatives generally granted to physicians.[77]

The privileges accorded to physicians, which might be referred to as full medical staff privileges, may be broken down into three basic elements as follows:

- *Admitting privileges*, which enable the practitioner to admit his or her patient to the facility for care.
- *Clinical privileges*, which give the person the right to practice in the hospital as an independent contractor.
- *Medical staff membership privileges*, which include the right to vote, hold office, and sit on medical staff committees.

In the context of most nonphysicians, the term "hospital privileges" often signifies only the second element, clinical privileges.

Privileges are generally granted by the hospital governing board based upon the recommendation of the medical staff. The scope of clinical privileges that may be granted to various categories of practitioners is delineated in hospital or medical staff bylaws.[78] In addition, the hospital, in granting privileges, may further specify or limit the scope of practice within the facility, based on the practitioner's training, experience, and competence.[79] The accreditation regulations of the Joint Commission on Accreditation of Hospitals (JCAH) are a major factor in determining hospital policies on privileges for nonphysicians. JCAH standards provide that only physicians and dentists can admit a patient to the hospital.[80]

In a case recently filed by the Ohio Attorney General, the State of Ohio alleged that the JCAH standards violate the Sherman Act by restricting access by psychologists to JCAH-accredited institutions.[81] In *Ohio, ex rel., Brown v. Joint Commission on Accreditation of Hospitals*, the Ohio Attorney General alleged that JCAH and other unnamed persons have "engaged in an unlawful combination and conspiracy to suppress and eliminate psychologists from competing as fully as their licenses permit."[82] The Ohio case challenges the JCAH standard's refusal to permit psychologists to admit patients for treatment.

Clinical privileges for nurse midwives or psychologists, however, do not appear to be inconsistent with JCAH regulations.[83] Authority for granting clinical privileges to nurse midwives can be found in the "Interpretation" to Standard I on the Medical Staff, which provides the following:

> The medical staff shall delineate in its bylaws, rules and regulations the qualifications, status, clinical duties, and responsibilities of specified professional personnel whose services require that they be processed through the usual medical staff channels.[84]

Nurse midwives seem to fall within the category of "specified professional personnel," and as such are permitted to perform the following:[85]

- The exercising of judgment within their areas of competence, providing that a physician member of the medical staff shall have the ultimate responsibility for patient care.
- Participating directly in the management of patients under the supervision or direction of a member of the medical staff.
- Within the limits established by the medical staff and consistent with the State Practice Acts, the writing of orders and the recording of reports and progress notes in patients' medical records.[86]

In no reported case has a successful suit been brought challenging the denial of privileges to a nonphysician provider on antitrust grounds. Moreover, for the reasons we discuss below, we believe that only rarely will future lawsuits challenging denials of privileges on antitrust grounds be successful. We suspect that it will be only in those instances where an anticompetitive purpose can be demonstrated, or where it can be shown that the hospital has delegated its decision-making authority to the medical staff, and that medical staff has acted arbitrarily, that privilege decisions will be reachable on anti-trust grounds.

In evaluating potential liability for a decision by a hospital to deny privi-leges to a class of nonphysician providers, it is useful to draw on the antitrust principles we analyzed in our prior discussion of insurance reimbursement. The liability of the hospital that makes the ultimate privileges determination, and of the medical staff that has made a recommendation for action by the hospital, should be analyzed separately. Under the principles of the *Colgate* doctrine, if a hospital determines not to grant privileges to nonphysician pro-viders, without some form of coercion by or conspiracy with the medical staff, the hospital's decision does not violate the antitrust laws.[87]

The liability of the medical staff poses more difficult questions. Absent coercive conduct or demonstrated purpose to restrain trade, a medical staff's recommendation to deny privileges to a class of nonphysician providers is not likely to trigger antitrust liability.[88] Applying that standard in our present context, a medical staff's recommendation to deny privileges to nonphysi-cians, standing alone, likely would not be proscribed under the antitrust laws without demonstrated anticompetitive purpose.

Perhaps the most difficult situation to evaluate is where it can be argued that joint or concerted action between the hospital and medical staff has oc-curred. For example, does antitrust liability exist, either for the hospital or the members of the medical staff, where the medical staff has made a recommen-dation to deny privileges to a class of nonphysician providers and the hospital has acquiesced in that decision because of a fear of incurring the opposition of the medical staff? An analogy can be drawn to the liability of a Blue Shield board dominated by physicians.

Applying this principle in the hospital privileges setting, it could be argued that where the recommendations of the medical staff are invariably implemented by the hospital, "physician control" of the hospital exists and the actions of the hospital should be viewed as those of competitors taking joint action, not a single entity taking unilateral action. In essence, the hospi-tal's action would be treated as the acts of the medical staff. Such a finding would not impose automatic liability under the law. Rather, it would only open the door to a rule of reason inquiry in which the anticompetitive effects of the denial would be measured against the procompetitive effects. Below we discuss those few instances in which, arguably, an anticompetitive purpose has been found. We then discuss some of the factors a court might consider in applying the rule of reason analysis to hospital privileges cases.

Proof of an anticompetitive purpose is one basis for establishing antitrust liability.[89] An example of a privilege case where an anticompetitive purpose was arguably present is the *Forbes Health System Medical Staff* case brought by the FTC.[90] In *Forbes* the FTC accepted a consent decree against the medical staff after alleging that the medical staff delayed processing requests for privileges from physicians who were affiliated with HMOs, with the purpose of denying them access to the hospital.

Another example of conduct with an anticompetitive purpose, although not directly a hospital privileges case, can be found in a second FTC case, *In the Matter of Hope, et al.*[91] In *Hope*, a hospital in a small Texas community attempted to hire a physician on a guaranteed-income basis. The doctors on the medical staff of the hospital allegedly responded to the hospital's action by threatening to refuse to provide emergency room coverage, which would have effectively terminated emergency room service. The evidence collected by the FTC included a letter allegedly sent by the medical staff to the new physician containing apparent threats that he would encounter difficulty in joining the medical society if he affiliated with the hospital on a guaranteed-income basis.

Evidence of clear anticompetitive intent of the type alleged in *Forbes* and *Hope* is seldom found. Indeed, as the professions grow accustomed to scrutiny under the antitrust laws and become more circumspect in their public actions, clear evidence of anticompetitive purpose will be increasingly difficult to prove.

The medical staff and the hospital governing board can probably raise a number of grounds upon which to justify their action as being procompetitive and thus not a violation of the rule of reason. For example, one of the primary justifications offered to explain the refusal to grant privileges to nurse midwives and other nonphysician providers is a desire to avoid or minimize malpractice liability. This concern has become more pronounced over the past 10 yr to 15 yr as a result of several cases that have held that hospital liability for the acts of persons functioning within the facility extends beyond responsibility for only the negligent acts of its employees.[92] In addition, there is case law that has held that hospital medical staffs can be held responsible for the negligent acts of individual physicians who are members of the staff.[93] Malpractice premiums and malpractice liability arguably can raise the costs of services and thereby affect the ability of physicians to compete with other physicians and hospitals to compete with other hospitals for patients.

Another basis cited for the denial of privileges to nurse midwives concerns the peculiar characteristics of teaching hospitals. Many of these hospitals claim that they are committed to high-risk care in obstetrics and "that normal maternity patients [are] admitted to satisfy the practice needs of the faculty" and, presumably, the students.[94] In addition, at least one teaching hospital has justified its denial of privileges to nurse midwives by stating "that all members of allied staff are full-time employees of the institution and have faculty appointments in the School of Medicine."[95] It can be argued that the restriction of privileges to instructors is necessary to permit the teaching hospital to compete for instructors.

Perhaps the most difficult assertion for a court to reckon with under the rule of reason will be assertions that restrictions on nonphysician providers are necessary to ensure the level of the quality of care provided. No one would argue, for example, that an antitrust violation exists where a hospital denies privileges to a class of professionals, such as lawyers, wholly untrained in the delivery of health services. Although the result of the hospital's action would be anticompetitive in the sense that it prevents lawyers from competing with physicians in treating patients in hospitals, the antitrust laws recognize that some restrictions are necessary to ensure that the quality of the product or service in question does not fall below acceptable levels.[96] The thrust of this doctrine is that some restrictions are permissible because they ensure that "better" competition can exist; that in essence, the restraints are not unreasonably anticompetitive.

Applying this principle to a factual situation not quite so ludicrous, the difficult nature of the questions facing the courts becomes apparent. For example, consider the case of nurse practitioners who engage in a family general practice. If the medical staff argued that where hospitalization is warranted for a patient, a physician should be responsible for the course of treatment, is the action of the hospital in denying privileges procompetitive (or at least not unreasonably anticompetitive), because it ensures that quality does not decline beyond acceptable minimums, or is it anticompetitive because it forecloses the nurse practitioner from the market?

How a court will approach these troublesome questions under the rule of reason remains a matter of speculation. It may be that courts will view total denials of privileges as impermissible, but sustain more carefully tailored restrictions (*e.g.*, requiring all courses of treatment to be authorized by the nurse practitioner's backup physician).

CONCLUSION

As we indicated at the outset of this discussion, our intention was to discuss some of the basic concepts that come into play in efforts to increase the autonomy of nonphysician providers through the antitrust and consumer protection laws. In each of the areas we discussed — state practice acts, third party reimbursement, and access to hospital privileges — the extent to which application of the antitrust and consumer protection laws can stimulate meaningful competition varies. Enforcement of these laws can assist in ensuring that competition between health care providers remains fair, within the general parameters established by legislative bodies.

We also attempted to show how various legal doctrines may perpetuate anticompetitive results. We believe that the necessary predicate for meaningful competition between physicians and nonphysician providers lies both in vigorous enforcement of the antitrust laws and fundamental legislative reform of practice acts, insurance acts, and guaranteed access to necessary health care facilities. The antitrust laws can implement these decisions and can serve as a prod for greater competition.

Federal antitrust enforcers such as the Department of Justice and the FTC, as well as state attorneys general, can serve as catalysts in bringing antitrust and consumer protection principles to the health services market. But in terms of long-range strategy, private enforcement efforts, such as the suit brought by the Virginia psychologists, will necessarily have to carry a large share of the burden. We do not suggest that law reform suits on these issues will ultimately be successful. But antitrust principles can be used in the health manpower market to increase the autonomy of provider groups who serve as alternatives to physician-directed care.

REFERENCES

1   The views we express in this article are those of the authors and do not necessarily represent the views of the Federal Trade Commission or any individual Commissioner. We would like to express our thanks to Arthur N. Lerner and Michael R. Pollard, attorneys at the Federal Trade Commission, for their assistance in helping us prepare this document. Their assistance does not necessarily mean they concur in the analysis we offer. We would also like to express special thanks to Elizabeth R. Hilder and Erica L. Summers, attorneys at the Federal Trade Commission, whose previous work provided the factual basis for portions of our discussion.

2   *See, e.g.,* In the Matter of Michigan State Medical Society, FTC Docket No. 9129 (Initial Decision June 19, 1981), (appeal pending), where the collection of proxies by a medical society, and the threat to collectively withdraw from participating status in a Blue Shield plan unless changes were made in reimbursement practices by Blue Shield, were found to be unfair methods of competition. Initial Decision at 74.

3   *See, e.g.,* In the Matter of Medical Service of Spokane County, FTC Docket C-2853 (Consent Decree, Dec. 1976).

4   *See, e.g.,* In the Matter of American College of Radiology, FTC Docket C-2871 (Consent decree, March, 1977).

5   *See, e.g.,* The Advertising of Ophthalmic Goods and Services, 16 CFR Part 456, (1978) [Federal Trade Commission issued a trade regulation rule preempting state laws and regulations which restricted advertising by eye doctors and opticians], *remanded,* American Optometric Ass'n v. FTC, 626 F.2d 896 (D.C. Cir.

1980); *see also*, American Medical Ass'n v. FTC, 638 F.2d 443, 449–50 (2d Cir. 1980); *cert granted*, 49 U.S.L.W. 3954 (June 23, 1981) [restrictions on advertising found in the Ethical Code of the American Medical Association were declared illegal].

6   15 U.S.C. §§ 1–7 (1973).

7   15 U.S.C. §§ 41–58 (1973), *as amended by* FTC Improvements Act of 1980, Pub. L. No. 96–252, 94 Stat. 274.

8   421 U.S. 773 (1975). Over thirty years earlier, in 1943, the Supreme Court held that the American Medical Association was subject to the Sherman Act but left open the question of whether a physician's practice of his profession constituted trade. American Medical Ass'n. v. United States, 317 U.S. 519, 528 (1943).

9   *Id.* at 786–88.

10   435 U.S. 679 (1978).

11   *Id.* at 681.

12   *Id.* at 692.

13   643 F.2d 553 (9th Cir. 1980), *cert. granted*, 49 U.S.L.W. 3663 (Mar. 9, 1981). (No. 80–419). For an excellent discussion of this concept, and the application of the rule of reason generally to health care questions *see* Pollard, Michael R. and Liebenluft, Robert F. FTC, Office of Policy Planning, *Antitrust and the Health Professions*, (July, 1981).

14   643 F.2d at 556–58.

15   The analysis of nurse practice acts is based on previous work done by FTC staff attorney, Erica L. Summers.

16   As of early 1979, this was the situation in both Indiana and Tennessee where the states authorized expanded nursing functions under their medical practice acts, thus leaving expanded practice nursing to be regulated exclusively by the medical boards. Kohn, Margaret. *School Health Services and Nurse Practitioners: A Survey of State Laws* 61 (Apr. 1979).

17   As of early 1979, fourteen states had given the nursing boards total authority to regulate expanded practice. *Id.* at 97–106. In practice, however, the board of medicine can sometimes thwart any regulations the board of nursing proposes by threatening to take legal action against the board of nursing for promulgating rules relating to the practice of medicine.

18   Eight states have utilized an approach whereby the two boards must jointly promulgate regulations. Another seven states have utilized an approach whereby the board of nursing has the authority to formulate the rules and regulations but only in collaboration with the board of medicine. *Id.* Trandel-Korechuk, Darlene, and Trandel-Korechuk, Keith. How State Laws Recognize Advanced Nursing Practice, *Nursing Outlook* (Nov. 1978) 713.

19   *See Hearings on Federal Trade Commission's Activities Concerning State Regulated Professions Before the Subcomm. on Consumers of the Senate Comm. on Commerce, Science and Transportation*, 97th Cong., 1st Sess. (1981) (testimony of American Nurses Association at 5).

20   The doctrine evolved from two cases decided in the 1960's: Eastern Railway Presidents Conference v. Noerr Motor Freight Inc., 365 U.S. 127 (1961); and United Mine Workers v. Pennington, 381 U.S. 657 (1965).

21   *See, e.g.*, Eastern Railway Presidents Conference v. Noerr Motor Freight, Inc., 365 U.S. at 138–45.

22   *See* California Motor Transport Co. v. Trucking Unlimited 404 U.S. 508, 512–

515 (1972). In that case a group of trucking companies agreed to oppose, regardless of the merits, virtually every application for operating rights filed by a group of competing companies before state and federal regulatory agencies. 404 U.S. at 509.

23   586 F.2d 530 (5th Cir. 1978), *cert. denied*, 444 U.S. 924 (1979).

24   *Id.* at 543 and n.6.

25   *Id.* at 542–45.

26   *Id.*

27   317 U.S. 341 (1943).

28   *Id.* at 350–52.

29   For a discussion of the state action doctrine, *see* Federal Trade Commission, Office of Policy Planning. *Report of the State Regulation Task Force.* 1978.

30   *See* California Retail Liquor Dealers Association v. MidcalAluminum, Inc., 445 U.S. 97, 105 (1980).

31   *See* City of Lafayette v. Louisiana Power & Light Co., 435 U.S. 389, 413 (1978).

32   In similar circumstances, the control of the activities of lawyers by a state supreme court was found sufficient to satisfy the "supervision" standard. *See* Bates v. State Bar of Arizona, 433 U.S. 350, 361–62 (1977).

33   United States v. Texas State Board of Public Accountancy, 464 F. Supp. 400, (S.D. Tex. 1978), *aff'd*, 592 F.2d 919 (5th Cir. 1979), *cert denied*, 444 U.S. 925 (1979).

34   464 F. Supp. at 404, *aff'd*, 592 F. Supp. 919.

35   15 U.S.C. §45 (a) (2).

36   *See* Statement of Basis and Purpose accompanying Trade Regulation Rule on the Advertising of Ophthalmic Goods and Services (16 CFR Part 456), 43 Fed. Reg. 23992, 24000 (1978).

37   In American Optometric Association v. FTC, 626 F.2d 896 (D.C. Cir. 1980), the Court set aside efforts by the FTC to preempt state advertising bans on eye doctors and opticians. At the same time the Court noted that the question of whether the FTC can preempt state laws was a difficult one, but offered no views as to whether the Commission possessed that authority. 626 F.2d at 910.

38   *See* Commission Statement of Policy on the Scope of the Consumer Unfairness Jurisdiction, 5 (Dec 17, 1980).

39   Federal Trade Commission, Bureau of Consumer Protection. *State Restrictions on Vision Care Providers: The Effects on Consumers.* 1980, 117.

40   In lieu of challenging these regulations, the Commission is considering requiring eye doctors to return eyeglass prescriptions to consumers after they are filled. *See* Advance Notice of Proposed Rulemaking, Eyeglasses II, 45 Fed. Reg. 79823, 79826, 79829. (Dec. 2, 1980). In this manner both the scope of practice limitation and the quality issue are avoided since the optician can compete for the replacement lens market simply by refilling the original prescription.

41   This is authorized by Section 6 of the FTC Act. 15 U.S.C. §46.

42   Pub. L. No. 96–252, 94 Stat. 274 (1980).

43   *See* H.R. 3722. The preamble to the bill states as its purpose, "To place a moratorium on activity of the Federal Trade Commission with respect to certain professionals and professional associations until the Congress expressly authorizes such activity."

44 *See, e.g.*, Miller & Byrne, Inc., *Review and Analysis of State Legislation and Reimbursement Practices of Physician's Assistants and Nurse Practitioners: Vol. I* at 129–30 (1978).

45 It may be, however, that these services are reimbursed indirectly. For example, an office visit to a physician may be reimbursed for and included within the physician's fee may be charges for this educational function, whether performed by the physician or the nurse. Nurse practitioners and nurse-midwives have frequently contended that reimbursement policies of this type, which typically cover expenses for "sick" care, but exclude coverage for "well" care of the type advocated by these practitioners, discriminate against their profession.

46 15 U.S.C. §1011 *et seq.* (1976).

47 15 U.S.C. §1012 (b) (1976).

48 438 U.S. 531 (1978).

49 *Id.* at 541.

50 *See* Hahn v. Oregon Physicians' Service, 508 F.Supp. 970 (D. Ore. 1981).

51 Kintner, Earl. *An Antitrust Primer.* New York: MacMillan, 1973, 37.

52 440 U.S. 205 (1979).

53 *Id.* at 220.

54 *Id.* at 211.

55 *See, e.g.*, Virginia Academy of Clinical Psychologists v. Blue Shield of Virginia, 624 F.2d 476, 484, (4th Cir. 1980), *cert. denied*, 49 U.S.L.W. 3617 (Feb. 24, 1981).

56 *See* Section on Concerted Refusals Deal, *infra*.

57 This doctrine emerged from the case of United States v. Colgate & Co., 250 U.S. 300 (1919) in which the Supreme Court referred to "the long recognized right of trader or manufacturer engaged in an entirely private business, freely to exercise his own independent discretion as to parties with whom he will deal." 250 U.S. at 307.

58 In a recent case, the Federal Trade Commission tried to challenge this doctrine. The FTC argued that a business entity holding a monopoly in a particular market has a legal duty to deal with customers in a separate market where the effect of the refusal to deal would be to create anticompetitive results in the second market and is not supported by any substantial business justification. The court of appeals rejected the FTC's challenge to this doctrine. *See* Official Airline Guides, Inc. v. Federal Trade Commission, 630 F.2d 920, 927 (2d Cir. 1980).

59 624 F.2d 476 (4th Cir. 1980), *cert. denied*, 49 U.S.L.W. 3617 (Feb. 24, 1981).

60 *Va. Code* §38.1–824 (1980 Cum. Supp).

61 624 F.2d at 478.

62 624 F.2d at 481, 484–85, *Va. Code* §38.1–817 (1980 Cum. Supp.) requires that the "majority of the [board of directors] shall be providers of health care services." The by-laws of one of the Blue Shield Plans in *Virginia Academy*, however, required that a majority of the board be physicians. 624 F.2d at 480.

63 For example, under Virginia's law, *Va. Code* §38.1–824, discrimination against podiatrists, chiropractors, optometrists, opticians and psychologists is proscribed. Our intent here is not to endorse laws of this type. Indeed, to the extent that some of these laws require that competing providers receive "equal dollar" reimbursement, these laws raise serious questions concerning efforts to contain costs.

64 45 *Fed. Reg.* 17019 (March 17, 1980).

65   Enforcement Policy of the Federal Trade Commission with Respect to Physician Agreements to Control Medical Prepayment Plans 9–10 (Oct. 1981).

66   *Id.* at 20.

67   Iowa Code §514.1 (Pkt. Part 1981–82).

68   Health Care Equalization Committee of the Iowa Chiropractice Society v. Iowa Medical Society, 501 F.Supp. 970, 989–91 (S.D. Iowa 1980).

69   *Id.* at 991.

70   *See* Ballard v. Blue Shield of Southern W.Va., Inc., 543 F.2d 1075 (4th Cir. 1976).

71   624 F.2d at 478.

72   FTC Docket no. 9129 (Initial Decision June 19, 1981).

73   *Id.* at 74.

74   *See* Virginia State Board of Pharmacy v. Virginia Citizens Consumer Council, Inc., 425 U.S. 748 (1976). (The Supreme Court held that speech which is motivated primarily by economic interests nonetheless enjoys the First Amendment's protection. *Id.* at 761–70.)

75   The discussion of the categories of hospital privileges is taken from previous work done by FTC attorney Elizabeth R. Hilder.

76   *See, e.g.*, Physician-Hospital Conflict: The Hospital Staff Privileges Controversy in New York 60 *Cornell L. Rev.* 1075 (1975).

77   *See, e.g.*, Staff Privileges for Nonphysicians, *The Hospital Medical Staff.* 7 (Feb. 1978), 16.

78   Joint Commission on Accreditation of Hospitals (JCAH). *Accreditation Manual for Hospitals, 1981 Edition* 95, 97, and 98. JCAH is the major accrediting agency for hospitals and accredits over 5,000 of the approximately 7,000 hospitals in the United States. American Hospital Association. *Hospital Statistics, 1979 Edition,* Table 10A, p. 186. Many third party payers require JCAH accrediation as a condition of reimbursement. JCAH-accredited hospitals are automatically deemed eligible for Medicare payments, while non-accredited facilities must establish their compliance with a set of federal standards.

79   *Id.* at 95.

80   The Accreditation Manual states: "The governing body must establish policies to ensure that only a member of the medical staff shall admit a patient to the hospital. . . ." JCAH, *Accreditation Manual for Hospitals, 1981 Edition* 56. According to the Manual, membership on the medical staff "shall be limited, unless otherwise provided by law, to individuals who are currently fully licensed to practice medicine and, in addition, to licensed dentists." *Id.* at 93.

81   Ohio, ex rel. Brown v. Joint Commission on Accreditation of Hospitals, Civil Action No. C2–79–1158 (S.D. Ohio, filed Dec. 14, 1979), complaint at paragraph 16.

82   *Id.* at paragraphs 7 & 18.

83   The fact that some JCAH accredited hospitals have granted clinical privileges to nurse-midwives lends support to this conclusion.

84   JCAH. *Accreditation Manual for Hospitals, 1981 Edition* 98.

85   Specified professional personnel are defined as: individuals who are duly licensed practitioners, members of the house staff, and other personnel qualified to render direct medical care under the supervision of a practitioner who has clinical privileges in the hospital, and who are capable of effectively communicating with patients, the medical staff, and hospital personnel. JCAH, *Accreditation Manual for Hospitals, 1981 Edition* 203.

86 *Id.* at 98.

87 *See* note 57, *supra.*

88 In *Virginia Academy* the Court held that the recommendations by the Neuro-psychiatric Society of Virginia (NSV) to Blue Shield suggesting that Blue Shield terminate direct payments to clinical psychologists was not illegal activity, absent any showing of coercive conduct.

89 *See* United States v. United States Gypsum Co., 438 U.S. 422, 436 n. 13 (1978).

90 Forbes Health System Medical Staff, 94 F.T.C 1042 (1979) (consent decree).

91 FTC Docket No. 9144, 46 Fed. Reg. 13235 (Feb. 20, 1981) (proposed consent order).

92 The precise scope of hospital liability to a patient injured in the course of treat-ment is unclear. The leading case is Darling v. Charleston Community Memorial Hospital, 33 Ill.2d 326, 211 N.E.2d 253 (1965), *cert. denied*, 383 U.S. 946 (1966). In *Darling* the Illinois Supreme Court held that the hospital had a duty to establish policies and procedures to monitor the quality of care provided in the institution. 211 N.E. 2d at 258. While some courts have extended the *Darling* holding, com-mentators have noted that the decision's psychological impact has been greater than its practical effect. Several courts have made reference to *Darling* in decisions upholding the authority of a hospital to discipline a physician for mis-conduct. Law, Sylvia and Polan, Stephen. *Pain & Profit: The Policies of Malpractice.* New York: Harper & Row, 1978, 57–58.

93 Corleto v. Shore Memorial Hospital, 138 N.J. Super. 302, 350 A.2d 534 (1975). Corleto also held that the hospital, its administrator, and its board of directors may be subject to liability. The liability, however, must be linked to their negligence in recommending or granting privileges to incompetent practitioners or to their allowing these practitioners to continue to practice once their inability is or should be apparent.

94 *See Hearings on Nurse Midwifery: Consumer's Freedom of Choice Before the Subcomm. on Oversight and Investigations of the House Comm. on Interstate and Foreign Commerce,* 96th Cong., 2nd Sess. (1980) (statement of Susan Sizemore, Transcript, p. 71). Ms. Sizemore also testified that, although the hospital claimed to be a high-risk refer-ral center, only 20% of the births in the preceding year were high risk. *Id.*

95 *Id.* at 70–71.

96 *See* Pollard and Liebenluft, *supra* n. 13, at 67.

7

PRESENT CONCERNS AND FUTURE ISSUES

The final part of the book is a summary of present and future issues of major concern to nurses.

Federal health policy has been important to nursing over the past 20 years as discussed by Aiken in Chapter 1. Chapter 24, written by Elliott and Osgood, discusses federal nursing priorities for the 1980s. Their analysis is particularly helpful in establishing priorities and underscoring the need for nurses to make greater investments in state level policy decisions and in private sector approaches to resolve the remaining issues of concern to nurses.

Fagin, in Chapter 25, provides a comprehensive review of nursing's unique contributions to the nation's health. Fagin's paper is a synthesis and summary of many of the issues raised in the volume. It represents nursing's immense progress in the 1970s and its potential in the 1980s.

Chapter 26, written by Moses and Levine, presents a statistical profile of nurses in 1980 and reports trends in nurses' employment and education since the 1970s. Answers are provided to many issues raised in recent years regarding the changing employment patterns of nurses.

The final chapter, by associate editor Susan Gortner, is a commentary on the themes discussed throughout this volume by various authors. Although the authors represent varying perspectives on the future of nursing, there is strong consensus that nurses will be even more important in the future than they have been in the past.

JO ELEANOR ELLIOTT
GRETCHEN A. OSGOOD

24

FEDERAL NURSING PRIORITIES FOR THE 1980S

A review of the report of the Surgeon General's Consultant Group on Nursing, *Toward Quality in Nursing*, suggests a striking similarity between the issues and recommendations identified in 1963 and the issues that are now a matter of public concern and spirited debate. This is not surprising; the issues addressed by that body were ones of long standing — little prior attention had been given to nursing as a national resource except during wartime emergencies.

Fewer than 20 yr of federal support could hardly be expected to solve problems so deeply entrenched in the health care delivery system and in the nursing profession, especially during a period of fundamental changes in society. Now, as then, hospitals are giving increasingly complex care to greater numbers of patients; skilled nursing homes are growing in number; and communities are acutely aware of the need for new and expanded programs for health promotion, disease prevention, and care of patients in their homes. In many institutions and regions of the country, the quality of care continues to suffer as inadequately prepared or overburdened nursing staffs are called upon to provide service beyond their capacity. There is concern with making the best possible use of the skills of nurses already in the work force and with the need for innovative approaches to staffing that would increase productivity and improve care in all practice settings. Even now, too few nurses have appropriate educational backgrounds for positions of leadership as teachers, administrators, or expert clinicians. In addition, there is a continuing need to

451

stimulate the conduct of studies focusing on clinical nursing practice and research to expand the scientific base of nursing knowledge.

EFFECTS OF FEDERAL SUPPORT FOR NURSE TRAINING

Recommendations responsive to these concerns were the cornerstone of the Nurse Training Act of 1964, the most comprehensive legislation ever enacted in support of nursing. Not all of the recommendations were reflected in the provisions of the act, and some underwent modifications during the course of the legislative process. Nonetheless, the authorizations were broad and well balanced and the sums appropriated were sufficient to launch a program with the potential for increasing the supply of well-prepared nurses for the nation. Three types of institutional support were authorized: matching grants to construct and renovate nursing education facilities; special project grants' for a number of purposes including curriculum revision, development and use of new instructional technologies, and projects to improve the teaching and clinical competencies of faculty; and grants to defray a portion of the cost of educating students in diploma programs. Student financial assistance was authorized through a program of low-interest loans and scholarships, and support was continued for professional nurse traineeships to prepare registered nurses for leadership responsibilities.

In 1968, 1971, 1975, and 1979 these authorizations were extended and amended in response to changing needs and federal priorities. Institutional support in the form of capitation grants for all three types of programs preparing nurses for entry into practice was authorized in 1971, and in 1975 support for advanced nurse training and for nurse practitioner training became separate provisions — each with its own authorization for appropriation. In all, the federal investment in nurse training from 1965 through 1980 has amounted to more than $1.5 billion.

Although it is estimated that this constitutes only about 10% of the total expenditures for nursing education, federal support has contributed to increasing the supply of nurses and improving the quality of educational programs. Indeed, the positive impact has far exceeded the dollar amounts expended. In some instances, a grant awarded to a single school involved collaboration with other educational or service institutions, and the project outcomes were shared by all. In other instances, grants produced models for competency-based curricula or for continuing education that were widely replicated. Federal support has also been instrumental in increasing the proportion of schools that have sought and achieved national professional program accreditation and in encouraging schools to recruit and retain members of minority groups in their student bodies.

CHANGES IN HEALTH CARE REQUIRING MORE AND BETTER PREPARED NURSES

If the concerns of the 1980s echo those of the 1960s, it is worth examining changes that have taken place in the health care arena, changes that are important in order to understand the continuing debate over the future federal role in support of nursing. First of all, it is important to remember that passage of the Social Security Amendments occurred just after the enactment of the Nurse Training Act of 1964. Changes in health care financing have enabled countless persons to make greater use of hospital services, and have stimulated rapid growth in the nursing home industry. Unprecedented advances in the basic sciences and the development of sophisticated technologies have made more complex therapeutic interventions possible, and the number of specialized intensive care units has multiplied accordingly.

The nature of the patient population has changed as well. Those admitted to hospitals have more severe illnesses and more complex problems, yet their hospitalizations are usually shorter, presenting nurses with a more dependent and more seriously ill patient population than in the past. In addition, nurses are assuming more responsibility for interventions that had earlier been the prerogative of the physician, and are expanding their roles in the areas of assessment and management of care. All of these changes require more nurses and better-prepared nurses.

The nurse training authorizations included provisions developed to address both the quantity and quality of the nurse supply. For example, matching grants were available for construction of new facilities or for renovating space that was unusable or unsuitable for teaching. This made it possible to increase enrollments, but it also allowed schools to add independent study laboratories and to supplement conventional teaching through use of new instructional technologies. The award of capitation grants required a commitment on the part of schools to increase their enrollments or engage in efforts to recruit and retain persons from disadvantaged backgrounds, to expand the types of clinical experience provided to students, or to provide programs of continuing education. Special project grants, as well, were geared to increasing the supply of well-prepared nurses.

A substantial federal investment has been made in projects to make the nursing work force more representative of the population it serves. In addition to stimulating recruitment of minorities, a number of projects have been developed to facilitate qualification of licensed practical nurses for licensure as registered nurses. Others have been designed for persons who wish to embark on a second career in middle life. To increase the nurse supply even further, a nationwide refresher training program was launched in 1968 in more than 40 states. In addition to adding nurses to the work force, the project produced a modular training program that has subsequently been used nationwide. Projects in support of continuing education have helped practicing nurses keep pace with the changing nature of practice, and have provided the professional stimulus that keeps nurses in the work force. They have also prepared nurses for new roles such as care of patients in hospice settings.

Support for programs of advanced nurse training, together with the availability of professional nurse traineeships, has helped to increase the number of nurses available to fill positions on faculties and in administration. It has also helped nurses to develop expertise in clinical fields for the direct care of patients. In addition, federal support has provided the incentive for schools to launch programs to prepare clinical specialists and to extend the programs to accommodate nurses living and working in areas remote from university campuses.

Programs in support of nursing research and research training, supported under another authority, have enhanced many of these achievements. Findings from projects in support of clinical nursing research have provided substance and content for programs of advanced nurse training. In settings where faculties have been engaged in exploratory research, federal support has often provided incentives to intensify research productivity.

ROLE OF NURSING IN HEALTH CARE DELIVERY

Nursing has begun a reexamination of its role in the health care delivery system. Since the mid-1950s, the Division of Nursing has supported studies of the concept of an expanded role for nurses in hospitals as well as in ambulatory and community settings. Interest in the preparation of nurses for primary care gained momentum as the results of the first formal program preparing school nurse practitioners at the University of Colorado became known. In his Health Message of 1971, President Nixon highlighted the significant contribution that specialized nurse practitioners could make in extending health care services, and the Nurse Training Act of that same year provided a broadened special project grant authority for this purpose. Subsequently, in 1975 support for nurse practitioner training became a discrete authority with authorization for appropriations.

Support for nurse practitioner training programs was the federal response to the need for greater access to primary health care. The underlying unstated assumption was the primary care services provided by physicians were adequate in every respect except quantity. The fact that the introduction of nurse practitioners into the health care delivery system was perceived as a means of reducing the drain on physicians while creating greater access to health care has led to a misconception that nurse practitioners are essentially "physician extenders." Hence, debate over the future role of the federal government in support of nurse practitioner training is certain to be considered in the context of forecasts of an adequate future supply of physicians.

CHANGES IN FEDERAL COMMITMENT

While all of the progress made during the last 2 decades in improving preparation for practice is not directly attributable to the availability of federal support, few would deny its importance as a catalyst for change. Nonetheless, in spite of increases in enrollment and increases in the number of nurses in the work force, reports of shortages continue. In vetoing extensions of the nurse training acts, three successive administrations have taken the position that no further federal stimulation of enrollments was warranted and that failure to limit growth could lead to an oversupply of nurses. Congress took this view into consideration, making modification primarily in the appropriations for the program that was authorized. Some members argued that the schools should take responsibility for further increases in the nurse supply. Others contended that simply producing more nurses would not alleviate the problem of achieving a more equitable geographic distribution. Still others felt that real or perceived shortages could be largely eliminated if inactive registered nurses rejoined the work force and if those who worked part time could be induced to return to full-time employment. Thus, the Nurse Training Amendments of 1979 (PL 96–76) instructed the Secretary of Health, Education, and Welfare to conduct a study to determine the need to continue a specific program of federal financial support for nursing education. The study is intended to determine why nurses do not practice in medically underserved areas and what actions could be taken to encourage them to do so, and what actions could be taken to encourage nurses to remain in or reenter the profession. In addition, the study will consider the need for nurses in the present health care delivery system and under certain specified modifications in the system; it will also address the need for nurses from each of the three types of programs preparing for licensure as well as for those with advanced preparation for primary care, clinical specialties, teaching, and administration. Finally, costs of the various types of nursing education are to be analyzed, and the availability of alternative financing sources is to be explored. A preliminary report of this study, conducted by the Institute of Medicine of the National Academy of Sciences, has been completed; the final report is scheduled for completion in January 1983.

Meanwhile, in 1981 three bills in support of nursing education, differing in the scope of legislative authorities and in the levels of authorization for appropriation, have been considered by the Congress. The signing of the Omnibus Budget Reconciliation Act (PL 97–35) in August 1981 authorized continued support for special project grants with emphasis on increasing nursing education opportunities for persons from disadvantaged backgrounds, increasing the supply and improving the distribution of nursing personnel, and upgrading the skills of vocational or practical nurses. Projects to retrain inactive nurses and to provide continuing education are also eligible for support. The law also authorizes continued support for advanced nurse training, professional nurse traineeships, and nurse practitioner training. Authority for capitation grants is not extended, reflecting the present administration's position that the nonfederal sector must now take responsibility for maintaining enrollments and for subsidizing the costs of any necessary increases. For those schools experiencing financial hardship or in danger of losing accreditation as a result of lack of further capitation grant support, a financial distress provision was included in the legislation.

The fact that programs are authorized does not necessarily ensure that funds will be appropriated to carry them out. Clearly, the present administration intends to curb federal spending and to place more responsibility for support of health programs in the nonfederal sector. The administration does acknowledge, however, the shortage of nurses in acute care settings and the need for working toward achievement of the goals outlined in Surgeon General Julius Richmond's report *Healthy People*. If funded, the presently authorized programs can help to improve the supply of well-prepared nurses, but federal efforts will have to be matched by efforts in the health care industry.

As the title indicates, the nurse training authorizations support the training of nurses; they provide for only tangential involvement in changing the practice environment. While the training authorities can be used to prepare nurses more adequately for practice settings, they are not designed to solve the complex and interrelated causes of the nursing shortage. Problems of dissatisfaction in the work setting and inability to exercise autonomy over practice must be addressed by the health care industry. A number of institutions have designed and implemented long-range programs that have significantly reduced staff turnover and improved the quality of patient care. These innovations need to be replicated and tested in other settings.

The federal government is unable to address directly the issue of salaries and their effect on nurses' work force behavior. However, the issue will be influenced indirectly by federal decisions regarding health care financing and delivery arrangements. For example, constraints on expenditures for Medicare and Medicaid and for federally aided health programs could encourage providers to limit salary expenditures.

Requirements for nursing personnel will also be influenced by federal health policy decisions. Participants at a recent federally sponsored workshop considered the criteria for the staffing of nursing homes, emphasizing therapeutic intervention rather than the provision of traditional, custodial care. They considered as outcomes of the envisioned staffing pattern such improvements in care as reduction of incontinence, maintenance of skin tone, reduction in number of contractures, improved oral care, closer monitoring of medication effects, earlier discharge, reduction in complications, increased surveillance of nutritional status, and improved family support services. In addition, they identified the need for increasing the number of well-prepared public health nurses to carry out programs of health promotion and disease prevention, and for providing nursing care and support services to the growing number of elderly and chronically ill living in their own homes or in congregate living facilities. These shifts in emphasis would require a different level of federal commitment, based on choices made by the American public regarding the allocation of national resources.

The 1980s promise to be a challenging, if difficult, decade. Decisions regarding future federal support for nursing will be profoundly influenced by societal decisions concerning the share of national resources to be invested in health care. Legislative authorities in support of nurse training are being carefully targeted, and appropriations are expected to be more limited than in previous years. This calls for careful planning by and close collaboration among the nursing profession, the federal and nonfederal sectors, and other interested groups. Nurses must be alert and prepared to respond to policy decisions that have implications for the provision of health care. In this context, the Division of Nursing will continue to serve as a catalyst and cohesive force in the federal government for programs to improve nursing education and practice nationwide.

REFERENCES

1   Surgeon General's Consultant Group on Nursing: Toward Quality in Nursing (PHS) Pub. No. 992. Washington, DC, US Government Printing Office, 1963

2   Healthy People: The Surgeon General's Report on Health Promotion and Disease Prevention, (PHS) Pub. No. 79-55071A. Washington, DC, US Government Printing Office, 1979

CLAIRE M. FAGIN

25

NURSING'S PIVOTAL ROLE IN AMERICAN HEALTH CARE*

Over the past 2 decades, the United States has experienced a three-fold escalation in the cost of health and medical care. Previous attempts to contain these explosive costs have largely resulted in failure. The decade of the 1980s promises to be a time of fiscal austerity. Tough social choices will have to be made about the allocation of public funds. Efforts therefore have intensified to find an acceptable way of maintaining a high standard of health care for all, but at costs the country can afford.

The purchase of health and medical care differs from the purchase of other goods and services in two important ways: The consumer is not necessarily able to judge the value of alternative health services, and consumers do not pay directly for the services they receive at the time the services are rendered. In a system where almost 90% of all services are reimbursed by third party payers, neither consumers nor providers — physicians and hospitals primarily — have any incentive to economize.

New proposals to contain costs focus on the value of encouraging the development of incentives for consumers to be more economical in their choice of health insurance and health provider. Nursing has, for the most part, been ignored in recent debates about competition in health care. In this paper I discuss the essentials of the "competition" proposals and the dilemmas such proposals present for nursing. Further, recent outcome studies of nursing care are analyzed from the perspective of the potential contributions of nurses to a more competitive and more cost-effective health care system. The paper concludes with recommendations for increasing nursing's contribu-

*Keynote Address, American Academy of Nursing Scientific Session, Washington, DC, September 21, 1981.

tions to the national effort to contain the rising costs of health care while maintaining high standards of health care for all Americans.

COMPETITION AND THE PARADOX OF NURSING

The new competition proposals follow past efforts to control the rising costs of health care: the development of health maintenance organizations (HMOs); a wide array of regulatory programs including state rate setting, certificate of need, mandated health planning, and peer review; the cost containment program known as the voluntary effort initiated by the hospital industry; and more recently, a variety of other programs that have required certain employers to offer multiple forms of health insurance and coverage, and insurer cost containment activities. While the rate of increase in health care costs has not been as extreme in the past 2 yr as it was formerly, there have been negative reactions toward the increased regulation of health care instituted to control costs. These objections to regulation have given rise to the current view that competition with minimal regulation and no addition to federal health financing in the national budget will be the cure for health care inflation.

The basic ideas for competition in health care were introduced by Enthoven in a proposal for a consumer choice health plan.[1] At present, many employers offer liberal health insurance benefits to their employees. Neither employer nor employee pays taxes on the funds invested in health insurance. Enthoven's plan would terminate the existing tax-free health benefit and provide the employees with a limited subsidy in the form of a tax credit for the purchase of what they see as the best deal in health insurance; hence there is competition between plans to enlist consumers. Competition proposals now before Congress seek to stimulate competition between various insurance plans, including HMOs, offered to employed persons.*

The current procompetitive proposals contain the following four basic elements:

*   Each consumer would have to be offered a choice among several competing health insurance plans.

*Procompetition legislative proposals have been introduced in the 97th Congress, sponsored by Senator Durenberger (R-Minn; S433), Senator Hatch (R-Utah; S139), and Congressman Gephard (HR850). Hatch's proposal is similar to the bill introduced last session by then Senator Schweiker and Gephard's bill, which was cosponsored by then Congressman Stockman. Currently, Durenberger is Chairman of the Finance Health Subcommittee in the Senate; Schweiker is Secretary of the Department of Health and Human Services; Hatch is Chairman of the Senate Labor and Human Resources Committee, which handles all health matters at the full committee level; and Stockman is the Director of the Office of Management and Budget. Obviously, these major proponents have tremendous political clout, and will play major roles in pushing competition in health care.

- Government and employers who offer financial assistance would be required to offer each consumer a set dollar subsidy towards the purchase of coverage of any of the competitors.

- Tax law would be changed and a tax-cap, or maximum tax deductible health benefit, would be set. Persons choosing a plan costing less could receive a tax-free rebate from the employer, and those selecting plans higher than the cap would pay taxes on the difference.

- Physicians, and possibly other providers, would be "competing economic units," each offering a specific range of health care services.

Those economists and others who take the procompetition stance believe that a large part of health care cost escalation is caused by the current structure of health care financing, which insulates the consumer from the expense of health care and rewards providers for inefficient use of resources. Nurses by and large would agree with this viewpoint. However, when one examines the so-called consumer choice procompetition bills, several important components of choice and competition seem to be lacking. The consumer, for example, is barely visible in any proposal, and competition, where it exists, is competition among the already present conglomerate of providers who cannot be assumed to be any more competitive under this kind of organization than under previous efforts.*

Physician services are at the core of all procompetition proposals. This is to be expected since physicians are the dominant providers, control their own and others' practice, serve as gatekeepers to the system, and drive the vast majority of health care costs. Nursing is not mentioned in the current bills in any way except in home health benefits. Major changes in the visibility of nursing in reimbursement patterns would have to be contemplated for nursing to have a visible role in legislation. Such changes, particularly in ambulatory care, are hindered by state law, regulations, and interpretation. Federal legislation cannot be expected to alter restrictive interpretation of nurse practice acts within states. However, federal legislation and subsequent regulations should be shaped to facilitate change.

In addition to the reimbursement issue, there are other issues that perpetuate nursing's invisibility on the current scene. The way in which nursing services are delivered prevents clients and colleagues from identifying a constant, accountable, and knowledgeable nurse provider. Further, deemphasis on specialized knowledge and skills in many service settings contributes to an imbalanced view of the nurse's role; that is, "a nurse is a nurse is a nurse."

In spite of these problems, the force of competition should facilitate

---

*Recent articles dealing with diagnostic related groups (DRG) and usual and customary reimbursement (UCR) indicate that these methods could provide the basis for extreme abuse. One could extrapolate from these to "consumer choice" if true competition does not occur.[2, 3]

change, especially where the competency and efficiency of nurses as health care providers can be documented. Thus, some recent studies on nursing efficacy are of particular interest.

NURSING CARE OUTCOMES

Over the past 20 yr data have accumulated indicating the importance of nursing and nursing care in affecting patient outcome in and out of hospitals.[4] I will summarize here some studies relating to advances in the public's health status through nursing intervention in ambulatory and institutional care. These studies show that nursing services can contribute immeasurably to the goals of a competitive delivery system.

AMBULATORY CARE

Positive outcomes of nursing care in community settings have been demonstrated from the beginning of community health work at the Henry Street Settlement in New York. However, I will focus here on the data from the past 20 yr. Some of these data relate to persons practicing in the roles commonly designated as nurse practitioners or nurse midwives, while others deal with various types of specialty nursing backgrounds.

In studies comparing the quality of nurse midwifery with routine obstetric practice as delivered by obstetric residents, nurse midwives achieved major reductions in prematurity and neonatal mortality, decreases in percent of low birth weight babies, and increases in the number of babies born symptom free. Similar outcomes between the two groups were found on other measures except that the resident group had a higher rate of forceps delivery and the nurse midwives a higher rate of compliance with appointments.[5] It has also been found that pregnant adolescents cared for by nurse midwives were less often anemic at delivery and had more normal spontaneous vaginal deliveries and larger babies than a comparable group of patients served by obstetric residents in a South Carolina project.[6] Cost savings resulting from nurse midwife care have been well demonstrated. In New York City the 6-yr study of comprehensive ambulatory maternity care shows savings from $885 to $1,840 when compared to normal birth charges in 13 Manhattan hospitals for a Medicaid population.[7] The noted epidemiologist C. R. Miller testified before the Subcommittee on Oversight and Investigation of the Interstate and Foreign Commerce Committee in December 1980, that all studies "confirm that the health benefits of care as rendered by nurse-midwives stand up to scientific scrutiny exceedingly well."[8]

While midwives are more successful than most other nurses in reaching the public interest, which includes the possibility for reimbursement, there are serious and growing barriers to midwifery practice. A precursor to some of the current conflicts was the experience of the nurse midwives in Madera County, California, in the early 1970s. A hospital clinic study of a nurse midwifery service in that county showed a marked decrease in prematurity among poor women and the reduction by more than 50% of neonatal mortality. Despite these positive outcomes, the nurse midwifery service ceased to exist after 3 yr when the California Medical Association refused to support a permanent change in legislation allowing nurse midwives to practice. Data for the 2 yr following termination of the service showed that prematurity had returned to the levels existing before the nurse midwifery program and neonatal mortality had tripled.[9] It is interesting to note that midwives practice in areas with the lowest population, lowest per capita income, lowest average hospital census, and the highest birth rates.[10] The evidence is clear that the positive outcomes of nurse midwife practice are staggeringly impressive. It should be evident that nurse midwives substitute for physician care — an already reimbursable service — at a lower cost and at equal or higher quality.

With regard to the nurse in primary care, a great deal of evidence shows successful outcomes as measured by standards of cost and quality. The most recent data summarizing all the studies that have been done indicate that nurse practitioners alter the production of medical services in a way that improves access and reduces cost. "In twenty-one studies comparing primary ambulatory care by nurse practitioners . . . with care by physicians there were essentially no differences between the two types of health providers in relation to outcome of illness and process of care."[11]

Examples of the varied clientele nurses serve with success are impressive. Data from research conducted at the Miami Center for Retarded Adults indicated that a nurse practitioner–staffed clinic is more cost-effective than an on-call physician who either visits the Center when needed or treats patients from the Center in his office. Off-site episodic treatment was reduced almost by one-half, and on-site episodic treatment almost tripled. Follow-up care also improved.[12]

Runyon's studies in Memphis of nurses' roles in the continuing clinical care of patients with selected chronic diseases have shown dramatic improvements in reducing diastolic blood pressures of hypertensive persons, reducing blood glucose levels of diabetic patients, and achieving a 50% reduction of hospitalization.[13]

In a study of home and nursing home care of chronically ill elderly persons, using nurse practitioners with physician backup, it was found that hospitalization frequency and length of stay were markedly reduced compared with similar populations receiving traditional care.[14] Martinson's studies of home care of dying children provide significant evidence of improved quality, improved satisfaction, and lowered costs.[15]

Even the report of the Graduate Medical Education National Advisory Committee (GMENAC), though guarded about the further production of nurse practitioners, concludes that they provide primary care without jeopardizing quality, are generally highly accepted by patients, and in some settings result in cost savings.[16]

Lest you assume the positive outcomes of nurse intervention in ambulatory and home care are related to a lower risk in the population served, a great deal of documentation shows that the patients first relegated to nurses in midwifery, primary care, and psychiatric nursing are the sickest, poorest, most complicated, and the most socially undesirable.[17]

NEONATAL MORTALITY

Numerous studies of the decline in neonatal mortality among low birth weight infants have attributed this decline to the "development of . . . medical technology for the successful management of premature infants and the consequent proliferation of this technology. Furthermore, although the effectiveness of neonatal intensive care has . . . been questioned . . . a number of studies evaluating specific intensive care units or regionalized perinatal networks do indicate a substantial benefit."[18]

These studies show declines in mortality ranging from 50% upward. While physicians and others have contributed to the development of such technology, nurses implement these developments through the 24-hr provision of neonatal care, and nursing must take a large share of the credit for the decline in neonatal mortality.

RENAL TRANSPLANT PATIENTS

Primary nursing was documented to be cost-beneficial in improving postoperative adaptation of renal transplant patients.[19] It was found that patients in the group receiving care from primary nurses required fewer days of hospitalization than a control group that received routine nursing care. In addition, a significant difference was found between the two groups in the number of complications after surgery. Patients receiving primary care were able to return to their homes and families an average of 28 days after transplantation, a full 3 wk before the control group. Because usual transplant patients require private rooms due to their immunosuppression, the reduction in length of stay results in substantial financial savings for patients and insurance providers.

CARDIAC PROBLEMS

Nationally there are more than 650,000 survivors of the 1 million myocardial infarctions per year. The majority of these people are in their most economically productive years, ages 40 to 64. Therefore, any program effective in reducing underemployment and social disruption potentially has large economic and social benefits.[20] During a 16-mo period, a study was done at Baltimore City Hospital of 102 sequential patients who had had myocardial infarctions. The effect of a coronary care unit–based nurse rehabilitator was examined in a prospective, randomized, controlled trial. The results of this study documented that the nurse rehabilitator, at minimal costs, was effective in increasing patients' return to work, improving knowledge of their disease, and decreasing their smoking. The importance of the smoking factor alone is an extremely important finding. The Framingham Study estimated that myocardial infarction incidents would be reduced 26% to 50% in a general population of adult males, depending upon the age when smoking was terminated.[21] Other studies have also indicated that increase in knowledge encourages myocardial infarction patients to assume responsibility for their own health, resulting in higher levels of posthospitalization performance.[22]

Although prevention and rehabilitation appear to have a far greater effect in cost saving than does dramatic technologic intervention, it is important to recognize that the coronary care unit is assumed to be responsible for a 33% reduction in in-hospital mortality.[23, 24] We must acknowledge and make known the effect of nursing on this extraordinary reduction in in-hospital mortality through the highly sophisticated technologic expertise of critical care nurses.

THE CHRONICALLY ILL

One final example concerns chronically ill patients. The Loeb Center for Nursing and Rehabilitation at Montefiore Hospital in New York City was established in 1963 to provide chronically ill patients a program of nursing care aimed at returning them to independent living as soon as possible. In the early 1970s the Department of Health, Education and Welfare (HEW) supported an evaluation of the Loeb Center. Patients were randomly assigned to Loeb or traditional care at Montefiore, and were followed for 18 mo after discharge. Loeb patients scored higher on assessments of functional status, experienced fewer hospitalizations and nursing home admissions, and incurred significantly lower overall costs (*see* Chap. 12).

SUMMARY OF NURSING CARE OUTCOMES

In summarizing outcome studies of nursing intervention in acute care, chronic care, primary health care, and health promotion, it should be clear that we no longer need to rely on feelings, impressions, and unsubstantiated opinions. A large amount of data attests to the phenomenal contribution of nurses in reducing morbidity and mortality, improving the capacity of people to function as productive members of society, enhancing quality of life by maintaining independent living, and reducing the overall costs of health care.

Data also indicate the increased incidence of iatrogenic complications from a variety of medical interventions.[25-28] In contrast, a recent study shows that increases in the number of nurses in communities are associated with improved health outcomes. In a study of the relative impact of community health resources — physicians, nurses, and hospital beds — on the community's health status, Miller and Stokes found that only an increase in nurses per capita was associated with declines in infant mortality and age and sex–adjusted death rates.[29] Thus, there is a clear cut case substantiating nurses' effectiveness in health care delivery.

The plethora of data about nursing contributions to health care outcomes is unknown to the public and barely known to nurses themselves. It is somewhat paradoxical that many nurses do not focus on these extraordinary contributions but are preoccupied with the quest for a unique definition of the nursing discipline.* It is no accident that this challenge often serves as a stumbling block isolating nurses from the economic and academic mainstreams. In academe, it takes the form of questioning why nursing should be considered a profession and what the unique body of knowledge is that constitutes the discipline. The concept "to nurse" applies to so many human caring activities that it presents an immediate hurdle to a group wishing to be identified as a learned profession. The noted philosopher Milton Mayeroff has commented, "We sometimes speak as if caring did not require knowledge, as if caring for someone, for example, were simply a matter of good intentions or warm regard."[30]

The data I have presented make clear that the range of caring functions undertaken by nurses is from the simple to the most complex. Nursing includes helping others do things they normally do for themselves in the activities of daily living; providing assistance — including technology — for

---

*I recommend the American Nurses Association's 1980 publication entitled *Nursing A Social Policy Statement*. This statement delineates the nature and scope of nursing practice and characteristics of specialization in nursing in the context of social policy.

maintaining, restoring, or replacing normal functions; applying sophisticated interpersonal and technologic treatment to enable people to cope with disease, and providing this care in a wide variety of settings that may influence the process in some way. Many aspects of nursing's caring role having to do with the presence, consistency, and continuity of care have remained constant. Other aspects having to do with advanced technology and knowledge have changed over the years. It is this amalgamation and breadth that form the basis for nursing's unique contributions and its requisite knowledge base.

No professional group can be said to "own" advances in knowledge of health and illness. Nursing draws its knowledge base from a variety of other disciplines that affect nursing phenomena. The scientific knowledge that provides a base for medical practice is also an amalgamation from a variety of disciplines. However, physicians have not had to defend their *unique* contributions or their *unique* body of knowledge to maintain their power in the total health–medical care system. While the data I have presented give ample evidence of nursing's unique contributions to health care, nursing as a discipline, in terms of its knowledge base, is no more and no less unique than any other applied social, medical, or engineering science.

MAXIMIZING THE UNIQUE CONTRIBUTIONS OF NURSING TO THE HEALTH CARE DELIVERY SYSTEM

How can we maximize the potential for nurses' contributions to the health care system at a time of growing concern and action to reduce health care spending? In examining previous proposals with regard to reimbursement for nursing services, it is apparent that, for the most part, nurses have recommended *expanding* the scope of services reimbursed by third party payers as well as adding categories of practitioners. Nurses have bemoaned the fact that health promotion and disease prevention services have not been included in benefit packages, and have recommended that other services such as home health care be expanded.

This approach for obtaining reimbursement for nurses has not been successful. What did achieve some success, however, was the direct reimbursement to some nurses offering services already reimbursed under current benefit packages, for example, normal obstetric services of midwives, psychotherapy by nurses, delivery of anesthesia by nurse anesthetists, and some primary care services delivered by nurse practitioners. A quest for direct reimbursement in ambulatory care that suggests *substitution* of nurses for other providers on the basis of cost, and both short-term and long-term quality, must be explored in relation to the supply of physicians in the United States in the coming decades. It should be clear that proposals for direct reimbursement for nurse providers who substitute for physicians imply head-on competition with physicians for the health care dollar. Since such reimbursement requires changes in legal and regulatory mechanisms, explicit recognition of this problem is essential and a conscious decision made whether to engage in such competition.

Proposing that nurses substitute for physicians to obtain third party reimbursement may be repugnant to some nurses. Therefore some greater explanation may be warranted. Reimbursable services are not necessarily medical services. Many reimbursable services fall in the area of overlap between nursing and medicine. Immunizations, for example, are a traditional responsibility of public health nurses; immunizations are reimbursable under some insurance policies. Normal obstetric care is reimbursed by most insurance packages but is considered within the established realm of nurse midwifery practice.

The strategy suggested here is meant to improve the economic viability of nursing practice, not to change the content or emphasis of nursing services. It is unrealistic for nurses to seek third party reimbursement for services such as health education and counseling; no provider is reimbursed for these services at the present time. The most sensible approach for nursing at present is to seek reimbursement for services that will substitute for those currently being provided. Nurses should continue to provide comprehensive nursing care as needed regardless of the availability of third party reimbursement. The proposal here is not to convert nurses to doctors but to generate for nurses the revenues to which they are entitled and that will enable them to offer consumers an alternative to expensive traditional medical services.

The data to support proposals that substitute nursing services for more expensive medical services are available and directly appropriate to the stated goals of procompetition reform. Indeed, cost control in health delivery stimulated by tax-caps and rebates to the economically minded consumer will depend to a great degree on two factors: opening the system to competition and reducing consumer dependence on health care providers. From the standpoint of opening the system, the studies cited earlier have shown that nurses are cost-effective providers of a wide variety of primary care services. Not only are their direct costs lower than those of physician providers, but the cost of ancillary services is greatly reduced when nurses are the primary carers. These cost benefits must be facilitated by new state and federal legislation. Barriers must be eliminated that prevent direct access to nurses for ambulatory services that can be provided more economically and with equal or better outcomes than traditional medical services. These services include health services for children and teenagers, prenatal and postnatal care, nurse-determined home care, and care of the elderly.

Nursing's use of the certification process to establish credentials for nurses seeking recognition by third party payers is essential. The National League for Nursing recommends that the appropriate educational credential for the nurse practicing independently and reimbursed directly by third party payers is the master's degree in clinical nursing. Most nurses, however, practice in group settings in collaboration with physicians, and alternative credentials may be appropriate. In any case, a standardized certification process should be developed with established qualifications of such nurses to protect the public and to simplify the process of direct reimbursement.

Regardless of the procompetition strategy eventually agreed upon, the system must be opened to true competition from properly credentialed nurses, home health agencies, and visiting nurse associations among others. It should be clear the consumer choice and competition among providers will rest in great part on the removal of restraints to access to appropriate practitioners.[31] In recognition of fiscal restraints, services to be reimbursed must be substitutive rather than supplementary. Further, nursing should be actively involved in the design of programs of health promotion and disease prevention that will ultimately reduce reliance on higher cost technologic interventions.

REIMBURSEMENT FOR NURSING SERVICES IN HOSPITALS AND OTHER INPATIENT SETTINGS

We have discussed several reasons for the limited public awareness of nursing's unique contribution to health care outcomes having to do with the reimbursement system, the organization of nursing services, and the mental associations to the nursing concept—associations made by nurses as well as the public. Lack of public access to nursing outcome data presented, and nursing's reluctance to make their contributions known add to nursing's low profile. An additional important factor in nursing's low profile is the way payment for institutional nursing services is handled in most settings.

Nursing service is an income-producing department in hospitals in that nursing care is specifically reimbursed by third parties. However, nursing service costs, as well as certain other service costs, have traditionally been lumped in the multipurpose category of routine operating costs of institutions. This practice has prevented true cost accounting, hampered the development of a financially responsive health care system, and prevented consumers from evaluating the services received in relation to their cost.

An example of the lack of knowledge among the public and nurses themselves about nursing cost is the confusion about nurses' income as it relates to solutions to the nursing shortage. An argument frequently presented in response to proposals to increase nurses' salaries is the negative effect such increases might have on cost containment priorities. The public has been in no position to either support or deny such views, and nurses have not been forthcoming with suitable responses. Not only is the public unaware of the percentage of daily rates they are paying for nursing, but nurses themselves are unaware that the salary expenses for nursing personnel have declined as a percentage of hospital expenses since 1968. Thus as the percentage of cost for technology has increased, it is nurses' incomes that have suffered.[32]

The cost of nursing services could be separated from other charges in the daily room rate for hospitals, and patients could be billed on the basis of the nursing effort required for their care (see Chap. 8). The patient's dependency level and the basic, technologic, rehabilitative, and supportive care required are the key considerations in classifying the patient for nursing. Such a classification system would also reflect the components of nursing practice affecting nursing care on a uniform basis.

Such billing for nursing care would permit patients, institutions, and providers to understand the cost–benefit of nursing care and allow prospective economic modeling of differing care environments and needs. Most important it would provide the public with a more accurate understanding of the costs and benefits of specific nursing care.

Finally, I want to offer some comments on the substitutability of alternate nursing services for higher cost hospital services. It has been shown that a variety of predominantly nursing interventions have low-cost–high-benefit results. Use of home care, skilled nursing facility care, nurse-aided family care, and nursing rehabilitative care with or without prior hospitalization should be part of benefit packages available to consumers. Changes in reimbursement policies to encourage such tested models must acknowledge that these services are not, for the most part, medical services.

SUMMARY AND CONCLUSIONS

There is a great deal of data that suggests the importance of restructuring nursing roles in competitive health plans. To maximize possibilities for the inclusion of nursing in federal legislation fostering competition, I have explicitly recommended third party reimbursement for nurses. In any competitive legislation adopted, nursing services should be included in the minimum benefit package and nurses permitted to compete on an equal basis with other providers. These recommendations acknowledge the constraining role of some state laws and regulations in the appropriate use and reimbursement of nurses. Nursing should give immediate attention, however, to removal of these constraints.

In the area of developing alternatives to high-cost technologic care, a clearinghouse for information must be established and necessary steps taken to formalize reimbursable substitutes for hospital and institutional care. Using health teaching, family support systems, home visiting, and other predominately nursing interventions under nursing management and design in consultation with physicians and appropriate others will bring about short-term and long-term cost savings.

In the area of long-term care, a variety of demonstrations will be conducted in the next 5 yr. The Robert Wood Johnson Foundation Teaching Nursing Home Program, cosponsored by the American Academy of Nursing, and the national study by the Health Care Financing Administration comparing long-term health care programs in patients' homes with those in nursing homes offer tremendous opportunities for maximizing nursing's potential. Successful achievements from these and other demonstration projects should be institutionalized in the health care delivery system.

If competition is to be the solution for controlling the major costs of the health care delivery system, hospitals will need to examine all cost and income variables with more discrimination than occurs at present. Specific billing for nursing care will permit patients, institutions, and providers to understand the costs and benefits of nursing care, and allow prospective economic modeling of different care environments and needs.

Nurses must recognize the threats and promises in seeking direct reimbursement. If reimbursement must be substitutive rather than additive, specificity with regard to services and credentialed practitioners is essential. A national network of state leaders should address state laws and regulations with consistent recommendations on this issue. New federal legislation should encourage states to examine and document the state laws and regulations that deny access to the market by credentialed practitioners such as nurse midwives and certified nurse practitioners.

Use of the term "competition" to describe current proposals will be merely rhetoric unless proposals are altered to include competition among a variety of credentialed providers. The data of the past 20 yr speak to the phenomenal contributions of nursing to health care outcomes. Whatever nursing is today, tomorrow it must comprise whatever nursing can do and can do effectively and competitively. The nursing leadership should fight whatever constrains nursing from its potential — be it law, insurance policy, or public image. The present push toward competition in health delivery should be seized on as an opportunity to lobby for legitimizing nursing's roles and realizing its potential.

REFERENCES

1 Enthovin AC: Consumer-choice health plan. New Eng J Med 298, No. 12: 650–658, 1978; 298, No. 13: 709–720, 1978

2 Finborg D.W: DRG creep. New Eng J Med 304, No. 26: 1,602–1,604, 1981

3 Roe BR: The UCR boondoggle. New England J Med 305, No. 1: 41–45, 1981

4 Georgopoulus BS, Mann FC: The Community General Hospital, New York. Macmillan, 1962

5 Slome C, Wetherbee H, Daly M, Christensen K, Meglen M, Thiede H: Effectiveness of certified nurse-midwives. Am J Obstet Gynecol, 124, No. 2: 177–182, 1976

6 Corbett MA, Burst H: Nurse-midwives and adolescents: The South Carolina experience. Journal of Nurse-Midwifery 24, No. 4: 10–17, 1979

7 Lubic R: Evaluation of an out-of-hospital maternity center for low-risk patients. In Aiken LH: (ed): Health Policy and Nursing Practice. New York, McGraw-Hill, 1981; unpublished data from the Maternity Center Association, New York, NY

8 Miller CA: Testimony to the Subcommittee on Oversight and Investigation of the Interstate and Foreign Commerce Committee, US House of Representatives, p 139. Washington, DC, Dec 18, 1980

9 Levy BS, Wilkinson FS, Moreen WM: Reducing neonatal mortality rates with nurse midwives. Am J Obstet Gynecol 109, No 1: 51–58, 1971

10 Langwell K, Wilson S, Dean R, Black R, Kwai-Fong C: Geographic distribution of certified nurse midwives. Journal of Nurse-Midwifery 25, No. 6 3–11, 1980

11 Sox HC: Quality of patient care by nurse practitioners and physicians assistants: A ten year perspective. Ann Intern Med 91: 459–468, 1979.

12 Hauri CM, Kline C: Cost effective primary care. Nurse Practitioner 4, No. 5: 54, 1979

13 Runyon JW: The Memphis chronic disease program: Comparisons and outcome and the nurses extended role. JAMA 231: 241–244, 1975

14 Master RJ, Feltin M, Jainchill J, Mark R, Kavesh W, Rabkin M, Turner B, Bachrach S, Lennox S: A continuum of care for the inner city. New Eng J Med 302: 1,434, 1980

15 Martinson IM: Taking the dying child home: What effect on patient family? Medical News, AMA 237, No. 24: 2,591–2,593, 1977

16 Graduate Medical Education National Advisory Committee: Report to the Secretary Department of Health and Human Services. Vol. VI: Nonphysician Health Care Provider Technical Panel, Washington, DC, US Department of Health and Human Services (Pub. No. (HRA) 81-656). Sept 30, 1980

17 Diers D: Nurse-midwifery as a system of care: Provider process and patient outcome, pp 73–89. In Aiken L (ed): Health Policy and Nursing Practice. New York, McGraw-Hill, 1981

18 Klineman JC, Kovar MG, Seldman JJ, Yound CA: A comparison of 1960 and 1973–74 early neonatal mortality and selective states. Am J Epidemiol 108: 454–469, 1978

19 Jones K: Study documents effect of primary nursing on renal transplant patient. Hospitals 49: 85–89, 1975

20 Posen MW, Stechmiller JA, Harris W, Smith S, Freed D, Voigt G: A nurse reha-
bilitators impact on patients with myocardial infarction. Med Care 15, No. 10,
830–837, 1977

21 Kannel WB, Gordon T: The Framingham study: An epidemiological investigation of cardiovascular disease. Section 6:26. Washington, DC, US Government
Printing Office, June 1968

22 Wagner NK, Mount ZF: An education algorithm for myocardial infarction. Cardiovascular Nursing 10:11, 1974

23 Luginbuhl WH, Forsyth BR, Hirsch GB, Goodman MR: Prevention and rehabilitation as a means of cost containment: The example of myocardial infarction.
Journal of Public Health Policy 2: 103–116, 1981

24 Beard OW, Hipt HR, Robins M, Taylor JB, Ebert RV, Beran LG: Initial
myocardial infarction among 503 veterans. Am J Med 28: 871–883, 1960

25 Shenker L: Clinical experiences with fetal heart rate monitoring of one thousand
patients in labor. Am J Obstet Gynecol 115, No. 8: 1,111–1,116, 1973

26 Goodlin RC, Haesslein HC: When is it fetal distress? Am J Obstet Gynecol 128,
No. 4: 440–447, 1977

27 Chan WH, Paul RH, Toews J: Intrapartum fetal monitoring: Maternal and fetal
morbidity and perinatal mortality. Obstetrics and Gynecol 40, No. 1: 7–13, 1978

28 American Academy of Pediatrics Committee on Drugs: Effect of medication during labor and delivery on infant outcome. Pediatrics 62, No. 3: 402–403, 1978

29 Miller MK, Stokes CS: Health status, health resources, and consolidated structural parameters: Implications for public health care policy. Journal of Health
Social Behavior 19, No. 3: 263–279, 1978

30 Mayeroff M: On Caring, p 13. New York, Harper & Row, 1980

31 Dolan AK: Anti-trust law and physician dominance of other health practitioners.
Journal of Health Politics Policy and Law 4, No. 4: 675–690, 1980

32 Michela WA: Changes in the distribution of selected hospital expenses. Hospitals. Journal of the American Hospitals Association 53, No. 3, 28–29, 1979

EUGENE LEVINE
EVELYN B. MOSES

26

REGISTERED NURSES TODAY:
A STATISTICAL PROFILE

INTRODUCTION

The annual estimates of the number of employed registered nurses in the United States has more than tripled in the 30-yr period 1950 to 1980 — from a little less than 400,000 to over 1 million. Relative to the population, the ratio has grown from 249 per 100,000 people to 506 per 100,000 over this period. Thus, the rate of growth in the number of nurses has been twice that of the population as a whole.

In spite of the substantial increases in the nurse supply, it has been widely held over this 30-yr period that the supply is not sufficient to meet all of the demands for nursing services. The existence of a nursing shortage has been claimed with increasing frequency during the past few years. Among the evidence offered for a shortage is an estimate of 100,000 vacancies for registered nurses in acute care hospitals, which has been widely quoted in congressional hearings, professional and popular journals, and newspaper articles.

The purpose of this paper is to analyze the current population of registered nurses in the United States. The main focus will be on the changes in the characteristics of the nurse population occurring in the last few years that could shed some light on reasons why the nursing shortage has seemed to become more severe in spite of substantial increases in the nurse supply.

The authors gratefully acknowledge the assistance of William E. Spencer, Statistician, Division of Health Professions Analysis, Bureau of Health Professions, United States Department of Health and Human Services, in the preparation of the statistical data from the 1980 study.

THE STUDY DESIGN

The primary data for this analysis will be the 1977 and 1980 sample surveys of registered nurses. Both surveys used highly refined sampling methodology. The 1977 survey was conducted by the American Nurses Association and the 1980 survey by Research Triangle Institute. Both were conducted under contracts with the Bureau of Health Professions of the Federal Government's Department of Health and Human Services. Both studies used the same survey design. The selection of the sample and the estimation of the universe parameters were the same in both. The survey design was initially developed by Westat, Inc., for the Division of Nursing in the Bureau of Health Professions.

The sampling design for these studies had to take into account several characteristics of the universe of registered nurses. For one, there is no single up-to-date listing of all registered nurses in the nation; there are instead 51 lists of licensees, one in each state and the District of Columbia. These lists cannot be tied together through licensure identification numbers from state to state; nurses often maintain licenses in more than one state, and a number of nurses are actually located in a state in which they are not licensed, while they maintain a license or licenses elsewhere. Moreover, nurses are predominantly female and therefore subject to name changes through marriage. They are also predominantly *employed* rather than *self-employed* and are thus subject to more business address changes than they would have if they were self-employed and had an established business office.

The sample for these studies is derived from the lists of licensees in each state board of nursing through the use of alphabetic segments. These segments consist of clusters of names that are alphabetically adjacent to one another. To allow for increased sample size in states with smaller populations than other states, higher proportions of the registered nurse licenses are selected in the smaller states than in the larger ones. Since each alphabetic segment represents a certain percentage of the entire registered nurse population, differing sampling rates can be achieved for each state from a combination of various segments. Each state's sample is "nested" into the others through the use of an overlapping alphabetic segment procedure, with the states having higher sampling rates having the broader alphabetic segment and those with lower rates a smaller portion of that broader segment. Names of nurses sampled from each state's registration files are then merged into a single file and duplications are purged. Subsequent elimination of duplicates are achieved when responses are received and licensing data from respondents are checked. Finally, the weighting procedure to develop the population estimates takes into account the multiple licenses some nurses may hold so that the estimates represent nurses rather than licenses.

In the 1977 study the sample consisted of 20,417 registered nurses following the "unduplication" of names before fielding the questionnaires. The final effective response rate was 82.2% after the subsequent deletion of duplicates from the responses received. For the 1980 study the sample size was doubled. A total of 39,573 nurses were surveyed with an effective response rate of 79.2%.

The data for both surveys were collected through mail questionnaires administered over a several-month period or telephone interviews, or both in some instances. In the case of the 1977 study, the nurses were asked to respond to a series of questions about their status in September 1977, so that is the date of the 1977 data. However, in this connection, it should be noted that the sample for the 1977 study was mainly selected in the early part of 1977 and therefore excluded nurses who were granted new licenses or reinstated licenses during the interval between sample selection and the mailing of the questionnaires. It is estimated that the total nurse population count for the September 1977 study might be understated by 15,000 nurses or about 1%.

The 1980 study asked for data for the month of November. The sample for that study was selected shortly before the time of the initial mailings and, thus, these data reflect all of the persons who had licenses to practice as registered nurses in at least one state or the District of Columbia in November 1980.

It should be noted that the data from the 1980 study are just beginning to be analyzed as this report is being written. The material contained in this report, therefore, represents a first view of the information. It is based primarily on selected, important, national statistics that were developed to provide an initial examination of the results. The actual numbers contained in this report for 1980 should be considered preliminary. The conclusions from these numbers, however, are considered to be reflective of what the final data are expected to reveal.

NURSE SUPPLY AND DEMAND

A shortage of nurses represents an imbalance between supply and demand wherein demand exceeds supply. Since the nurse supply has grown so remarkably in the past few years, a continuing shortage can be explained by demand growing even more. Demand is composed of a number of factors of which the population — potential users of nursing services — is one rather gross indicator. In the past 30 yr, while the nurse supply has more than tripled, the nurse–population ratio has only doubled in size, suggesting that this demand factor only partially explains the increases in supply and the continuing shortage. However, the population has not only grown, it has aged, and with more older persons there is greater use of nursing services. Moreover, other demand factors have exerted important influences in recent years, including the growth in labor-intensive technology in hospitals. And, fundamental to all expansions in the health care industry are the recent rises in *per capita* income and in private and public cost-based third party reimbursement, which has expanded the use of health care.

Not all of the causes of the nurse shortage are on the demand side of the supply–demand equation. Shortages could arise from such supply side factors as decreasing "productivity" of nurses, which could result in a diminished output of nursing services even while the supply is increasing. That is, while the total number of nurses has increased, more could be working part time or fewer could be providing direct patient care. Moreover, some potentially available nursing services might be lost through misuse of employed registered nurses. Also, there is the possibility that more nurses might be available today but greater proportions of the total nurse population have chosen not to work or to work in other fields.

This report will examine some of these supply side assertions. (The issue of misuse is not addressed here.) It will see whether these assertions can be supported by changes and trends in the registered nurse population between 1977 and 1980. The report is organized into two sections. The first will describe briefly how the demographic characteristics of registered nurses have changed from 1977 to 1980 and the implications of these changes, if any, in understanding the reported imbalance between supply and demand. The second will present some of the suppositions about supply side causes of this imbalance and examine the extent to which they are upheld by the 1977–1980 data.

CHANGES IN DEMOGRAPHIC CHARACTERISTICS OF THE REGISTERED NURSE POPULATION 1977 to 1980

The total number of nurses licensed to practice in November 1980 was estimated to be 1.62 million, compared to 1.4 million in September 1977, an increase of about 15%. The number of employed registered nurses grew at an even greater rate, from slightly less than a million in September 1977 to about 1.24 million in November 1980, an increase of about 24%. During this 3-yr period, the growth rates for both the registered nurse population and the working supply far exceeded the growth rates of the total population in the United States, which increased only 3%.

The 3-yr increase of about one-quarter million employed registered nurses exceeds the growth during the previous 5-yr period by 50,000 nurses. However, the entire decade of the 1970s is characterized by substantial increases in the numbers of registered nurses. In part, these increases have reflected the large increases in the number of graduates from basic nursing educational programs that occurred in the first half of the decade. Annual increases in graduations during this period varied between 10% and 15% according to the data obtained by the National League for Nursing (NLN) in their annual surveys of schools of nursing. In the 1970–1971 academic year, there were 46,455 graduates from basic nursing educational programs in the United States. By 1974–1975 the number of graduates reached 73,915, a 59% increase. The latter part of the 1970s showed a decline in the rate of growth in the number of graduates with a reversal of the growth trend in the overall numbers of graduates toward the close of the decade. Thus, the number of graduates peaked at 77,874 in 1977–1978, and by the end of the decade it was 75,523. Admissions to basic nursing educational programs, which had about doubled from the mid-1960s to the mid-1970s, were also showing signs of some decline in overall numbers toward the latter part of the 1970s, portending further decreases in the annual number of graduates in the near future.

The growth in the numbers of basic nursing education admissions and graduations are in a large measure owing to changes in the associate degree and baccalaureate programs. Diploma programs have been declining for a long time. These declines persisted during the rapid growth period of the early 1970s as well. Total admissions to diploma programs today are less than half of what they were in the 1950s, despite the substantial increase in total admissions to basic programs, and the number of diploma programs are about a third of what they were at that time. In the 1979–1980 academic year 33% of the 106,000 admissions to basic nursing education programs were to baccalaureate programs, 51% to associate degree programs, and 16% were to diploma programs. These changes in the mix of graduates will cause radical changes in the composition of the future registered nurse population.

Looking only at new entrants into the registered nurse population, however, does not allow for a complete evaluation of trends in this population. A review also must be made of the composition and work behavior patterns of all the nurses.

Table 26-1 reveals a number of interesting changes in the characteristics of the registered nurse population from 1977 to 1980. The median age of all registered nurses declined from 39.8 yr to 38.4 yr. Among employed nurses there was a similar decline—from 37.7 yr to 36.3 yr. The median age of registered nurses *not* employed in nursing rose from 46.1 yr in 1977 to 47.1 yr in 1980.

The percentage of males among the registered nurses increased from 1.9% to 2.7% in the 3 yr. Because men tend to have higher participation in employment than women, 3.0% of the employed registered nurses in 1980 were men, compared to 2.1% in 1977.

TABLE 26-1 Statistical Profile of Registered Nurses, September 1977 and November 1980*

Characteristic	Total Registered Nurses		Total Employed in Nursing		Total Not Employed in Nursing	
	1977	1980	1977	1980	1977	1980
Total number	1,401,633	1,615,846	978,234	1,235,152	423,400	379,712
Median age	39.8	38.4	37.7	36.3	46.1	47.1
Percentage male	1.9	2.7	2.1	3.0	1.4	1.6
Percentage minority	6.2	7.0	7.5	8.2	3.5	3.4
Percentage married	72.4	70.8	68.9	68.1	80.5	79.8
Percentage married with children at home	45.7	47.5	43.8	46.3	50.1	51.6
Percentage whose basic nursing education was:						
Diploma	74.8	63.4	71.4	59.6	82.6	75.7
Associate degree	11.3	18.5	13.7	21.2	5.8	9.7
Baccalaureate or higher degree	13.7	17.3	14.6	18.5	11.4	13.6
Percentage whose highest nursing related education was:						
Diploma	67.0	54.6	63.4	50.9	75.1	66.4
Associate degree	11.3	17.7	13.5	20.0	6.0	10.1
Baccalaureate	17.5	22.1	18.5	23.2	15.4	18.4
Masters or doctorate	4.1	5.1	4.4	5.3	3.3	4.4

*Percentages included on this table are derived from the segment of the total population indicating the particular characteristic being studied.

Among the registered nurses employed in nursing in 1980, 8.2% were from minority groups, compared to 7.5% in 1977. The higher participation rate of minority nurses in nursing leads to a fairly low percentage of minority nurses among the registered nurses *not* employed in nursing—3.5% in 1977 and 3.4% in 1980.

The percentage of married nurses among *all* registered nurses declined from 72.4% to 70.8%. At the same time, however, the percentage of the registered nurses who were married and had children living at home increased. Among the employed registered nurses, the percentage who were married and had children at home increased from 43.8% in 1977 to 46.3% in 1980.

As suggested by the changing mix of new graduates, the educational preparation of registered nurses shows remarkable changes since 1977. There has been a significant decline in the percentage of nurses whose basic educational preparation and whose highest educational preparation was a diploma in nursing. Among those employed in nursing the percentage of those whose basic preparation was in a diploma program declined from 71.4% to 59.6%. This was offset by increases in the percentage of nurses with associate degree and baccalaureate basic preparation, with the greatest rate of increase in those with associate degree preparation—from 13.7% to 21.2%.

Among those not employed in nursing, the percentage of nurses whose basic preparation was an associate degree also increased between 1977 and 1980—from 5.8% to 9.7%. Three-quarters of all nurses not employed in nursing in 1980 received their basic preparation in diploma programs, but this has declined from 82.6% in 1977. Thus, the diploma-prepared nurse is becoming less prominent among both categories—those employed and those not employed in nursing.

As Table 26-2 shows, the diploma graduates among the registered nurse population are on the average considerably older than the graduates from the other basic nursing educational programs. The median age of the diploma graduates was 44 yr as compared to 31.5 yr for the associate degree graduates and 30.2 yr for the baccalaureate graduates, which provides additional evidence of the effect of the movement away from the diploma program to associate degree and baccalaureate program as the entry into nursing. These data also suggest that the large decrease between 1977 and 1980 in the percentage of registered nurses coming from diploma programs will continue into the future.

Of interest as well in these data is the finding that the median age of the nurses who were originally associate degree graduates is higher than the median age of those who were initially baccalaureate graduates. This difference occurs despite the fact that the associate degree program is the newest of the

TABLE 26-2 Selected Statistics on Registered Nurses from Each Type of Basic Nursing Educational Program, November 1980

Characteristic	Diploma	Associate Degree	Baccalaureate*
Total number	1,023,898	298,208	280,560
Median age	44.0	31.5	30.2
Percentage male	1.6	5.8	3.8
Percentage minority	5.1	10.9	9.9
Percentage who obtained post RN-degrees in nursing	13.9	8.9	13.1
Percentage employed in nursing	71.9	87.6	81.6

*Includes those whose basic nursing education was a master's degree.

three types of basic nursing educational programs, having first produced graduates in the early 1950s. Associate degree programs are far more likely to have students from older age groups than are the baccalaureate programs. They also tend to have a higher proportion of minority students, thus, perhaps, accounting for the 5.8% minority complement among associate degree registered nurses, compared to 3.8% among the basic baccalaureate graduate registered nurses. Associate degree graduates are also more likely to be employed in nursing. The study showed that they were less likely to go on for additional education after having achieved licensure as a registered nurse. When the additional education that the registered nurses had received was taken into account, the associate degree nurses represented 17.7% of all the registered nurses and 20% of those employed in nursing.

When all the formal academic nursing-related education of registered nurses is considered, it is seen that nearly three nurses out of every ten who were employed in nursing in 1980 had attained a baccalaureate or higher degree. In 1980 the *number* of employed nurses who held at least a baccalaureate degree was nearly 130,000 greater than in 1977. The 3-yr increase in the number alone is equal to the *total* number of employed nurses who held a baccalaureate degree or higher in 1972. In 1952, the earliest year for which data on the educational preparation of nurses are available, fewer than one nurse in ten had a baccalaureate or higher degree.

In summary, the changes in the characteristics of the registered nurses noted in the 1977 and 1980 comparisons are as follows:

Increases in
- Total number of registered nurses
- Number of registered nurses employed in nursing
- Ratio of employed registered nurses to population
- Number and percentage of minority nurses
- Number and percentage of male nurses

- Number and percentage of nurses with children at home
- Number and percentage of nurses with baccalaureate and higher degrees
- Median age of nurses not employed in nursing

Decreases in
- Median age of total registered nurses and those employed in nursing
- Percentage of married nurses among those not employed in nursing
- Number and percentage of nurses whose basic education preparation was a diploma in nursing
- Number and percentage of nurses whose highest educational preparation was a diploma

The next section will provide a more intensive examination of the changes in the characteristics of nurses between 1977 and 1980 in the light of some of the possible explanations for the current imbalance between the registered nurse supply and demand.

WHAT THE DATA REVEAL ABOUT POSSIBLE EXPLANATIONS OF THE IMBALANCE BETWEEN SUPPLY AND DEMAND

In the numerous discussions of why a shortage of registered nurses has intensified recently, a number of supply side causes have been advanced. The more widely held of these will now be questioned.

ARE FEWER NURSES WORKING IN NURSING?

As pointed out earlier, the estimated number of registered nurses employed in nursing in November 1980 was 1,235,152, about 24% more than the number estimated in the September 1977 study. The 1980 study also showed an unprecedented activity rate for registered nurses: 76.4% of the total number of registered nurses were employed in nursing in November 1980. In September 1977 69.8% were employed. As will be seen in Table 26-3, these increases in the percentages employed were evident in all age groups, and most particularly among nurses in their 30s and 40s, the ages at which women are usually assumed to be home raising families.

The study itself does not provide any specific explanation for these increases. A more in-depth analysis of the study data may at some point provide some important insights. The report on the 1977 study suggested that a factor in a married nurse's decision to participate in the labor force was the anticipated family income, *excluding* the nurse's wage. The 1980 study, while

TABLE 26-3 Estimated Percentage of Registered Nurses Employed in Nursing by Age
Group, September 1977 and November 1980

Age Group	September 1977	November 1980
All registered nurses	69.8	76.4
Under 25	93.1	95.3
25–29	82.8	87.6
30–34	70.7	80.6
35–39	70.2	77.1
40–44	73.4	78.3
45–49	71.7	78.2
50–54	71.5	75.2
55–59	65.5	66.3
60–64	46.8	51.4
65 and over	19.4	24.8

it looked at the nurse's salary, did not attempt to determine family income, but that question might be kept in mind as attempts are made to examine how many nurses will and do participate in the work force.

It is important to consider that these activity rates relate to those who have licenses to practice as registered nurses. Higher activity rates can be obtained if fewer numbers of nurses not employed in nursing maintain licenses. The rather sizable increases in the number of employed nurses coupled with the decrease in the number who were not employed in nursing suggests that this may be a partial explanation for the high rates of employment. While definitive information on those who drop their licenses and the reasons for doing so are not available from this study, a comparative review of these data with the data from the 1977 study can provide some clues.

An initial examination of the data, taking into account mortality rates, suggests that those dropping their licenses are most likely to come from the older age groups. Since it is possible to reinstate a license if it is dropped and there are no data on reinstatements, only the net effects can be determined. However, these net effects do provide some interesting data. In this first examination, there were four age groups of nurses that showed actual net losses, taking into account mortality but not examining the effects of the new licensee additions to the registered nurse population. Not unexpectedly, the largest of these net losses occurred among those who would be 65 yr old or more in the November 1980 study. That group appeared to lose almost four out of ten of those who were licensed in 1977. Much smaller but still rather significant net losses were noted for those who would be between the ages of 60 yr and 64 yr and between 55 yr and 59 yr in 1980. The other age group that showed a net loss was the 45 yr to 49 yr one. These data suggest then that significant drops in licensure may start occurring somewhere after the age of 40 yr. Of course, since new licensees were not taken into account in this first analysis, it is possible that significant losses might be determined for the younger age groups after such refinement can be made. However, given the relatively large net gains noted for these younger age groups, it does not seem too likely. In general, then, these data show that, while some of the increase in the activity rates may be due to nurses dropping all their active licenses, there did not seem to be a sufficiently large enough loss to account for all of the increase, with the possible exception of the rates for the oldest age groups.

Another interesting statistic is the number of nurses not employed in nursing who were seeking work. In 1977 this group was estimated to be 42,028 nurses, approximately 3% of total number of registered nurses. In 1980 this group had declined to an estimated 31,652 nurses, slightly less than 2% of the total. About one out five of these were seeking employment for less than a week and more than half for no more than a month. From these data it can be seen that the low unemployment rate of 1977 has declined even further in 1980, indicating continuing strong demand for nurses relative to supply.

ARE NURSES LEAVING NURSING TO WORK IN OTHER FIELDS?

An often expressed explanation of the nursing shortage is attrition from the profession because of economic reasons, "burnout," and attractions of other fields of work. Data on the total number of registered nurses who are not employed in nursing and the number of these who are working in other fields are available from the sample surveys. As indicated above, the surveys do not directly measure the extent to which nurses have dropped their licenses and are no longer working as nurses. It may be possible to study the characteristics of nurses who do drop their licenses, but the reasons for their dropping their licenses and whether or not they become active in other fields cannot be determined from the data collected in the sample surveys.

A possible proxy for a measure of the exodus from nursing is the count of registered nurses who are employed in a field other than nursing. In 1980 there were an estimated 73,934 registered nurses in this category. Thus, the registered nurses who were employed in another field represented 4.6% of total registered nurses, and 19.5% of the registered nurses not employed in nursing. In 1977 a total of 61,929 registered nurses were working in another field, 4.4% of total registered nurses and 14.6% of the registered nurses not employed in nursing. Thus, there was a small increase in the number and proportion of nurses who were working in other fields, but not enough to suggest a significant exodus from the profession. Furthermore, 32% of the 73,934 were estimated to be employed in a health-related field. Both in 1977 and 1980 the vast majority of registered nurses who were not employed in nursing were not working for pay at all.

The educational backgrounds of these registered nurses who were employed in another field provides further insight into this category of nurse. Nurses with doctorates were most likely to report that they were employed in a field other than nursing. Out of the 4,000 doctorally prepared nurses with licenses to practice nursing, some 780, or 19.5%, were estimated to be employed in some other field. Those with a master's degree in another field related to nursing were more likely to be employed in a non-nursing occupation than were those with a master's degree in nursing. About 9% of the registered nurses with master's degrees in other fields were employed in an occupation other than nursing while only about 3.5% of those with a master's degree in nursing were so employed. A similar picture was noted for those whose highest preparation was a baccalaureate degree.

ARE MORE NURSES WORKING PART TIME?

In 1977 68% of all employed registered nurses worked full time. In 1980 the rate was 67% (Table 26-5). Given the higher overall activity rate in 1980, there was actually a higher proportion of *all* registered nurses with licenses to practice who were employed in nursing on a full time basis: 51.2% in 1980 compared to 47.5% in 1977. On a full time equivalent basis, the number of employed registered nurses increased from about 821,000 in 1977 to about 1,025,000 in the 1980 study, representing a 25% increase in the full-time equivalent supply of registered nurses.

Table 26-5 shows a comparison of the full-time rates for the various fields of nursing for 1977 and 1980. There are slight decreases for many fields of nursing, including hospitals and nursing homes, but these do not significantly affect the full-time equivalency data.

Although the proportion of persons doing part-time nursing has not significantly increased since 1977, a large number of registered nurses are represented in that group. The 395,615 part-timers in 1980 are more than the *total* number of registered nurses employed in 1950 (375,000).

Full-time nurses differ from those employed part time in many ways. One of these is educational preparation. As Table 26-6 shows, as educational preparation increases a higher proportion of nurses tend to work full time, rather than part time.

ARE FEWER NURSES WORKING IN HOSPITALS?

Many recent studies express the concern that nurses are leaving hospital employment because of work pressure, poor salaries, and lack of career advancement. Nevertheless, the total number of nurses employed in hospitals increased approximately 35% from 1977 to 1980 while the total of all employed nurses increased 26%. This has occurred despite a decline in the

TABLE 26-4 Estimated Number and Percentage of Registered Nurses Employed in Each Field of Employment on a Full-time or Part-time Basis, November 1980

Field of Employment	Total*	Full time		Part time	
		Number	Percentage	Number	Percentage
Total registered nurses employed in nursing	1,235,152	826,937	67.0	395,615	32.0
Hospital	810,851	556,286	68.6	249,976	30.8
Nursing home	98,851	53,144	53.8	45,163	45.7
Nursing education	45,114	34,440	76.3	10,553	23.4
Public/community health	80,522	62,857	78.1	16,454	20.4
Student health services	43,540	31,194	71.6	11,995	27.5
Occupational health	28,112	22,726	80.8	4,287	15.2
Physician's or dentist's office	70,177	39,691	56.6	30,084	42.9
Private duty	19,617	5,239	26.7	14,053	71.6
Other self-employed	10,332	3,471	33.6	6,750	65.3
Other	21,076	15,256	72.4	5,747	27.3
Missing	6,959	2,631	37.8	556	8.0

*Includes those for whom full-time or part-time employment was not available.

TABLE 26-5 Estimated Percentage of Registered Nurses Employed in Each Field of Employment on a Full-time Basis. September 1977 and November 1980

Field of Employment	1977	1980
Total, all fields	68.0	67.0
Hospital	70.6	68.6
Nursing home	57.6	53.8
Nursing education	80.3	76.3
Public/community health	78.3	78.1
Student health services	71.7	71.6
Occupational health	76.4	80.8
Physician's or dentist's office	56.0	56.6
Private duty	27.5	26.7
Other self-employed	31.3	33.6

number of patients per day in all hospitals and a modest 4.5% increase in the average number of patients per day in the community hospitals. In 1980 hospitals employed an estimated two-thirds (65.6%) of all employed nurses, while nursing homes, another field that is said to have severe retention problems, employed 8% of the total (see Table 26-4). Thus, nearly three-quarters of employed nurses worked in inpatient settings.

Included in these counts are a number of nurses who are employed by agencies providing temporary nursing services, mainly to hospitals and nursing homes. This is a rather new phenomenon and considered by some to be a response to the nursing shortage. In 1980 a total of 37,162 nurses were estimated to be working in these agencies, of whom 18,077 considered such employment their primary position; 19,085 were estimated to have employment in a temporary agency as a secondary position.

While hospital employment increased 35% since 1977, other fields of nursing have had little or no growth. Nurses in the major ambulatory care areas of office nursing, public health, occupational health, and school nursing increased roughly 5% over the 3-yr period, just a little more than the percentage increase in total United States population.

TABLE 26-6 Estimated Percentage of Registered Nurses Employed Full Time by Highest Educational Preparation

Highest Educational Preparation	Percentage Employed Full Time
Total	67.0
Diploma in nursing	60.6
Associate degree in nursing	71.8
Baccalaureate in nursing	72.3
Baccalaureate in other field	80.0
Master's in nursing	80.2
Master's in other field	86.0
Doctorate	92.7

ARE FEWER NURSES WORKING AS BEDSIDE NURSES IN HOSPITALS?

While some analysts of the nursing situation grant that there has been a significant rise in the number of employed registered nurses, they claim that fewer are providing "hands-on," direct patient care. Direct patient care, particularly in hospitals, which is sometimes labeled bedside nursing is said to be an area where dissatisfaction is highest because of work pressures, inadequate incentives, and the availability of more attractive job opportunities that draw nurses away from the patient's bedside.

In 1977 a total of 414,986 nurses were classified as either general duty nurses, staff nurses, charge nurses, or team leaders in a hospital, positions that are squarely in the realm of bedside nursing; in 1980 583,410 nurses were in these positions (Table 26-7). This is a 41% increase, compared to a 22% increase in other nursing positions in hospitals.

In recent years, moreover, a number of new position categories have been established that require higher academic credentials than general duty and staff nursing and that are also heavily oriented toward direct patient care. These new positions showed large growth in hospitals between 1977 and 1980. The number employed in hospitals in 1977 and 1980, respectively, are as follows: clinical Nursing Specialist, 5,910 and 13,175; nurse clinician, 4,018 and 4,451; nurse practitioner or midwife, 3,296 and 5,500.

In all fields of nursing there has been a considerable growth in positions such as these, which are concerned with direct patient care. Table 26-8 shows that the percentage increase in these categories far exceeds the growth in other nursing positions.

The data in Table 26-8 are shown according to position titles and do not indicate how the nurses actually spend their time on the various activities that make up their jobs. In both the 1977 and 1980 studies respondents were asked to estimate how much time is spent in the major work areas such as direct patient care, consultation, supervision, and teaching. Preliminary analysis of these data indicates a small but not particularly significant drop-off in the percentage of nurses who spend a majority of their time in direct patient care (Table 26-9). This decline is hardly enough, however, to offset the large increase in the number of nurses providing direct patient care. Thus, both in terms of the position titles and of the functional responsibilities, the majority of the registered nurses were engaged in direct patient care.

HAVE MORE NURSES RETURNED TO SCHOOL?

In 1980 a total of 161,732 registered nurses were enrolled in a formal education program, 10% of all registered nurses. Of these, 31,245 were enrolled full time, less than 2% of the total. In 1977 an estimated 165,979 nurses were

TABLE 26-7. Field of employment and type of position of employed registered nurses, November 1980

Field of employment	Total	Administrator or assistant	Consultant	Supervisor or assistant	Instructor
Total registered nurses employed in nursing	1,235,152*	59,804	7,879	73,904	58,594
Hospital	810,851	22,437	1,084	46,969	15,567
Nursing home	98,851	19,354	1,043	14,196	1,938
Nursing education	45,114	3,791	81	344	36,314
Public health/ community health	80,522	7,302	1,948	7,163	680
Student health service	43,540	1,121	122	357	1,265
Occupational health	28,112	1,038	578	1,173	223
Physician's or dentist's office	70,177	1,274	293	1,977	544
Other	51,025	3,173	2,691	1,498	1,886
Missing	6,959	316	41	231	178

* Individual items may not add up to totals because of rounding.

enrolled in a formal education program, almost 12% of all nurses. Moreover, a higher number in 1977 — 35,989 — were enrolled full time. The data thus indicate that there has actually been a small decline in the number and proportion of nurses who are attending school. Also, of those attending school, only about 10% were not employed in nursing. Among the full-time students, less than one-quarter were not employed at all in nursing.

ARE NURSES UNDERPAID?

In the November 1980 study the average annual salary of all registered nurses working on a full-time basis was estimated at $17,393. In September 1977 the average was $12,948. The average annual percentage increase between 1977 and 1980, therefore, amounted to 10.3%. This increase is somewhat higher than that shown for all nonagricultural workers in private industries or white collar workers in general over this same period, although not equivalent to the recent "double digit" inflationary rate changes in the consumer price index.

Table 26-10 shows that some variation does exist in salaries depending upon where the nurse works and the type of position filled. Contrary to the often stated belief, the hospital staff nurse is not at the lowest level in the array of salaries paid to nurses. Staff nurses in nursing homes, public health agencies, student health services, and physician's offices had lower average salaries than the hospital staff nurse, with the physician's office nurse showing the lowest average salary.

In nursing, however, unlike a number of other professions where there

TABLE 26-7.

Head nurse or assistant	General duty/ staff nurse	Nurse practitioner/ midwife	Clinical nursing specialist	Nurse clinician	Nurse anesthetist	Other	Missing
87,292	800,369	16,212	18,465	7,840	14,168	84,175	6,451
72,427	583,410	5,500	13,175	4,451	11,584	32,687	1,561
5,581	52,943	84	154	38	—	3,346	173
226	2,254	93	401	134	250	1,042	184
2,441	46,490	4,129	1,990	672	55	7,556	93
462	37,424	1,009	256	246	—	1,257	21
1,850	19,712	279	260	359	32	2,403	205
3,039	46,204	4,042	1,725	1,654	387	8,352	688
1,054	9,816	1,076	477	285	1,802	27,183	96
213	2,117	—	27	—	57	349	3,430

may be gradations of positions, there is not much difference in average salaries paid to those in positions that are essentially first-level, such as the hospital staff nurse, and to those in positions requiring additional education or experience as well as having additional responsibilities. Thus, the study showed that nurses in administrative positions in hospitals earned only 50% more than the staff nurse at the bottom of the hierarchy. Nurses in such specialized direct patient care positions as the clinical nursing specialist, nurse

TABLE 26-8 Distribution of Employed Registered Nurses by Primary Position Held, September 1977 and November 1980

Type of Position	September 1977	November 1980	Percent change 1977–1980
All registered nurses employed in nursing	978,234	1,235,152	+ 26.3
Administrator or assistant	47,563	59,804	+ 25.7
Consultant	4,639	7,879	+ 69.8
Supervisor or assistant	66,883	73,904	+ 10.5
Instructor	48,369	58,594	+ 21.1
Head nurse or assistant	84,770	87,292	+ 3.0
General duty/staff nurse	622,170	800,369	+ 28.6
Nurse clinician	7,045	7,840	+ 11.3
Nurse practitioner/midwife	9,634	16,212	+ 68.3
Clinical nursing specialist	8,065	18,465	+129.0
Nurse anesthetist	13,046	14,168	+ 8.6
Private duty nurse	28,563	22,277	− 22.0
Other	36,460	61,898	+ 69.8
Not reported	1,026	6,451	+528.7

TABLE 26-9 Estimated Percentage of Registered Nurses in Selected Positions Who Spent the Majority of Their Time During a Usual Work Week in Direct Patient Care, September 1977 and November 1980

Registered Nurse Positions	September 1977	November 1980
All registered nurses employed in nursing	57.1	55.8
Private duty nurse	96.9	83.7
General duty nurse	84.8	80.5
Staff nurse	81.4	81.5
No position title (only nurse on staff)	66.9	59.6
Team leader	60.0	59.7
Nurse practitioner	83.1	78.3
Nurse anesthetist	89.2	80.6
Public health nurse	61.2	58.8
Charge nurse	49.4	50.3
Nurse clinician	54.5	57.5
Clinical nursing specialist	66.2	55.5
Nurse midwife	74.6	83.1
Head nurse	36.9	31.2
School nurse	55.9	45.7

clinician, and nurse practitioner had average salaries that exceeded that of the hospital staff nurse by only about 20%.

SUMMARY AND CONCLUSIONS

Data from the 1980 sample survey of registered nurses, when compared to the findings in the 1977 study, show substantial increases in the total nurse population and in the supply of nurses, both in terms of total number employed and number of full-time equivalencies. While the proportion of nurses whose responsibilities are in direct patient care is about the same in both studies, the actual number of those providing such care has significantly increased. The increases noted here far surpass the overall increase in the general population of the United States or in patients in community hospitals between 1977 and 1980.

Data from the 1980 study suggest that nurses are participating in the work force at greater rates and are remaining for, perhaps, longer, more continuous periods. While a greater proportion of the nurse population has achieved a higher level of academic preparation, nurses are not withdrawing from employment to attend schools at higher rates than previously, nor does it seem that they are withdrawing from nursing to pursue other occupations at any great rate.

Furthermore, while graduations from and admissions to schools of nursing tend to be declining, such factors as the age distribution of the nurse population and the high proportion of working nurses in that population suggest

TABLE 26-10 Estimated Average Annual Salaries of Registered Nurses Employed Full
Time in Selected Nursing Positions, September 1977 and November 1980

Nursing Positions	September 1977	November 1980	Average Annual Percentage Increase
All full-time registered nurses	$12,948	$17,393	10.3
Hospital			
Administrator	17,532	24,620	12.0
Supervisor	14,196	19,820	11.8
Clinical nursing specialist	14,472	19,412	10.3
Nurse clinician	14,400	19,675	11.0
Head nurse	13,464	17,719	9.6
Staff nurse	12,252	16,451	10.3
Nursing home			
Administrator	14,064	17,304	7.2
Staff nurse	10,572	14,332	10.7
Nursing education			
Instructor	13,752	18,766	10.9
Public health			
Administrator	14,664	20,829	12.4
Supervisor	14,064	17,961	8.5
Staff nurse	12,096	15,068	7.6
Student health			
Staff nurse	11,244	14,578	9.0
Occupational health			
Staff nurse	13,368	18,710	11.6
Physician's office			
Staff nurse	9,720	11,938	7.1
Nurse practitioner/midwife			
All settings	14,220	19,395	10.9

that there will be continued growth in the registered nurse supply. This, though, would be in a large measure dependent on the maintenance of the high activity rates. Those activity rates may be very directly related to the present inflationary conditions in the country and of a need to boost family incomes to compensate for increases in the cost of living.

The changes in the population and characteristics of registered nurses outlined here offer no explanations as to why shortages should have intensified in recent years. Thus, it is necessary to look elsewhere in seeking answers. One possible source of explanation is the productivity of nursing resources both in a qualitative and quantitative sense. Head counts of registered nurses do not reveal how much care is actually delivered to consumers of nursing services. Increases in numbers of nursing personnel could well be offset by decreases in productivity. For example, if new graduates need long periods of "internship" before they can function with full effectiveness, head counts can seriously overstate the amount of nursing services actually delivered.

Among the reasons for the current concerns about a nursing shortage, the key explanatory variable could be increased *demand* for registered nurses. Demand increases consist of a variety of factors such as increases in case load and mix and increases in the technological and clinical complexities of the care provided. Fundamental to all this has been the increased availability of funds through the cost-based reimbursement system.

As to the future, it is expected that the supply of registered nurses will continue to grow. The amount of growth will be heavily influenced by many factors — economic, social, psychological, and political. The current uncertainties surrounding these factors make forecasting into the future a rather risky enterprise.

REFERENCES

National League for Nursing, Division of Research, *NLN Nursing Data Book 1980*, Pub. No. 19-1852, 1981.

National League for Nursing, Division of Research, *State-Approved Schools of Nursing,—R.N.*, 1981, Pub. No. 19-1853, 1981.

Roth, Aleda, et al. *1977 National Sample Survey of Registered Nurses*, Stock No. HRP 0900603, National Technical Information Service, Springfield, Va., 1978.

Brum, Joan D., "Wage Increases in 1980 Outpaced by Inflation." *Monthly Labor Review*, May 1981, U.S. Department of Labor.

Division of Health Professions Analysis, BHPr, HRA, DHHS, *Source Book—Nursing Personnel*, DHHS Publication No. (HRA) 81-21, 1981.

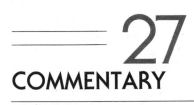

SUSAN R. GORTNER

27
COMMENTARY

How will nursing practice be characterized in the next decade? In the opinion of the majority of authors of this volume, the answer to this question will be determined by whether there is a renewed societal mandate for nursing services in an era of continued high costs and risks and whether nursing services can substitute for other needed services. The experience of the last 20 yr of heavy federal subsidy of health manpower training are now past history; the consequences of such subsidies include an admirable increase in the number of the major health professionals but also unfortunately, a limited understanding and documentation of how these persons might best be used to improve access, as well as quality, of health services. In part, this limitation is a function of the authorizing legislation for physician and nurse training that did not, at the onset, examine use and practice setting issues. In part, it is a function of professional arguments for self-regulation and autonomy. In part, it is a result of a generation of technologic advances that now require a health care bureaucracy for their management and that have almost disenfranchized professional nursing, according to Norris.[1]

Aiken has analyzed the evolution of public policy in nursing, citing the early and continued support by nursing of efforts to increase consumers' access to health care. Shortages in numbers and kinds of professional nurses became apparent during World War II. Federal efforts to redress the situation used the mechanism of training subsidies to alter the educational mix in the work force and to enlarge career opportunities for nurses with preparation in primary care. Such expanded roles for nursing altered the relationships between medical and nursing politically, economically, and clinically, and prompted a decade of evaluative studies, many of which form the data bases from which our authors speak.

Schramm and Fagin address the nursing shortage from economic and professional perspectives. Both agree that competitive market considerations do not prevail in nursing for a number of reasons, including the monopsonistic power exercised by hospitals, the monopoly on health care services and reimbursement held by medicine, the nontransferable nature of nursing work, and the underpricing of that work. Fagin speaks cogently to the spiral effect of the inpatient nursing shortage, addressing needed solutions with regard to employment conditions, educational opportunities and career advancement, entry level credentialing, and improved public views of nursing services. These are solutions proposed again and again by our authors, to which might be added the equivocal effects (as noted by Schramm) of governmental intervention in the marketplace to alleviate shortages.

The situation confronting hospital nursing is very well depicted by McClure. She cites three major intertwined developments: the increased knowledge level required of the nurse (as a result of the increased acuity of patients in inpatient settings); the increased demand for professional nurses in face of a declining national supply; and the change to primary nursing as a system of care. The care-giving and coordinating activities of the hospital nurse are two central areas of responsibility that can be in conflict with one another. To avoid such conflict, McClure argues that top-level administration must make clear to respective department heads that a high degree of responsiveness to patient needs is expected; such responsiveness would mean taking corrective action where there were systematic failures in the system. Authority for patient care must be delegated to those who are faced with daily responsibilities and accountability for such care. Our authors repeatedly comment on the continual presence of nursing in the hospital care sytem, in contrast to the intermittent care given other providers. Yet nursing's basic presence is represented inappropriately in room and board charges to patients, rather than in specified services. Walker has made an excellent case for disaggregating nursing services from room charges and billing separately to reflect the quality and quantity of professional nursing rendered. Such accounting would value professional nursing as a marketable and essential health care service, and go a long way toward recognizing the knowledge and skills that are needed to provide physical assessment, medications and treatments, ambulation, teaching and counseling, coordination of inpatient care, support to family and friends, and discharge planning.

Nursing is an increasingly scarce hospital resource, as budgeted vacancies nationwide show. Given the prospect that many American hospitals will become giant intensive care settings, requiring even greater numbers of skilled personnel, the need for a well-educated, experienced, and stable nursing staff grows. In a number of institutions across the country — among them some of our prominent teaching hospitals — the proportions of nurses with baccalaureate and master's degrees are increasing in response to the acuity levels of the inpatient populations. While salaries for clinical specialists with master's degrees may be competitive, compression at the base or first level staff is generally acknowledged as the biggest salary problem. There remains a question among some of our authors whether there should be a salary differential based on experience and education. McClure argues for such a differential; Clifford indicates that there is none at Beth Israel. Many settings are examining merit and promotion avenues to reward competence in direct care and to keep the highly skilled professional at the bedside. The innovations in staffing reported by several of our authors and in the major professional journals reveal impressive results in terms of reduced turnover rate and increased satisfaction for practitioners. The 10-hr day, 4 day week, and the 12-hr shift, allows some relief from burnout and increasing opportunity to see immediate outcomes of one's services. Other variations in work schedules have increased retention of nursing personnel and therefore may be a solution to turnover. Not examined systematically as yet is the impact of such schedules on patient welfare and satisfaction. While such rotations have worked well in intensive care situations, patient dissatisfaction with periodic loss of continuity with primary nurses may militate against their success on regular units with alert post-surgical patients, for example. Thus the desire of the consumer for highly individualized, continuous, competent nursing care may collide with the desire of the nurse to have relief from the provision of such care on a continous daily and weekly basis. The nature of the work is among the most difficult and demanding, physically and emotionally.

Given recognition of this fact, opportunities for innovation abound. It is no accident that a number of our authors are associated with the nursing departments of teaching hospitals in major medical centers. Historically, these settings have taken the lead in establishing optimal environments for care and for teaching and research. In keeping with university traditions, learning, discovery, and collegiality are important values. Nurses in the 1980s will require these values to stay in the inpatient setting and to practice effectively. Most certainly good patient management will need nursing judgment at every level of activity.

Some inpatient settings have heavily invested in the clinical specialist model of care, matching clinical expertise with patient and unit requirements, to everyone's satisfaction.[2] Some settings have increased continuing education opportunities, established nursing research units to study clinical problems, secured travel funds to send staff to professional meetings, and encouraged discussion between medicine and nursing on selected case management and institutional policies along the restructuring lines noted by Jacox. These features will become more frequent in the next decade, as will models of collaborative practice within the inpatient setting, some on the order of the recently published guidelines.[3, 4]

Finally, the next decade may well see the reentry of academic nursing to the inpatient unit and the ambulatory clinic. For nearly a generation many of the best prepared nurses have chosen teaching rather than practice and have therefore been "lost" to practice. As more well-prepared nurses enter practice, as institutions examine "unification" structures and other means for bridging the gap, and as more academicians carry joint responsibilities as associate directors or clinical associates with some patient contact, the opportunities for establishing practice environments supportive to nursing are enlarged. Initiative, inquiry, knowledge, and skill are virtues of the academician as they are of the clinician. It is impossible to educate differentially for these characteristics in nursing, or to expect different behaviors in different settings. The cooperation now occurring between academic and clinical nursing is one of the most encouraging signs for the next decade. So is the talent being displayed in nursing administration on behalf of nursing needs and resources, and the gradual recognition by patients and by other professionals of the patient advocacy position nursing holds and promulgates. Where such advocacy supports patients' rights to determine their treatment course, or at least share in decisions, it provides an indirect means for influencing patient management. Perhaps a new social contract between hospital administration, medicine, and nursing can be drawn to provide the direct means, as proposed by Aiken, for hearing nursing's recommendations on patient care as well as other matters.[5] Certainly the return of the "traditional nurse" is neither desired nor advised, despite the reflections of interested onlookers.[6] Rather, the die is cast in favor of increased nursing autonomy on behalf of patients and, not infrequently, at their insistence.

Nonhospital nursing in homes, schools, clinics, and the community has developed increasing professional identity as a result of historic roots in public health and the recent training and practice of nurse practitioners. A number of our authors have spoken to the prospects for nurse-rendered primary care in the 1980s. Ford draws on her long association with nurse practitioners to comment on their evolution and contributions and suggests that the practitioner is a model for all nursing. Lewis uses a similar time frame of experience to analyze the future for practitioners as the number of physicians increases. To break the chain binding nurse supply to physician supply, he proposes demonstration of the services practitioners in nursing can provide that physicians will not or cannot. Among these have been services to the structurally underserved, as well as to those in need of pre-hospital or post-recovery care. Complementary nursing services to those of medical services can be developed, according to Lewis, if greater attention is paid to the variation in the effectiveness and quality of medical services and if the strengths of consumer groups are well used. This last may become nursing's most potent ally in the decade to come, as it was midwifery's in the last, according to Diers. Repeatedly in inpatient and outpatient settings, consumers are critical of fragmented and impersonal medical services and of the inability of nurse providers to initiate actions that would directly meet client needs. While standing orders and protocols may allow for such action in primary care settings, only in those units dealing with intensive or critical care is the authority of nursing on a comparable level to that of medicine. An interesting study might be to explore the reasons for this situation and why there is apparent increased need for medical oversight and presence with decreased acuity of illness.

Loeb Center for Nursing is an important exception to this last statement. Since its inception as a comprehensive nursing facility, its performance data have shown excellent patient care outcomes at considerably lower *per diem* costs than the parent institution, Montefiore Hospital. Because of quality and effectiveness, Loeb stands a model of nurse-rendered service for a high-risk group — but a model that has not been replicated as rapidly as some would have thought. Medicare is an important source of revenue, and it, as well as other income sources, may provide a partial explanation for Loeb's longevity. The particular usefulness of nursing service in the rehabilitation of the elderly and the chronically ill is another known factor in Loeb's success. It is precisely that service that Reif and Estes feel is paramount for those in need of long-term care. While Loeb's patients are institutionalized, many thousands of others would benefit from expanded home health services and from frequent assessment and counseling in day centers or free-standing clinics run by nurses. Although small in number, these facilities generally have provided top-quality care at low costs. They have yet to benefit from stable financing and from physician approval and support. The medical monopoly is such as to make short lived most attempts to organize nonphysician-rendered health services. Authority has come slowly for third party reimbursement of nursing service; it can be expected to continue to grow slowly.

Just as the body of evidence showing nursing to be a high-quality service is limited, so is the documentation of the quality of physician services limited. Some of our authors suggest that we be less reticent in depicting our claims of worth and in providing examples of physician unworth.

For example, the known performance of nursing in increasing access and expansion of services, particularly in primary and outpatient settings, can be better publicized. Nurse performance, according to LeRoy, can be superior in symptom relief, diagnostic accuracy, and in that most important outcome variable, patient satisfaction, to that of physician performance. If one accepts the premise that physicians and nurse practitioners are not interchangeable, then, attention can be devoted to the combination of services that can improve access and reduce production costs. Luft makes a good argument for renewed national interest in health maintenance organizations (HMOs) to reduce medical costs. He predicts that increased HMO growth would lead to reduced hospitalization rates, and decreased reduction in nurse staffing because of the need for less intensive nursing. On the other hand, if McClure's predictions are correct, hospitals are becoming more intensive, rather than less intensive, and staffing needs remain acute, if not downright critical. In HMOs, in traditional public and community health activities, in school health, and now in home health, long-term, and hospice care, nursing flourishes because of its foundation in supportive and nurturant activities and because well care, rather than acute and illness care, is emphasized. Yet, it has been precisely in the area of actue illness, particularly dramatic, high-cost illness, that nursing's special and unique performance in providing high-quality technical services and concern for the psyche, as well as the soma, have been best dramatized and understood, both by physicians and by the public.

To what extent hospital-rendered care will continue as the model pattern for the next decade is not known. All evidence suggests that conversion to alternative care models will come slowly and will be linked inexorably to the dollar and how investments of plant, personnel, and equipment can be refinanced. Some sort of national health insurance may be with us by the end of the decade; in all probability it will incorporate nonphysician services where cost and quality are concerns. In the ambulatory arena, nurse practitioners and nurse midwives (and their antecedent school and community health practitioners) have well demonstrated their work in quality, client satisfaction, and reduced service costs. In the hospital arena, such demonstrations to date have been sparse, because incentives have not been present to finance them or to disturb what has been a profitable and prestigious care system based on full occupancy, high-cost illness and treatment, and adequate access. The last — access — may mean providing sufficiently safe service to a full population of very sick people. Frequently, numerical coverage is marginal, but the quality is so good that tragic errors have not yet occurred. They will occur unless medical admissions and surgeries are scheduled not on availability of beds but on availability of specialized nursing personnel for the treatment and recovery period.

Perhaps Clifford's impressive model for the development of nurse autonomy and the control of nursing practice within the inpatient setting may be an approach of value in resolving the above concerns for hospital nursing. The nursing structure noted in Clifford's chapter is patterned after academic and medical governance models, which channel professional power according to professional capability and competence. The levels of nursing practice identified by Clifford recognize differentials in education and experience but are now characteristic of a number of university hospital settings. Lodging of nursing practice policy in a professional nursing structure must be recognized and incorporated into hospital governance. It provides an important option to industrial models, allows for incorporation of collective bargaining, and is an alternative to the development of non-nursing unions and a weakened national professional organization.

The National Commission on Nursing of the American Hospital Association recently has published the reported testimony obtained during a number of hearings nationwide. Increased decision making and authority for nursing within the inpatient setting is a major recommendation of the Commission. It will remain to be seen how these recommendations can be implemented, and at what political as well as social cost to administration and physician control. In her chapter on role restructuring, Jacox makes a telling argument in support of valuation of hospital nursing. All those who have thoughtfully examined the structure of the nurse's role understand that restructuring will require readjustment of roles of others in the hospital, including those of physicians, pharmacists, radiologists, and technicians. Innovative strategies for reducing stress in intensive work situations have been employed in industry for some time; rotations off and away from intensive care settings, increased opportunities for education flexitime, innovative staffing arrangements, and increased salaries are among the solutions.

The American Academy of Nursing Task Force on Hospital Nursing is examining those organizational and administrative characteristics of hospital settings that have provided a successful solution to the dilemma of the work place for nursing. Although not scientific in its approach, such anecdotal and descriptive information will do much to provide illustration of organizations that have surmounted some, if not all, the barriers to retention and satisfaction for professional nursing in the hospital situaiton. These descriptions coupled with increased research on hospital-rendered services may allow us to maximize economic and professional features important to the retention of nursing as a major service within hospitals in the last part of this century.

Another task force of the Academy is studying issues in long-term care, particularly with respect to the Loeb model and other examples for innovative care to the elderly and the chronically ill. Other activities of the Academy address public means for depicting the scope and capabilities of modern nursing.

Perhaps the greatest issue confronting nursing in the 1980s is its substitutability for medically rendered services. This issue is put clearly by Fagin in her final chapter. Substitutability is bound to generate controversy not only from physicians and others concerned with health care policy but from nursing itself, which has long maintained its unique and distinct ethos and activities apart from medicine. There is considerable data that suggest that nurses can substitute selectively for physicians at lesser costs and equal, if not greater, quality. The proposal is for reimbursement of services that will substitute for those currently being provided; Fagin's intent is not to convert nurses to doctors but to generate for nurses the revenues to which they are entitled and that will enable them to offer the American public an alternative to expensive and traditional medical services. The financial constraints of the next 5 yr, coupled with the changing political philosophy, will bring a real test of this proposal. It will certainly require greater involvement and review of public policy on the part of professionals. It offers a challenge to us all, and it is hoped that the views of the authors of this volume can provide guidance on the strategies for the decades ahead.

REFERENCES

1   Norris, Catherine M. The impact of the nurse on the practice environment and consumer health. In *Power: Nursing's challenge for change*. Papers presented at the 51st Convention, Honolulu, Hawaii, June 9-14, 1978. Kansas City: ANA, 1979, 96-109

2   Shurkin, Joel, & Levinson, Arnold H. Nursing: Does moving forward mean also taking a look back? *UCSF Magazine*, February-June 1981, *4*(1-2), 2-19.

3   Devereux, Pamela McNutt. Does joint practice work? *Journal of Nursing Administration*, 1981, *XI*(6), 39-43.

4   Mauksch, Ingeborg G. Nurse-physician collaboration: A changing relationship. *Journal of Nursing Administration*, 981, *XI*(6), 35-38.

5   Aiken, Linda. Nursing priorities for the 1980's: Hospitals and Nursing Homes. *American Journal of Nursing*, 1981, *81*(2), 324-331.

6   Newton, Lisa H. In defense of the traditional nurse. *Nursing Outlook*, 1981, *29*(9), 348-354.

ADDITIONAL READING

American Academy of Nursing. Aiken, Linda (ed.). *Health policy and Nursing Practice*. New York: McGraw-Hill, 1981.

American Academy of Nursing. *Nursing's influence on health policy for the eighties*. Kansas City: AAN, 1979.

American Nurses' Association. *Nursing: A social policy statement*. Kansas City: ANA, 1980.

National Commission on Nursing. Initial Report and Preliminary Recommendation. Chicago: The American Hospital Assoc., September, 1981.

INDEX

Numbers in italics indicate a figure; t following a page number indicates tabular material.